Service Delivery for Vulnerable Populations

New Directions in Behavioral Health

Steven A. Estrine, PhD, is the founder and President of SAE & Associates. He has over 35 years of experience as a high-level administrator, strategic planner, and program developer in mental health and substance abuse for the most vulnerable, at-risk population across the lifespan. Estrine has held positions as Director of Adult Psychiatric Services of the New York State Office of Mental Health, Director of Public Sector Psychiatry at New York Presbyterian Hospital, and Director of Program Development at North Shore-Long Island Jewish Health Systems. Dr. Estrine's primary interests are in programs that address the needs of vulnerable, at-risk populations across the lifespan.

Robert T. Hettenbach, MPS, is Senior Vice President for Business Development at PSCH in the Greater New York Area. He has over 36 years of experience in health, mental health, and managed care. As a senior administrator within the North Shore/Long Island Jewish Health Care System, Hettenbach helped develop their managed care network, has been the Executive Director of a local community hospital responsible for quality care, finances, and regulatory compliance. Accordingly, he has developed a unique understanding of the integration of behavioral health with primary care, and the impact of mental illness on the management of chronic and acute medical conditions. Hettenbach also directed New York State's Office of Mental Health's New York City Regional Office, with oversight of eight state hospitals, and responsibility for the licensure of all inpatient and outpatient programs and the distribution of millions of dollars in funding for community-based programs serving the seriously mentally ill.

Heidi Arthur, LMSW, is Vice President for Program Development and Grant Writing at SAE & Associates. Arthur has over 15 years of experience in human services project design, implementation, and administration. At SAE, her work has yielded more than $25 million for programs benefiting children families, and adult populations. Arthur has previously held grants management positions for both the New York City Department of Health and Mental Hygiene and the New York State Office of Mental Health. She has also developed and implemented a community-based outreach initiative for pregnant and parenting substance abusers, a child welfare training curriculum for workers serving those who are pregnant, and a school-based curriculum for acquaintance rape education.

Maria Messina, PhD, is a consultant and program evaluator at SAE & Associates. Messina is a medical anthropologist with more than 16 years of experience in public health, specializing in ethnographic and ethno-epidemiological research including HIV risk environments, behaviors, and sero-sorting/sero-disclosure practices among men having sex with men (MSM) in New York City (NYC); crystal methamphetamine use and HIV risk among MSM in five U.S. cities; crack injection practices and health risks among homeless street youth in NYC; risk and protective factors for drug use among youth in the barrios of Caracas, Venezuela; residential therapeutic community drug treatment among male and female homeless or formerly incarcerated adults in the NYC public shelter system and adjudicated and nonadjudicated adolescents in the United States and Canada; and HIV prevention among YMSM and MSM in the House/Ball and Kiki communities. Messina speaks French and Arabic and is a Fulbright scholar and a Social Science Research Council Fellow for her research in North Africa on gender, sexuality, and Islam.

Service Delivery for Vulnerable Populations
New Directions in Behavioral Health

Steven A. Estrine, PhD
Robert T. Hettenbach, MPS
Heidi Arthur, LMSW
Maria Messina, PhD

Editors

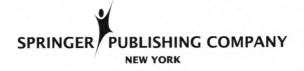

SPRINGER PUBLISHING COMPANY
NEW YORK

Springer Publishing Company, LLC
11 West 42nd Street
New York, NY 10036
www.springerpub.com

Acquisitions Editor: Jennifer Perillo
Project Manager: Judith Estrine
Senior Production Editor: Diane Davis
Cover Design: Steven Pisano
Composition: Techset Composition Ltd.

ISBN: 978-0-8261-1855-4
E-book ISBN: 978-0-8261-1856-1

10 11 12 13/ 5 4 3 2 1

The author and the publisher of this work have made every effort to use sources believed to be reliable to provide information that is accurate and compatible with the standards generally accepted at the time of publication. Because medical science is continually advancing, our knowledge base continues to expand. Therefore, as new information becomes available, changes in procedures become necessary. We recommend that the reader always consult current research and specific institutional policies before performing any clinical procedure. The author and publisher shall not be liable for any special, consequential, or exemplary damages resulting, in whole or in part, from the readers' use of, or reliance on, the information contained in this book. The publisher has no responsibility for the persistence or accuracy of URLs for external or third-party Internet web sites referred to in this publication and does not guarantee that any content on such web sites is, or will remain, accurate or appropriate.

Library of Congress Cataloging-in-Publication Data
CIP data is on file at the Library of Congress.

Special discounts on bulk quantities of our books are available to corporations, professional associations, pharmaceutical companies, health care organizations, and other qualifying groups.

If you are interested in a custom book, including chapters from more than one of our titles, we can provide that service as well.

For details, please contact:
Special Sales Department, Springer Publishing Company, LLC
11 West 42nd Street, 15th Floor, New York, NY 10036-8002
Phone: 877-687-7476 or 212-431-4370; Fax: 212-941-7842
Email: sales@springerpub.com

Printed in the United States of America by Hamilton Printing.

*This book is dedicated to the memory of
three extraordinary mentors*

Morton Wallach, MD

Robert N. Butler, MD

Myrna I. Lewis, PhD

Contents

Contributors

Charles Amrhein, PhD, is the clinical director of the Bronx TASC Mental Health Court Program and teaches doctoral students in clinical psychology at the John Jay College of Criminal Justice and forensic psychiatry fellows at the Albert Einstein College of Medicine.

Virginia Barber-Rioja, PhD, is currently the clinical director of Queens TASC Mental Health Diversion Program, an alternative to incarceration program that works in collaboration with the Queens felony and misdemeanor Mental Health Courts. She obtained her PhD in clinical-forensic psychology at John Jay College of Criminal Justice of the Graduate Center (City University of New York).

Andrea Blanch, PhD, has worked in public mental health systems for over 30 years. She is currently the director of the Center for Religious Tolerance, and consults widely on issues of culture, violence and trauma-informed care.

Ann Boughtin, MS/MPA, has held executive positions in government and the private sectors, leading major service design initiatives for behavioral health systems of care, as well as managed care operations with a focus on Medicaid and high need individuals.

Susan M. Bowler, PhD, has 20 years experience in policy and system development in child, youth, and family services in Rhode Island. She is a leader in the Advanced Youth Forum, which is seeking to fully integrate economic development, employment support, and clinical/social services to assist the highest risk youth to succeed in the market economy.

Michael Cheng, MD, is a child/family psychiatrist at the Children's Hospital of Eastern Ontario in Ottawa, Canada, as well as an Assistant Professor with the University of Ottawa, and is the cofounder of eMentalHealth.ca, an initiative of the Provincial Centre of Excellence for Child and Youth Mental Health.

Judith Estrine is a writer and editor with over 15 years of experience in the field of gerontology.

Paul Feuerstein, President/CEO of Barrier Free Living, was, over the past 24 years, instrumental in developing the largest domestic violence program in the country for victims with disabilities.

Nina Rose Fischer, LMSW, PhD, has 18 years of experience in program development. Her doctoral dissertation is on transitioning and stabilizing high needs youth in child welfare and juvenile justice in the community.

Henrietta Fishman, LCSW, is the U.S. Department of Veterans Affairs Network 3 Manager of Residential Treatment and Homeless Veterans Treatment Programs.

Frank Guida, PhD, a psychologist who received his degree from the University of Chicago, is a program evaluator for a number of federal and international agencies, including the Substance Abuse and Mental Health Services Administration (SAMHSA), the National Institute on Drug Abuse (NIDA), U.S. Department of Education, U.S. Department of Labor, National Science Foundation, and the Chilean Ministry of Education.

Benjamin Henwood, LCSW, is a mental health services researcher pursuing a PhD in social work at New York University. He helped start and served as the Clinical Director of Pathways to Housing in Philadelphia and is now working to develop an integrated primary care model within their behavioral health services program.

Nancy Hepler, PhD, is an independent Behavioral Health Researcher and Evaluator with a long time affiliation with Meharry Medical College in Nashville, Tennessee.

Sel J. Hwahng, PhD, is a Visiting Scholar and Adjunct Professor at the Center for the Study of Ethnicity and Race at Columbia University and was Research Investigator on the New York City Transgender Project at National Development and Research Institutes, Inc.

Mohamed Kanu, PhD, MPH, is Assistant Professor & Interim Director of the MPH Program at Tennessee State University College of Health Sciences.

Kenneth A. Knapp, PhD, is an economist and gerontologist whose research projects have included public policy issues in health and long-term care, housing, and work and retirement.

Edie Mannion, MSW, is co-founder and director of the Training and Education Center, a program of the Mental Health Association of Southeastern Pennsylvania.

Charlotte Muller, PhD, is Professor Emerita of Economics at City University of New York Graduate School (CUNY).

Nora O'Brien-Suric, PhD, is a gerontologist with over 20 years experience in the field of aging. She is a senior program officer at The John A. Hartford Foundation.

Jill Wolski Ordoñez, PhD, is the Director of the United Way 2-1-1 and CONTACT Lifeline in Albany, NY, programs of Family and Children's Service of the Capital Region.

Dick Orndoff, MEd, has been an Executive Manager in both the public and private sectors, working in managed care and behavioral health services, where he led corporate operations and product development.

Harvey Rosenthal, has over 35 years of experience working to provide or promote public mental health service innovations and legislative and social policies that promote the recovery, rehabilitation, rights and community integration of people with psychiatric disabilities, most notably as executive director of the New York Association of Psychiatric Rehabilitation Services (www.nyaprs.org).

Jan L. Roth, PhD, has over 30 years experience in local and state, public and private sectors serving persons with intellectual and developmental disabilities.

Lisa Schmidt, PhD, is a Clinical Assistant Professor at Drexel University's Department of Behavioral Health Counseling and has extensive experience as both an educator and provider of psychiatric rehabilitation services.

Sandra A. Smith, MPH, PhD, is Director of the Center for Health Literacy Promotion, Seattle, WA, and author of the Beginnings Guides curriculum for promoting health literacy in parents.

Phyllis Solomon, PhD, is Professor of Social Work, School of Social Policy and Practice and Professor of Social Work in Psychiatry, Center for Mental

Health Policy and Services Research, Department of Psychiatry, both at University of Pennsylvania.

Peggy Swarbrick, PhD, OT, CPRP, is Director of the Institute for Wellness and Recovery Initiatives, Collaborative Support Programs of New Jersey, and part-time Assistant Clinical Professor for the Department of Psychiatric Rehabilitation at the University of Medicine and Dentistry of New Jersey.

Denise Torres, PhD, is a licensed clinical social worker with over 20 years of direct practice, administration, and research experience.

Sam Tsemberis, PhD, founded Pathways to Housing, a nationally acclaimed consumer-driven stable housing initiative in 1992 after years working as a member of a psychiatric street outreach team to house New York City's chronically homeless street population.

Anthony Vavasis, MD, is the Clinical Director of Medical Services and former Clinical Director of the Health Outreach to Teens Program at Callen-Lorde Community Health Center in New York City.

Foreword

Attempts to relieve human misery are often difficult, unrewarding, arduous, and frequently unsuccessful. However, as communication becomes virtually instantaneous with the harnessing of cyberspace, innovative ideas that offer hope have come to the fore. Traditional and time-honored interventions have had their place historically, and indeed, they are what most students are exposed to in their formal training. In contrast, the editors of this textbook address with a fresh eye a wide variety of problems that affect individuals as well as society. Their approach is national in scope and culturally sensitive in outlook.

As a practicing psychiatrist for over 40 years, with extensive experience directing psychiatric hospital units for adolescents and adults, and teaching trainees in child and adult psychiatry, I know that as students embark on careers in their respective fields of behavioral and social sciences they will benefit greatly from exposure to the creative ideas expressed herein.

The editors and contributing authors have significant professional experience and credentials in the delivery of human services. This comprehensive textbook is addressed to students and trainees, as well as complementing and enhancing the knowledge base of practicing behavioral health professionals and administrators who are seeking new ideas to improve the quality of life for the consumers they serve.

Mark R. Novick, MD

Assistant Clinical Professor
Department of Psychiatry and Behavioral Sciences
Albert Einstein College of Medicine
Bronx, New York

Preface

Service Delivery for Vulnerable Populations: New Directions in Behavioral Health was written with the aim of introducing innovative approaches to program design, service delivery, and evaluation to graduate students in social work, psychology, and other students of behavioral health. We also hoped to provide public sector professionals around the nation with new material with which to address the pressing needs of their vulnerable populations. With an understanding of the overlapping complexity of the issues being addressed and sensitivity to the realities that one size does not fit all situations, the editors engaged 33 specialists in behavioral health and allied fields from venues around the nation, with years of experience and a deep breadth of knowledge in their area of expertise. Their task was to offer new strategies, program initiatives, and concepts, as well as to review available research and literature and present a historic overview.

This book is the result of their efforts. It explores the needs of adults, children, youth, families, and older persons who are coping with mental illness, substance abuse, HIV/AIDS, and those with co-occurring combinations of these disorders, for whom state and local systems by and large have failed. As anyone who has worked in the behavioral health field is aware, too often these problems are compounded by the effects of social problems such as poverty, homelessness, criminal justice involvement, racism, and cultural barriers, as well as chronic co-occurring medical conditions that often go untreated.

In this era of increasingly competitive funding, research documents the success of coordinated systems of care. In order to establish credibility and obtain government and private funding, it is critical that programs offer dynamic approaches, incorporate evidence-based practices, and target the specific, often unique, needs of the people to be served. We believe that this book answers the need for a broadly focused text that will make a significant contribution to students of behavioral health and the providers, consumers, and key stakeholders within the behavioral health community.

Service Delivery for Vulnerable Populations is organized around nine broad issues. Following are brief reviews of what the reader will find in each category.

Section I: *New Directions in the Treatment of Persons with Psychiatric Disabilities* begins with a comprehensive review of the evolving definition of the term "serious mental illness" and its impact on health-care policy, program development, and treatment. The concept of recovery and its impact on the consumers' role in the management of his/her illness and the treatment staff's knowledge about consumers and their needs are explored. Observations are made of how evidence-based psychosocial strategies and services are transforming how people with psychiatric disabilities are being helped to recover and lead fulfilling lives, including a description of these practices. The chapter concludes with identification of future directions in the development of new funding, services, and approaches.

Section II: *New Directions in Services for Children, Youth, and Families* addresses the impact of co-occurring needs and the barriers to access to care for children and youth with multiple mental health and/or substance abuse needs that are related to stigma, cultural and developmental factors, and fractured systems, as well as the opportunities for engagement that exist when services are driven by families and youth. The prevalence of children with complex behavioral health needs within the Juvenile Justice and Child Welfare systems is examined. The Systems of Care approach is explained and the Wraparound model is described and illustrated as a best practice guide to individual service delivery for children and youth with multiple needs whose care requires attention from a range of systems.

Section III: *New Directions in Services for LGBTQ Individuals* provides a chapter devoted to a summary of the special needs of LGBTQ youth and one relating to LGBTQ adults. Dr. Maria Messina and coauthors describe research reflecting a growing body of evidence that LGBTQ youth have health-care needs that are different from their heterosexual, gender-conforming peers. Authors integrate the resulting consequences of the historical lack of access to appropriate care among LGBTQ youth and the consequences of lack of access among LGBTQ youth to appropriate care. Many of the conclusions proposed in the chapter on sexual minority youth, such as a more comprehensive sexual behavior assessment, improve the health care of all youth, irrespective of identity. In their chapter on LGBTQ adults, Messina et al provide a comprehensive overview of behavioral risks and factors in order to determine the most sensitive and effective service delivery strategies for issues such as abuse/victimization, HIV/STIs, behavioral health, substance use, domestic violence, gender transitions, and aging.

Section IV: *New Directions in Housing and Homelessness* directs its attention to the quintessential victims in American society, where homelessness often serves as a shorthand for minorities and those suffering from a range of physical and emotional problems. This section focuses on factors that negatively affect the residential stability of three unique target populations—persons with psychiatric disabilities and often a co-occurring substance abuse problem, veterans, and older adults. Dr. Sam Tsemberis, founder of Pathways to Housing, the nationally recognized program for homeless individuals, discusses his concept of the unconditional provision of housing for persons with psychiatric disabilities, without the contingency of treatment participation. Tsemberis and the coauthor explain that residential stability is the *sine qua non* for successful treatment engagement and adherence, and evidence is offered to support the efficacy of this consumer-driven approach to reduction of homelessness among those with psychiatric disabilities. Henrietta Fishman's chapter on veterans speaks to the causes of homelessness among veterans as compared to non-veterans; the changing demographics of homeless veterans; veterans' perceptions of their needs, and how to address the issue of homelessness effectively among this cohort. It discusses the "New York experience" as a model for the provision of services to homeless veterans. The final chapter in this section focuses on elements that affect housing security among older persons and the special vulnerability of older women, as well as insights on helping people age in place by incorporating mental health interventions with other wraparound services to address issues such as depression and loneliness, which many older persons attempt to hide. The chapter discusses the integration of a full array of ongoing, specific medical, psychiatric, and social services into elder-friendly housing to address issues relating to the various iterations of elder abuse, depression, alcoholism, substance abuse, and HIV-AIDS that occur in this population.

Section V: *New Directions in Services for Older Adults* discusses two complex issues relating to needs of the growing demographic of older adults—behavioral health and elder abuse. Drs. Guida and Estrine address behavioral health, unique substance use issues, and medical comorbidities that are faced by persons aged 50 and older, with emphasis on minorities and women. Included are several innovative evidence-based practices. The following chapter relates to the prevalence and various forms of elder abuse and factors that make older adults particularly vulnerable. The section concludes with a description of an innovative program designed to address the emerging silent social epidemic of elder abuse.

Section VI: *New Directions in Services for Refugees* examines the impact of trauma on refugee populations. The recent groups of refugees and immigrants, unlike earlier immigrants, are maintaining their cultural identity rather than assimilating completely. These new patterns of assimilation, coupled with frequent traumatic histories of newcomers, are extremely challenging to social services. Nationally recognized expert in refugee trauma, Dr. Andrea Blanch identifies the scope and varied precipitants of trauma experienced by refugee populations and the role that population-based cultural values, norms, and beliefs play in informing the experience of trauma. Dr. Blanch presents innovative models of trauma treatment for refugee populations, including those derived from the application of current models of trauma treatment and those developed from and informed by the unique culture and experiences of the refugee population.

Section VII: *New Directions in Services for the Disabled* explores the related themes of persons with intellectual and developmental disabilities, autistic children, and disabled women who are victims of abuse. The high prevalence of domestic abuse among women with disabilities, historic changes in the treatment of developmentally disabled individuals, and innovative strategies to promote the quality of life are reviewed by experts with years of experience working with developmentally and physically disabled individuals. Dr. Jan Roth discusses the most salient change in care for people with developmental disabilities since the latter third of the 20th century, which is the move from large institutional settings to smaller community residential housing. Paul Feuerstein provides personal experience working with disabled victims of domestic violence. The authors bring a refreshing combination of profound understanding and boots-on-the-ground practicality to these largely ignored Americans.

Section VIII: *Critical Considerations in Service Delivery* addresses the linked subjects of jail diversion models and that of program evaluations with vulnerable populations. Drs. Amrhein and Barber-Rioja describe the history underlying the nation's overreliance on the criminal justice system. They detail the role it plays as the nation's largest provider of psychiatric services and the impact of deinstitutionalization, mandatory drug sentencing, and the movement to create a problem-solving court on the situation. They also highlight the importance of jail diversion strategies and program models embedded in the criminal justice system that provide diversion pathways, such as the mental health court and the Treatment Alternative to Street Crime (TASC) model.

Section IX: *Emerging Issues in Service Delivery* is a grand finale, a look at where the field of behavioral health is heading as we discard old systems and ways of thinking and move forward in the 21st century. "New Mental Health Meets New Media" explores innovative communication strategies, consumer-oriented and new media in origin designed to increase a behavioral health consumer's access to health care. Explaining how chat rooms, email, video, social networking, message boards, and texting, as well as the internet, offer increased access to services, Drs. Jill Ordoñez and Michael Cheng then describe how these new approaches to communication can help consumers overcome the stigma and shame often associated with traditional behavioral health services. Crisis intervention and information and referral services are cited as adaptable to this new media environment.

In Chapter 19: *Health Literacy and Human Service Delivery*, Dr. Sandra Smith examines the meaning, measure, and practice of health literacy, while assisting the reader in navigating through conceptual models, research approaches, and intended outcomes, and provide a window into the emerging role of person-centered health care. Teaching functional skills to behavioral health consumers, rather than relying performance levels on standardized health literacy tests has been shown to improve access to health care, enabling individuals to exert better control over the process and improve their overall health.

Chapter 20: *Transformative Impact and Initiatives of the Mental Health Consumer/Survivor Movement* provides a historical perspective of attitudes toward and perceptions of individuals labeled as suffering from or diagnosed with "mental illness" to the more current practice of neutrally regarding these diverse individuals as "consumers" or simply people who have "psychiatric disabilities." Executive Director of the New York Association of Psychiatric Rehabilitation Services (NYAPRS), Harvey Rosenthal explains that fundamental to understanding this transformation are the values and philosophical meanings expressed through the human and patient's rights movements. Alternatives to traditional treatments, research on the adoption of the recovery model used in substance abuse treatment, and self-directed service designs where individuals receive support to develop their own wellness goals, are also included.

Chapter 21: *The Future of Managed Behavioral Health Care* describes how managed care organizations balance the needs and interests of key stakeholders: payers, members, and providers. The role that each stakeholder plays in the managed care model shapes the operation of the managed care organization to coordinate quality care, manage the healthcare benefit, and maintain a network of providers, while monitoring clinical outcomes. This chapter describes the history of managed behavioral health care, particularly Medicaid managed care and provides operational information regarding the functions of managed care organizations, plan design, reimbursement and payment structures, and emerging trends.

Finally, a word about the terminology used in this text. The editors have made every effort to insure that the cultural values, norms, and beliefs of the consumers who are referenced in this book are referred to in a respectful and culturally competent manner. Any perceived shortcoming is unintentional.

Steven A. Estrine, PhD
Robert T. Hettenbach, MPS
Heidi Arthur, LMSW
Maria Messina, PhD

Acknowledgments

We acknowledge the support of Sheri Sussman and Jennifer Perillo at Springer Publishing, Sheri for first approaching us with the concept and Jennifer for her enthusiasm and skill in shepherding us through the process. Thanks to the research assistance of Brigid Lang, Scott Henkle, and Julia Page. A note of appreciation to Marilyn Kamile who contributed to the editing process, and to Charlotte Muller, who provided a much appreciated voice of reason. Thanks to Amanda Joan Monier of the John Jay College of Criminal Justice and Kimberly Nessel of the Bronx TASC Mental Health Court program for their thoughtful feedback on jail diversion models and to Mona Rae Mason, who provided relentless support for early development of the chapter on adult LGBTQ individuals. We also acknowledge Clair Horn at Aging in America and the social workers at the Hebrew Home for the Aged in Riverdale for their willingness to share their insights during the early stages of the book's development. We are most grateful for the support of staff at SAE & Associates. Finally, a special note of thanks to Judith Estrine, without whose efforts this book could not have come to fruition.

Acknowledgment

Service Delivery for Vulnerable Populations

New Directions in Behavioral Health

I. New Directions in the Treatment of Persons with
Psychiatric Disabilities

CHAPTER ONE

Defining Severe Persistent Mental Illness

Implications for Knowledge, Needs, and Services

Denise Torres

INTRODUCTION

The persistence of "a tower of Babel" (Bachrach, 1988) regarding the definition of serious mental illness (SMI) despite ongoing attempts to standardize the term reflects its very political and social nature. Although it may appear to be an issue of interest for only researchers and academics, how SMI is defined has real-world impacts on program development and practice. As health and social service delivery incorporates the concept of recovery and related evidence-based practices (EBPs), program design and service delivery will need to fundamentally change. This chapter will review the history of the terms associated with SMI and discuss their implications for knowledge about consumers[1] and their needs. The contentious history of the term will be used to discuss the concept of recovery, resistances to it, and the need to reformulate our understanding of SMI if we are to transform the mental health service delivery system.

---

[1]Consumer is used as a general term encompassing individuals receiving services within the health and social welfare system, recognizing the terminology is fraught with debates and political implications (Koyangi, 2007).

COMPETING DEFINITIONS OF SMI

The terms *serious mental illness* (SMI), *serious and persistent mental illness* (SPMI), and *chronic mental illness* (CMI) are frequently used interchangeably, although each comes from a different time period and reflects the ideological forces and economic factors that were at play as much as professional and scientific knowledge. That is, the election of a social designation of consumer groups is informed by different ways of *knowing and seeing* (Bogdan & Taylor, 1989), which shape and in turn are shaped by policies and practices (Anderson, 1997), with consequences for consumer voice and perceived capacity and culpability (Blau, 2003).

Definitional Sources in the United States

There is an absence of international consensus regarding what constitutes SMI (Ruggeri, Leese, Thornicroft, Bisoffie, & Tansella, 2000), and no comparable World Health Organization (WHO) term exists (Slade, Powell, & Strathdee, 1997). The different ways of knowing and seeing SMI have been informed primarily by the need to create policies and categorize individuals for purposes of service eligibility and access. As Goldman and Grob (2006) note, "mental health policy is shaped by the definition of mental illness associated with the policy" (p. 737). The following is a short discussion of the policy and social contexts relating to commonly used terms.

Chronic Mental Illness

Chronic mental illness (CMI) is one of the earliest terms used to categorize individuals who experience long-term functional impairments due to a mental health disorder. It is ideologically linked to historical debates regarding custodial versus community-based care models and "embodied the view that these people would not improve and required long-term custodial care" (Chinman, Weingarten, Stayner, & Davidson, 2001). During the 1950s, the issue saw a resurgence as mental health consumers recently released from facilities took on the labels of "survivors," "ex-patients," and "former inmates" (Campbell, 1992) and aligned with other stigmatized groups to strategically argue for full civil rights (Mizrahi, Lopez-Humphries, & Torres, 2009). The issue was temporarily put to rest by the passage of the Mental Retardation Facilities Act, which funded community mental health centers (CMHCs) that were designed to increase access to services (PL-88-164, 1963),[2] and by the legal gains achieved by various constituencies during the civil rights era.

> In the mid-70s the issue again took root: In 1977, President Carter established the President's Commission on Mental Health (henceforth "Commission") which was charged with "recommending how the mental health needs of the Nation can be met and identifying the relative priority of those needs." Ultimately, the Commission's report became the foundation for the Mental Health Systems Act of 1980 (PL 96-398), although most of the provisions would be undone by the Omnibus Reconciliation Act of 1982.
> — *PL 97-35, 1981*

In the same year, the American Psychiatric Association (APA) issued a position statement citing the "deinstitutionalization programs of the past" for the failures of the period, and a strong psychiatric patients' liberation movement argued against the label "chronic" (Chamberlin & Rogers, 1990).

Legislatively, CMI is addressed in the State Comprehensive Mental Health Services Plan Act of 1986 (PL 99-660), which focused on "establishing and implementing a community-based system of care for chronically mentally ill individuals." One aim was to correct the lack of mandated coordination between state hospitals and the CMHCs (Grob, 2008). Notably, during this time a surge in homelessness was burdening hospitals and treatment facilities (Neibacher, 1990). Given that many homeless persons had mental disorders, "deinstitutionalization"[3] was assumed to be the cause (Goldman & Morrissey, 1985; Hopper, 1988; Snow, Baker, Anderson, & Martin, 1986) and, by implication, the CMHCs. While the act did not define CMI, it required that states develop definitions and enumerate persons with SMI. Subsequent legislation specifically mandated "replacing references to chronically mentally ill individuals [in PL 99-660] with references to individuals with serious mental illnesses" (PL 101-639, 1990).

---

[2]The act was informed by *Action for Mental Health*, a report issued by the Joint Commission on Mental Illness and Health, which had been contracted under the Mental Health Study Act of 1955 (Pub. L. 84-182) although it did not fully implement the report's recommendations (Koyangi, 2007). Grob (2008) asserts this was due to the influence of the NIMH, in particular Dr. Felix, which developed the concept of CMHCs.

[3]Deinstitutionalization is used here as it is commonly understood (i.e., a time-limited exodus), recognizing that the social problems associated with it are derived from various economic, political, and social forces.

Serious and Persistent Mental Illness

The term serious and persistent mental illness (SPMI) was promulgated by the National Institute of Mental Health (NIMH) during its efforts to formulate a consensus definition (Grob, 2008; Schinnar, Rothbard, Kanter, & Jung, 1990). The definition issued in 1987 is the most frequently cited, and defines SPMI as a function of the 3Ds or:

> *Diagnosis:* A major mental disorder according to DSM-III-R: a major affective, non-organic psychotic disorder or a disorder that may lead to a chronic disability such as a borderline personality disorder. *Disability:* Severe recurrent disability resulting from mental illness. The disability results in functional limitations in major life activities. Individuals must meet at least two of the following criteria on a continuing or intermittent basis: (1) Is unemployed, is employed in a sheltered setting or supportive work situation, or has markedly limited skills and a poor work history (2) Requires public financial assistance from out-of-hospital maintenance and may be unable to procure such assistance without help (3) Has difficulty in establishing or maintaining a personal social support system (4) Requires help in basic livings skills such as hygiene, food preparation, or money management (5) Exhibits inappropriate social behavior which results in intervention by the mental and/or judicial system; *Duration:* Treatment history meets one or both of the following criteria: (1) Has undergone psychiatric treatment more intensive than outpatient care more than once in a lifetime (e.g. crisis response services, alternative home care, partial hospitalization, or inpatient hospitalization) (2) Has experienced an episode of continuous, supportive residential care, other than hospitalization, for a period long enough to have significantly disrupted the normal living situation.
>
> —*Slade et al., 1997, p. 178*

Preference for this definition derives from its limitation of SPMI to "major Axis I" disorders and more demanding duration and disability criteria.

Serious Mental Illness

In 1993, the term "serious mental illness" became the official federally legislated term through the Alcohol, Drug Abuse, and Mental Health Administration (ADAMHA) Reorganization Act of 1992 (PL102-321). The act restructured the federal behavioral health service delivery system by establishing the Substance Abuse and Mental Health Services Administration (SAMHSA) and, for the first time, requiring an explicit definition of SMI for adults and serious emotional disturbance for children.

IMPLICATIONS OF OPERATIONALIZING SMI

Although the SAMHSA and NIMH definitions share the three criteria of diagnosis, duration, and disability/impairment, there is significant divergence in how these are operationalized. This reflects a consensus regarding the need for the 3Ds and also continued uncertainty over the specific character, relative importance, or the nature of interrelationships among them (Bachrach, 1988; Schinaar et al., 1990; Slade et al., 1997). The lack of resolution to these fundamental differences influences knowledge of SMI and mental health services for individuals with SMI.

Prevalence

It is difficult to ascertain how many persons in the United States are living with an SMI at a particular point in time. Schinnar, Rothbard, and Kanter (1991) noted that the lack of a single definition prevented a meaningful national estimate derived from state-level data. Compounding this, much of the research and attention has been focused on the disorders themselves rather than on impairment following from these disorders. Understanding how many individuals have a specific diagnosis does not offer much insight into the prevalence of SMI: disorders are frequently mild, remit, or attenuate over the treatment and life course (Kessler, Chiu, Demler, & Walters, 2005, p. 617).

Morbidity and Mortality

On average, public mental health service recipients die 25 years earlier than the general population (Parks et al., 2006). In an early review including over 20 studies, Felker et al. (1996) found that the standardized mortality ratios were more than double that of the general population. Black and colleagues (1985) found that suicide and accidents were significant factors in the higher-than-expected mortality rates. In a 16-state study, suicide accounted for 30% of excess mortality (Parks et al., 2006).

Comorbidity

It has been noted that "rates of disease for the population with SMI exceed those of the non-SMI population in every disease category" (Parks et al., 2006, p. 14). Felker et al. (1996) found that 50% of persons with SMI had a known medical problem, another 35% had an unknown medical problem, and 20% had medical issues that may exacerbate mental disorders.

Frequent comorbid issues include obesity, nicotine dependence, substance dependence, sedentary lifestyle, cardiovascular disease, metabolic syndrome, diabetes, cancer and cerebrovascular diseases, and comorbid mental disorders (Dickerson et al., 2006; Parks, Svendsen, Singer, & Foti, 2006), of which many are related to or have complex interplays with psychiatric medications (Parks et al., 2006).

Comorbidity is related to increased mortality, poorer health status, and greater disability, with each added comorbid mental disorder increasing the odds of a medical disorder being classified as severely impairing (Druss et al., 2007). Individuals with comorbid conditions (both behavioral and health) tend to use more intense levels and more numerous services, complicating care coordination, which increases the risk of poorer care (Gijsen et al., 2001). In one study, poorer continuity was related to higher hospital costs and lower community costs, and greater continuity was linked to better consumer outcomes (Mitton, Adair, McDougall, & Marcoux, 2005). Hence, case management services that assertively link consumers, such as Assertive Community Treatment (ACT), and that bring intensive and multidisciplinary community-based services to consumers, have repeatedly had positive impacts on service coordination and outcomes for individuals with SMI (Dixon, 2002; Goldman et al., 2002; Gonzalez & Rosenheck, 2002). ACT model enhancement using higher levels of psychiatric nursing care has demonstrated significant improvements in health and community functioning over ACT-as-usual (Kane & Blank, 2004).

Comorbid mental disorders: Kessler and colleagues (2005) found that greater than 40% of 12-month cases were comorbid (Kessler et al., 2005). Affective, anxiety, and psychotic disorders frequently occur in combination. One study found that social phobias were comorbid with major depressive disorder (MDD) in approximately 20% of respondents, were frequently present with other anxiety disorders, and when participants had both an anxiety disorder and social phobia the rate of MDD was 65.2% (Ohayoon & Schatzberg, 2010). Others have found that from 7% to 70% of persons with schizophrenia have comorbid depression, which increases the risk for rehospitalization and suicide (Delahanty et al., 2001). Issues of trauma and posttraumatic stress disorder (PTSD) are of significant concern because comorbidity is present in greater than 80% of diagnosed cases and complicates treatment (Dadíc-Hero, Toríc, Ruzík, Medved, & Graovac, 2009). For example, individuals having comorbid depression are associated with poorer outcomes than those without PTSD (Quarantin et al., 2009).

Co-occurring disorders (COD): Public mental health facilities in the United States reported that 24% of consumers with SMI also had a substance-related disorder (Lutterman, Berhane, Phelan, Shaw, & Rana,

2009). More than 21% of adults with SMI reported a dependency on alcohol or illegal drugs even as the prevalence of COD may be increasing, especially for specific minority populations (Compton, Kevin, Conway, Stinson, & Grant, 2006). Although the reasons for COD are complex, research indicates that self-medication with substances is common when individuals have PTSD (Leeies, Pagura, Sareen, & Bolton, 2010), mood (Bolton, Robinson, & Sareen, 2009), and other anxiety disorders (Bolton, Cox, Clara, & Sareen, 2006). In fact, an important finding from a number of studies indicates that the onset of a mental disorder frequently precedes substance disorder (CSAT, 2007).

Consumers who do not receive integrated treatment but instead receive segregated or serial services disengage from care, which is associated with an increase in relapse, an increase in symptoms, and poorer health outcomes (Drake, Mueser, Brunette, & McHugo, 2004). Integrated Dual Disorders Treatment (IDDT) demonstrates that services focusing on providing concurrent and integrated treatment improves both mental health functioning and reductions in substance abuse (Drake, Essock, Shaner, Carey, Minkoff et al., 2001; Drake, Mueser, Noordsy, Drake, & Fox, 2003). Although it has become clear that concurrent mental health and substance abuse treatment improves outcomes, an analysis of participants in the National Surveys on Drug Use and Health found that 46% of those with COD and 65% of those with multiple substance and multiple mental health conditions did not receive any treatment (Harris & Edlund, 2005). The continued lack of treatment and integrated service reflects the segmentation of addiction and mental health into distinct silos (Horvitz-Lennon, Kilbourne, & Pincus, 2006) as well as an underutilization of EBPs because of providers' and organizations' entrenched beliefs and modes of service delivery, resistance from threatened organizational structures, outdated reimbursement rules, lack of provider training, and a dearth of resources (Corrigan et al., 2008; Drake & Bond, 2008; Rogers, Vegare, Baron, & Salzer, 2007).

Issues of Significance

Culture, "race,"[4] and ethnicity: The importance of culture, race, and ethnicity—as well as language (IOM, 2009)—in informing the social context of service delivery is underscored by the disparities in access and

---

[4]The initial bracketing of the term recognizes that there is wide debate regarding the social construction of race as a biological category although given the history of oppression it is meaningful as a social category. In the United States, race and ethnicity are

outcomes for individuals of color and socioeconomic groups not only in mental health but also in primary health care (Smedley et al., 2002; USDHHS, 2001). It has been noted that "the sources of these disparities are complex, are rooted in historic and contemporary inequities, and involve many participants at several levels" (Smedley et al., 2002, p. 1).

At the research level, considerations of culture, race, and ethnicity were historically absent from discussions on mental illness. In the 1970s, the works of Kleinman and others brought the issue of culture to the fore, resulting in numerous studies specifically dedicated to understanding mental disorders within a cultural context. Even as progress was being made, Kleinman (1988, p. xi) noted that "The concept of culture is treated in most psychiatric textbooks as unessential to mental illness and psychiatric treatment." This failure arises, in part, from assumptions that mental illnesses are primarily "brain diseases," and by extension that SMIs are a product of specific pathologies rather than complex expressions of biological, social, and psychological factors.

Even after the Surgeon General (1999) and Institute of Medicine (Smedley et al., 2002) issued reports documenting differential access and outcomes for persons of color in mental health and physical health, respectively, culture, race, and ethnicity remain "impractical." Bass, Bolton, and Murray (2007, p. 918) appropriately warn that "the recognition of the effect of culture on the understanding of mental illness cannot be an after-the-fact consideration ... Without such knowledge, we will continue to be stuck with the 'unsure of culture appropriateness' caveat as a limitation in research." In 2001 SAMHSA developed cultural competence standards for mental health services with underserved racial ethnic groups, which include African Americans, Hispanics, Native Americans/ Alaska Natives, and Asian/Pacific Islanders. Also, the American Association of Community Psychiatrists (2008) issued a position statement on diversity that offered cultural diversity that included "issues of race, ethnicity, gender identity, language, age, country of origin, sexual orientation, religious/spiritual beliefs, social class, and physical disability." Nevertheless, culture as a concept continues to be poorly defined, remains difficult to operationalize, and research still "relies on an outdated definition of culture," which views culture as received rather than

---

defined legislatively for political and economic reasons with the Office of Management and Budget (OMB) using five racial and one ethnic category (see IOM, 2009 for discussion).

negotiated through daily routine social interactions (Lopez & Guarnaccia, 2000, p. 573).

At the service level, research continues to find that the differences in general prevalence and overrepresentation among high-needs groups may be a function of access to quality care (Alegria et al., 2008; Cook, McGuire, & Miranda, 2007; Cooper, Beach, Johnson, & Inui, 2006; Wells, Klap, Koike, & Sherbourne, 2001) including differential access to case management (Barrio et al., 2003), medications (Knudsen, Ducharme, & Roman, 2007), and frequently based on the diagnosis that individuals of color are given (Elway, Ranganathan, & Eisen, 2008; Keyes, Hatzenbuehler, Alberti, Narrow, & Grant et al., 2008).

At the diagnostic level, within the context of the larger conflict of the definition of SMI, it is important to recognize that the disorders upon which any definition is built are themselves issues of debate and inherently social. The IOM (2009, p. 22) notes:

> With depression there is not even a real scientific definition of the focus of the disease—"mood"—and no accurate way to measure how it changes, nor is there a core understanding of how serotonin impacts the brain as a whole to alter mood.

In fact, studies indicate that the diagnostic criteria used may underestimate the rate of depression among African Americans (Coyne & Marcus, 2006) and their exposure to stress (Turner & Avison, 2003). A vital issue is the difference between disorders as disease and illness: The sociologic and anthropologic literature emphasizes that within the Western medical paradigm, disease is viewed as pathology or maladaptation in biologic and psychophysiologic processes, whereas illness is the expression of reactions to disease, distress, and discomfort shaped by personal, interpersonal, and cultural frames (Gaines, 1992; Kleinman, Eisenberg, & Good, 2006). Differences in vantage points are important, given that research on the nature of consumer–physician encounters suggests that consumers anticipate biased, stigmatizing, and/or nonresponsive provider interactions that may reduce help-seeking (Doescher, Saver, Franks, & Fiscella, 2000; Johnson, Roter, Power, & Cooper, 2004; Saha, Arbelaez, & Cooper, 2003).

Beyond the potential of race, ethnicity, and culture to serve as indicators of social disadvantage and systemic oppression (Smedley et al., 2002; USDHHS, 2001), ethnographers, sociologists, and ethnopsychiatrists have underscored that the expression of illness and the socially sanctioned mechanisms for help-seeking will differ (Gaines, 1992; Kleinman, 1988; Kleinman, Eisenberg, & Good, 1978; Lopez & Guarnaccia, 2000). For example, Alverson and colleagues (2007) identified ethno-cultural differences among Americans of European, African, and Puerto Rican descent in how consumers "en-story" or communicate their experience of illness and disability. Studies have consistently documented the underutilization of mental health services among racial and ethnic "minorities" (Neighbors et al., 2007; USDHSS, 2001; Wang et al., 2005), with a recent study indicating that among African Americans, beliefs related to the natural remission of mental distress may partially explain the lower utilization rates (Anglin, Alberti, Link, & Phelan, 2008).

Family Involvement

Just as treatment has focused on the index condition a consumer might have, it has focused on intrapersonal issues rather than interpersonal relationships. Indeed, *families have historically been viewed as problems rather than assets* (Fisher, Benson, & Tessler, 1990), with many professionals seeing families as obstacles to progress, and to believing consumers would benefit from being separated from them (Kim & Salyers, 2008), perhaps deriving from strongly held theories of "dysfunctional families" or more sophisticated iterations of the schizophrenic-genic mother/parent. It is not surprising, then, that families frequently perceive they are being blamed for their family member's illness or treatment trajectory (Fisher et al., 1990).

Research has begun to examine family needs and preferences, and researchers have found that the stigma related to having a member with SMI is a barrier to engagement in treatment despite high levels of unmet need (Drapalski et al., 2008). For example, some researchers have found that the stigma related to medication with Latinos is a significant barrier (Interian, Martinez, Guarnaccia, Vega, & Escobar, 2007). While needs were as complex and unique as the families themselves, researchers underscored respondents' need for information about the disorder, discussion and engagement in care planning, and advocacy related to services (Drapalski et al., 2008).

As sources of caregiving and instrumental supports, families experience a great deal of burden related to the ill family member (Shankar & Muthuswamy, 2007). This is especially true for communities of color who may have a preference for more communal approaches. For example, the Latino concept of *familismo*, which emphasizes loyalty to the family, interdependence among family members, and cooperation, encourages members of both the nuclear and the extended family to help one another in times of need and can serve as a buffer against stress (Organista, 2007). Guarnaccia (1998) found that African-American families have denser, larger social networks and rely on them for help to a greater degree than families of European descent, exemplifying how caregiving and cultural attributes can support consumers' engagement in treatment. Within some Asian cultures, SMI is considered punishment for offenses committed by the consumer; perceived as a family problem, recovery requires members to call upon obligations and make sacrifices for the wellness of the entire family (Hsiao & Van Riper, 2010). Despite families experiencing a great deal of stress, Doornbos (1996) reports that they desire and do develop coping skills when engaged by providers.

Efforts that perceive families, as consumers define them, as important instrumental and affective supports have proven to be effective and underscore the need to engage "families" in consumer service planning (Corrigan, Mueser, Bond, Drake, & Solomon, 2008). One such EBP, family psycho-education, has demonstrated consistent reductions in hospitalizations (Dixon et al., 2001; Pharoah, Rathbone, Mari, & Streiner, 2004).

Homelessness

The successful characterization of homeless persons as mentally ill draws on the reality that research consistently reports approximately *"one-third to one-half of homeless people had severe psychiatric disorders"* (McQuiston, Finnerty, Hirschowitz, & Susser, 2003, p. 669). This sizable cohort struggles with a complex interplay of SMI, including comorbid substance or trauma-related disorders (Bassuk, Dawson, Perloff, & Weinreb, 2001; Burt et al., 1999; Koegel et al., 1996; Najavits, Weiss, & Shaw, 1997; Smith, Meyers, & Delaney, 1998; Tsemberis & Eisenberg, 2000). One study indicated that almost half of those with SMI also experienced some sort of victimization (Lam & Rosenheck, 1998). In addition to finding more victimization among homeless persons with mental disorders, they experience more problems with health (Sullivan, Burnam, Koegel, & Hollenberg, 2000). This was supported in a New York City study which found that 69% of all hospital admissions from the shelter system were related to substance disorder or mental illness (Kerker et al., 2005).

Individuals who are homeless and have SMI have been known to travel the "institutional circuit" (Hopper et al., 1997) among acute facilities, shelters, the streets, and transitional residences, which contributes to their poor health status and their depiction as treatment resistant (Drury, 2003). Historically, technologies that were effective in engaging homeless people with SMI in treatment and housing were associated with increased costs (Rosenheck, 2000), although current EBPs such as ACT and Housing First/Pathways to Housing are proving to be cost effective (Tsemberis & Eisenberg, 2000; Tsemberis, Gulcur, & Nakae, 2004; Tsemberis, Moran, Shinn, Asmussen, & Shern, 2003).

Unemployment and Underemployment

· The unemployment rate among individuals with SMI has *been estimated to be as high as 85%,* with long-term unemployment associated with a diagnosis of psychosis, severe symptoms, and a history of multiple hospitalizations (Goldberg et al., 2001). SMI is also significantly associated with reduced earnings whereas there is no statistically significant reduction in wages for individuals who have ever had a mental disorder (Kessler et al., 2008). Kessler and colleagues estimated the cost burden of lost productivity at $193.2 billion for the total population, with 75.4% attributable to reduced earnings and 24.6% attributable to a diminished probability of employment.

Approximately *50% of U.S. employers surveyed expressed reluctance to hire individuals with psychiatric histories* and 75% expressed reluctance to hire individuals with histories of substance use who are currently taking antipsychotic medication (Scheid, 1999). Thus, despite federal legislation that prohibits discrimination based on disability, individuals with SMI continue to experience direct and indirect discrimination because of attitudes, structural disincentives, and generalized policy neglect (Stuart, 2006).

In a recent multisite randomized trial, researchers found that persons with schizophrenia were less likely to be competitively employed but fared better when enrolled in evidence-based supportive employment programs even when "at study baseline, individuals with schizophrenia had significantly higher levels of symptoms, greater number of months hospitalized over their lifetimes, younger ages of illness onset, lower education, poorer work histories, and lower work motivation than those without schizophrenia" (Cook et al., 2008, pp. 43–44). In addition, supported employment models designed to place first/fast track employment appear more effective than models emphasizing training first (Corrigan &

McCracken, 2005). Hence, evidence-informed supported employment programs can assist a wide range of individuals with SMI and may be especially beneficial in improving competitive employment rates among those with clinical issues that have historically impeded workforce retention (Bond, Drake, & Becker, 2008; Drake & Bond, 2008; Rosenheck et al., 2006).

Criminal Justice Involvement

Some suggest that individuals with SMI have not been treated in the community but instead the institutions in which they are warehoused has changed; specifically, Lurigio and Swartz (2006) state that prisons, jails, and detention centers have become the *de facto* treatment setting given their overrepresentation in criminal justice settings. A U.S. Department of Justice report on the mental health status of U.S. prison and jail inmates reported that more than 700,000 inmates reported symptoms of mental disorder or a history of treatment for mental disorder in the past year (Bureau of Justice Statistics, 2006). Specifically, the Department of Justice found that 56% of state prisoners met the definition of SMI, with 43% reporting a history or symptoms of mania, 23% reporting symptoms or a history of major depression, and 15% having experienced psychotic symptoms such as hallucinations or delusions.

The complex interaction between SMI and incarceration is exacerbated by issues of recidivism, gender, and homelessness (Braithwaite, Treadwell, & Arriola, 2005) so that consumers experience a revolving door with high rates of recidivism (Lamb & Weinberger, 2001; Lovell, Gargliardi, & Peterson, 2002). As early as 1995, Roesch, Ogloff, and Eaves underscored the need for collaborative approaches, especially bridging researchers to criminal justice systems, in order to improve the identification, prevention, and treatment of individuals with SMI. A SAMHSA study examined collaborative jail diversion models for SMI consumers with forensic involvement. The study found that aggressive linkages to services and implementing nontraditional models of care were central to decreasing recidivism (Steadman et al., 1999). In particular, Lamb, Weinberger, and Gross (2004) spoke to the need for mental health professionals to work with police departments to prevent the unnecessary criminalization of consumers with SMI. More recently, Loveland and Boyle (2007) explored the effect of different models of case management and found that intensive models that provided integrated addiction treatment led to a reduction in arrests and incarceration. The proliferation of drug treatment and mental health courts and other programs address these issues.

Stigma

Stigma is embedded in the systems from which consumers seek services, and this exacerbates the barriers they must overcome. Stigma, or the loss of social status and discrimination generated by negative stereotypes that have become linked in a particular society to a particular human attribute such as mental illness (Link & Phelan, 2001), impacts individuals as soon as they have officially been labeled by the treatment establishment (Link, Cullen, Struening, Shrout, & Dohrenwend, 1989), especially among individuals with COD (Link, Struening, Rahva, Phelan, & Nuttbrock, 1997; Luoma et al., 2007; Semple, Grant, & Patterson, 2005). For example, the public image of individuals with SMI as violent is perpetuated in our language, media (Wahl, 2006), and research (Lidz, Banks, Simon, Schubert, & Mulvey, 2007) although *they are more likely to be victims of violence rather than perpetrators* (Choe, Teplin, & Abram, 2008; Teplin, McClellan, Abram, & Weiner, 2005). In fact, even the most well-meaning professionals and advocates stigmatize consumers by judging their capacity to recover and by limiting consumers' decision making instead of allying with them (Wagner & Cohen, 1991). Such subtleties of bias reinforce professional power and control of oppressed and stigmatized communities (Forest, 2003) and inform consumers' experiences of their illnesses and its consequences and whether they use available services (Rüsch et al., 2009).

RECOVERY IN CONTEXT

The President's New Freedom Commission on Mental Health (2003) emphasized the need to transform how mental health services are delivered and insisted that consumer voice and participation was necessary in creating this change. Despite resistance, the Recovery Movements, which encompass a number of ideological stances, have been central in maintaining momentum toward systemic change. Yet, the definitional debate surrounding SMI impacts how recovery is incorporated into systems change and, in point of fact, whether it is viewed as a legitimate intervention. If SMI is a function of specific disorders, then it will be conceived as severely limited, whereas if SMI is fundamentally the embodiment of the interplay between social, psychological, and biological processes, it has much greater potential. The arguments around recovery are examined here in order to make these issues explicit and to assist program planners in understanding the implications of the various choices on program design and delivery.

Defining Recovery: More Debate

The concept of recovery as used by consumers in mental health movements has a long history. Although it has been suggested that recovery is a new paradigm that began in the 1970s (Allott, 2003; Anthony, 1993; Schiff, 2004), it has also been noted that consumers and advocates have been questioning psychiatric practices and the custodial care of individuals with SMI for hundreds of years (Chamberlin, 1990; Chamberlin & Rogers, 1990; Roberts & Wolfson, 2004; Van Tosh, Ralph, & Campbell, 2000). Some suggest that increased interest in recovery stems from cross-cultural and local research findings that between 25% and 65% of study participants with SMI recover from mental disorders, in particular schizophrenia (Davidson, O'Connell, Tondora, Styron, & Kangas, 2006; Jacobson & Greenley, 2001). However, others attribute it to the strength of the psychiatric patients' liberation movement that began in the 1970s and took root in the 1980s (Anthony, 1993; Frese & Davis, 1997; Schiff, 2004; Van Tosh & del Vecchio, 2000; Van Tosh et al., 2000). Chamberlin (1990), recognized as the psychiatric patients' liberation movement founder, places the consumer movement within an evolving—and uncompleted—consciousness-raising process begun during the Civil Rights Era.

Similarly, there continues to be some disagreement regarding the appropriate term for consumers themselves. For many in the consumer movement, it is ultimately a political statement that speaks to consumer control and ownership of the defintions and processes (Schiff, 2004).

Given the politics inherent in the concept, depending on whether one questions survivors, ex-patients, consumers, professionals, former substance abusers, or other constituencies, the definition of recovery itself will differ (Davidson et al., 2006). Roberts and Wolfson (2004) suggest that the different definitions are captured by two competing streams: The first emphasizes both clinical and social functioning, which approximate what is understood as "cure" and the second focuses on personal and subjective elements that speak to accommodations to the illness. Davidson et al. (2006) suggest that much of the confusion results from the various uses of the term "recovery" as related to physical conditions, trauma, substance use, and SMI. They elaborate that the emphasis on a return to a normative state is dominant in discourses related to physical disability and rehabilitation.

The term recovery was coined by substance self-help groups (White, 1998, 2000) and, therefore, the addiction-based definition emphasizes abstinence from substances through admission of the substances' impact on the individual's life and maintaining sobriety through vigilance and community support. And, lastly, they suggest that the mental health usage of the term reflects the individual reclaiming life and creating a narrative that is not defined by the disease or by others.

The most frequently cited definition is that offered by Anthony (1993). He states that recovery is:

> a deeply personal, unique process of changing one's attitudes, values, feelings, goals, skills and roles. It is a way of living a satisfying, hopeful, and contributing life even with limitations caused by the illness. Recovery involves the development of new meaning and purpose in one's life as one grows beyond the catastrophic effects of mental illness.

However, many consumers have viewed this definition as a subversion of the lived meaning of recovery owing to its emphasis on limitations (Fisher & Chamberlin, 2004). In the competing National Empowerment Center (NEC) definition, they emphasize consumer control and full recovery regardless of continued symptoms or the use of medication (Ahern & Fisher, 2001; Fisher & Chamberlin, 2004). A definition deemed more acceptable to many across disability communities is that offered by SAMHSA (2005):

> Mental health recovery is a journey of healing and transformation enabling a person with a mental health problem to live a meaningful life in a community of his or her choice while striving to achieve his or her full potential.

In this definition, focusing on a transformative journey, choice and meaning are viewed as promoting increased awareness and reducing stigma and discrimination (NCD, 2008).

Recovery: Principles and Models

Regardless of the definition, however, there are some key components recognized as necessary in recovery approaches. SAMHSA (2005) offers the following 10 components as essential to recovery in mental health: (1) self-direction; (2) individualized and person-centered; (3) empowerment; (4) holistic; (5) nonlinear; (6) strengths-based; (7) peer support; (8) respect; (9) responsibility; and (10) hope.

Ahern and Fisher's (2001) Empowerment Model is based on the experiences of persons with different diagnoses and is meant to capture the general process of recovery from SMI. These models are described in Table 1.1.

TABLE 1.1
Recovery Models in Serious Mental Illness

Fisher and Ahern (2002)		Andresen, Oades, and Caputi (2003)		Young and Ensing (1999)	
Stage	Theme	*Stage*	Theme	*Stage*	Theme
Emotionally Distressed	Loss/Stress	*Moratorium*	Denial, hopelessness, Self-protectiveness to envision themselves differently	*Initiating Recovery & Overcoming 'Stuckness'*	Accepting the illness, motivation for change, and finding sources of hope and inspiration
Severe Emotional Distress (SED)	Insufficient supports & coping	*Awareness*	Emerging hope of a different experience		
Mentally Ill	Mentally Distressed	*Preparation*	Taking stock of values, limitations and strengths; Developing skills; Reconnecting	*Regaining What Was Lost*	Empowerment and self-definition (i.e., taking responsibility for recovery, behaviors, and empowering attitudes, gaining insight about self and the relationship between self and illness, and taking care of self, being active, and reconnecting socially)
Recovery & Healing emotionally	Recovery from mental illness through self-management & social role	*Rebuilding*	Taking responsibility; Forging of positive identity		
Balanced & Whole	Sufficient supports & coping	*Growth*	Resiliency despite setbacks; positive sense of self; integration of illness; identity as a meaningful experience	*Improving Quality of Life*	Attaining a sense of well-being, finding meaning and purpose, using creative capacities, and improving the standard of living

Recovery as a Process

Essential to an understanding of recovery is acknowledging it as a self-ascribed, nonlinear process including, for some, the continued presence of symptoms, use of medication, and limitations or impairments (Fisher & Chamberlin, 2004; Roberts & Wolfson, 2004). The relationship a consumer has to the symptoms and/or limitations is telling; in a qualitative study of recovery narratives among individuals with schizophrenia, Shea

(2010) found that a sense of *living with* rather than "*engulfment*" *by* the disease was central. Thus, the central issue from the standpoint of the consumer is in distinguishing the disorder or disease from the personal experience of it as an illness. Indeed, how consumers interpret their experience of SMI has significant consequences for recovery: Studies examining narratives of people in recovery have found that the transformation from an illness-dominated sense of self to one that is viewed as competent and as having agency is critical to the recovery process (Mancini, 2005; Mancini & Lawson, 2009; Mancini & Rogers, 2007; Ridgway, 2001).

Yet, the recovery movement is clear that the process of recovery is an individual transformative process that is not easily reduced or necessarily viable for others. What has been found is that the active management of the recovery process for consumers is an opportunity to reclaim their voice and power within *all* the systems that comprise their lives so that they can fully participate in society and perform roles other than "client." Approaches that engage individuals in such active efforts around disorders that can be disabling are understood as "recovery management models." These models emphasize fostering consumers' capacity to overcome stressors and achieve wellness-enhancing goals (Brown et al., 2008), including the development of *recovery capital* or the institutional and social resources (e.g., social networks, employment, education, and self-determination) that sustain recovery and promote inclusion in society (Granfield & Cloud, 2001). Recovery management stresses problem solving and normalizes the varied trajectories in recovery, which demedicalizes the illness experience and recovery process (Ellison & Dunn, 2006). The Empowerment Model and recovery management models appear to share recognition that a consumer's capacity to maintain wellness and *an experience* of being in recovery or recovered is dependent less upon the resurfacing of symptoms than upon the marshalling of supports and strategies during the inevitable situational stressors and crises in life.

Recovery's Evidentiary Base

The emerging evidence base for consumer-directed and consumer-delivered approaches comes from many fields, including mental health, education, and addictions. Within mental health several meta-analyses have demonstrated that self-help programs had positive outcomes as compared to no treatment (Gould & Clum, 1993; Kurtzweil, Scogin, & Rosen, 1996; Scogin, Bynum, Stephens, & Calhoun, 1990). One-to-one peer support programs have produced improvements in many areas of functioning (fewer crisis events, fewer hospitalizations, improved social functioning, reduction in substance abuse, and improvements in quality of life) as compared to those not receiving peer-delivered services (Klein, Cnaan, & Whitecraft, 1998; Resnick & Rosenheck, 2008; Salzer, 2002). Also, case management delivered by consumers has been found to be as effective as professional services (Chinman, Rosenheck, Lam, & Davidson, 2000; Dixon, Hackman, & Lehman, 1997; Solomon & Draine, 1995). Researchers have found that relationships built around mentoring and coaching for information, affiliation, and instrumental supports impact service retention, likelihood of employment, and retention in employment (Bauldry & McClanahan, 2008). There is evidence that consumer programs increase empowerment and participation, and impact service utilization (Forquer & Knight, 2001; Rogers et al., 2007; Trainor, Shepherd, Boydell, Leff, & Crawford, 1997). More recently, consumer-run self-help groups and individual support within a chronic management program based on the Flinders model were found to improve illness self-management and quality of life (Lawn et al., 2007) in employment (Bauldry & McClanahan, 2008).

Peer Support

Peer support incorporates life-meaning and spirituality (Laudet, Morgen, & White, 2006) and has been found to be positively associated with changes across nine areas of recovery and empowerment (Corrigan, 2006). The value of peer support derives from the powerful effects that social relationships are now widely recognized as having on both physical and mental health (Berkman, Glass, Brissette, & Seeman, 2000). As with individuals with SMI, assertive linkage, rather than passive referrals, and utilization of various supports improved outcomes for individuals with severe substance-related disorders (Scott, Foss, & Dennis, 2005; White & Kurtz, 2006). Thus, rather than seeing self-help and community supports as after-care once abstinence is achieved, they are themselves legitimate pathways to recovery.

RECOVERY-ORIENTED SYSTEMS OF CARE

Within the addictions sector, the drive toward Recovery-Oriented Systems of Care (ROSCs) and the evidence supporting it are instructive to mental health planners and administrators. The development of ROSCs began as substance treatment was reconceptualized from an acute model of stabilization and abstinence to that of a chronic care model wherein substance disorders are recognized as having different trajectories (White, 2005, 2006, 2008). The central elements in ROSCs are the same components identified by SAMHSA as components of mental health recovery (Bellack, 2006).

Informing ROSCs is the recognition that formal treatment too often views relapse as failure on the part of consumers rather than as an indication that the appropriate combination of services and supports matching the particular cultural, spiritual, and racial/ethnic needs of a consumer has yet to be identified (White & Kurtz, 2006). The underutilization of alternative pathways to recovery is especially problematic for persons of color given that they receive a lower quality of care; even when socioeconomic factors or access-related factors are controlled (Smedley et al., 2002), they appear to respond differently to standard treatments (Le Fauve et al., 2003; Venner et al., 2006).

Recovery and System Transformation

As repeatedly emphasized in multiple federal reports encouraging systems transformation (Smedley et al., 2002; USDHSS, 2001), providers, policy makers, and program planners need to fundamentally reframe their understanding of recovery and its role in improving the lives of consumers with SMI. A decade ago, Norcross (2000) suggested that "A massive, systemic, and yet largely silent revolution is occurring in mental health today and is gathering steam for tomorrow: self-help efforts without professional intervention." Nevertheless, achieving this transformation is fraught with tension. The movement to a consumer-directed system will be difficult within a mental health system that is run by professionals who have the power to establish etiology, define nosological systems, and determine illness course. Just as the concept of EBP has altered the structure and thinking of the health and social service systems, it is (hopefully) causing us to question our individual and institutional roles in favoring certain professional technologies while resisting more "exotic" or less established ones (e.g., our historic dismissal of medicinal herbs).

Recovery, Communities, and the Embodiment of Social Factors

The attractiveness of the Empowerment Model of Recovery (Fisher & Ahern, 2002) derives from an understanding of the vulnerability of all individuals to mental illness and to SMI when faced with loss, trauma, and stress in an environment without sufficient supports, both before and after formal diagnosis. That is, whether a mental disorder becomes disabling is not solely a function of a disease but a product of the availability of social and institutional supports in combination with individual coping capacities.

Mechanic and Tanner (2007) note that today health and social services are much more cognizant of the poverty issues and "upstream factors" that contribute to the inequalities and inequities as experienced by and embodied among these populations and groups, but policy and programming are hampered by assessments of blame typically focused at the individual level. They also note that as we further empirically substantiate "that neighborhood and community context affects health and welfare beyond personal characteristics and resources, it makes clear the need to design improved interventions at the community level" (Mechanic & Tanner, 2007, p. 1228). The development of approaches, such as ROSCs and livable communities, offers the promise of such community efforts.

Beginning in 2004, the National Council on Disability (NCD) developed a model for individuals with disabilities that incorporates consumers' preferences for independent living and those environmental factors that facilitate autonomy (NCD, 2004a, 2004b, 2006, 2007, 2008). Based on these findings, the NCD developed a number of models of livable communities and has offered one specifically for the needs of individuals with psychiatric disabilities. Six essential elements of communities were identified across the models: (1) affordable, appropriate, and accessible housing; (2) accessible, affordable, reliable, and safe transportation; (3) work, volunteer, and education opportunities; (4) access to health and supportive services; (5) participation in civic, cultural, social, and recreational activities; and (6) adjusting the physical environment to ensure inclusiveness and accessibility (NCD, 2008). For individuals with SMI, and individuals with psychiatric disabilities who experience homelessness, criminal justice involvement, and substance dependence, a key issue is housing.

Although access to affordable housing is a concern among all disabled populations—and increasingly an issue for all Americans—the hindrance for individuals with SMI is that housing continues to be viewed within custodial terms. In 1999, through Executive Order 13217 and the Supreme Court decision in *Olmstead v. L.C.* the federal government underscored the right to housing in the least restrictive setting for individuals with mental disabilities in accordance with the American with Disabilities Act (ADA) (PL 101-36). Both the executive order and the decision affirmed that "Unjustified isolation or segregation of qualified individuals with disabilities through institutionalization is a form of disability-based discrimination."

Yet, consumers with SMI continue to be perceived as unable to participate in community life. And, the issue of housing and institutionalization is a central fulcrum in the definitional debate regarding SMI and in society's appropriate response. The concept of ontological security—that is, a place engendering feelings of well-being, safety, constancy, and security (Neale, 1997; Padgett, 2007) for individuals with SMI, and for recovery communities in general—connects the experiential sense of belonging to social interaction within spatial and ideational communities. The relevance is that communities provide individuals with some measure of ontological security, the capacity to create meaningful narratives, perform daily routines, and provide direction. Linking this more explicitly, recovery provides a social network that offers rules, repertoires, and shared views. It serves as a counterforce or counter-discourse to biomedical explanations and directives and to moralistic or etiological discourses that frame consumers as disempowered by, and eternally subject to, their condition or vulnerability.

The lack of social integration among consumers with SMI is captured by Fisher (2009), who writes: "For most of us consumer/survivor/ex-patients (c/s/x's) our central issues are discrimination, helplessness, and isolation." Much of current social and health programming, however, pays insufficient attention to assisting consumers to meaningfully connect with others in terms of both physical and emotional/psychological space: Interventions are *directed at* or *provided to* individuals with SMI rather than engaging them as full partners. And, while shelter has been increasingly recognized as necessary, it is assumed that it is also sufficient in the creation of ontological security, although this is not the case. This is wonderfully captured by Ware, Hopper, Tugenberg, Dickey, and Fisher (2007), who suggest that without consequential civic activities, relationships, respect, and political voice consumers "living outside the hospital may be described as *in* the community, *but not of it*" (p. 474) (emphasis added).

Communities and social networks are critical to recovery because it is through them and within them that consumers can strengthen their capacity to create empowered, hopeful narratives that are syntonic with their experiences. Indeed, social networks are crucial to the management of crises in that they provide *havens* or a sense of belonging and being assisted, *bandages* as they provide routine emotional support and coping under stressful conditions, *safety nets* that lessen the impact of acute crises and chronic difficulties, and *social capital* (Wellman & Gulia, 1999). Hence, interventions that include volunteerism, mutual aid, citizen participation, and organizational decision making have been shown to have positive outcomes as consumers take on "valued roles" (Brown, Shepherd, Merkle, Wittuk, & Meissen, 2008; Brown, Shepherd, Wituk, & Meissen, 2007; Petersen & Zimmerman, 2004; Rowe et al., 2007) and acquire recovery capital (e.g., social networks, self-determination, employment, etc.).

In terms of program development and planning, constructing more socially integrated interventions requires maximizing collaborative and coalitional approaches to service design and delivery. The emerging evidence from mental health and drug treatment courts as well as ROSCs demonstrates that approaches which capitalize on existing services and create *interventive communities* that promote consumer education around a range of available services and support, and that respect consumer choice, work. Indeed, these strategies recognize that service aversion and treatment ruptures are inherent within a system that is fragmented and poses barriers to access and quality care. As new models are created, further exploration and development of the inclusive livable community framework may prove useful in that it can serve as a "unifying and universal construct" (NCD, 2007) for all individuals with disabilities. Individuals with SMI will remain socially isolated—as well as persons in other "vulnerable populations" —if we continue "segregating people by their disabilities into specific housing and other ... programs [which] is discriminatory, creates barriers to services, and divides the disability community, as well as creating 'disability ghettoes'" (NCD, 2000, p. 46). Furthermore, if we are to truly benefit from evidence-based and promising practices funders, program planners and administrators need to break down the barriers and silos created by different disability sectors, to develop cross-disability coalitions to advocate for such communities, to promote cross-fertilization, and to transfer innovations and models that may be relevant across multiple sectors (NCD, 2004b).

Recovery, Language, and Stigma

Today, the continued variable and interchangeable use of the three terms underscores the fact that consensus has yet to be reached in defining SMI (Parabiaghi, Bonetto, Ruggeri, Lasalvia, & Leese, 2006). Beyond custom, "the often chronic and persistent nature of mental illness" (Woodward et al., 2008, p. 1297) may reinforce and justify perpetuation of the use of CMI and SPMI despite a federally legislated definition. The observation in practice, research, and life is that many individuals with SMI have an illness experience that is nonlinear, burdensome, and unrelieved—both to the person and their families and to society. For example, some have recently constructed operational definitions of CMI in research with individuals who are also homeless (Koegel, Burnam, & Farr, 1998; Sullivan, Burnam, Koegel, & Hollenberg, 2000; Wolf, Burnam, Koegel, Sullivan, & Morton, 2001). Such terminology prevails because it can quickly and easily capture and communicate a complex individual process that, while unique, is not exceptional.

Although the use of CMI and SPMI may make it easier to communicate a complex phenomenon, their use has consequences for individuals living with SMI. In particular, it is noted that the term "chronic" can serve as coded language or as a "demeaning euphemism" (Chinman et al., 2001) for individuals with SMI or particular diagnoses. In normalizing the term chronic, Bachrach noted, "I think the only one that is really bizarre is SPMI, which stands for severe and persistent mental illness. In discussions I have heard people with illnesses referred to as speemies" (Talbott, 2000). While the categorization of individuals to a single term or acronym may economize attention and simplify understanding, it also stereotypes, devalues, and dehumanizes those to whom it is applied—which impacts consumers' willingness to enter care (Grossman, 2004). This is apparent with other stigmatized service groups, especially individuals experiencing homelessness and persons with substance disorders, who are similarly characterized as "chronic," reinforcing characterizations of individuals and populations as "difficult," hopeless and unresponsive to interventive strategies and services. While professionals may use chronic, "speemies," and other terms to facilitate communication, they preserve distance between "us" and "them," perpetuate stigma, and ultimately require a redoubling of efforts to connect with and be purposefully used by those seeking service.

CONCLUSION

Transforming the mental health system requires that we incorporate and embrace inclusive approaches. The persistence of definitional dilemmas for SMI and recovery highlights the fundamental ideological, epistemological, and methodological schisms among those in the biomedical and social sciences. Yet, as more individuals are affected directly or impacted politically, economically, or in their own communities, the public will look to professionals and policy makers for answers. And, of course, as is currently the situation, they will hold those working in these arenas accountable if our attempts at system transformation fail. Hence, it is critical to integrate family members, consumer allies, and communities in the change process.

Current research efforts will hopefully advance our comprehension of how folk and popular technologies work and can contribute to our understanding and treatment of SMI and, more importantly, can engage consumers (and allies) in meaningful, culturally appropriate ways that develop their sense of integrity and self.

REFERENCES

Ahern, L., & Fisher, D. (2001). Recovery at your own PACE. *Journal of Psychosocial Nursing, 39,* 22–32.

Alegria, M., Chatterji, P., Wells, K., Cao, Z., Chen, C., Takeuchi, D., et al. (2008). Disparity in depression treatment among racial and ethnic minority populations in the United States. *Psychiatric Services, 59*(11), 1264–1272.

Allott, P. (2003) Services run by Experts by Experience. Published as part of the e-conference 'The importance of Values in Mental Health' delivered in March, jointly by NIMHE, the Mental Health Foundation, Sainsbury Centre for Mental Health and the University of Warwick (www.connects.org.uk/conferences) .

Alverson, H. S., Drake, R. E., Carpenter-Song, E. A., Chu, E., Ritsema, M., & Smith, B. (2007). Ethnocultural variations in mental illness discourse: Some implications for building therapeutic alliances. *Psychiatric Services, 58*(12), 1541–1546.

American Association of Community Psychiatrists. (2008). Position statement on Diversity. Retrieved from http://www.communitypsychiatry.org/publications/position_statements/AACPPositionStatementDiversity.pdf

Anderson, H. (1997). *Conversation, language and possibilities: A postmodern approach to therapy.* New York: Basis Books.

Andresen, R., Oades, L.G., & Caputi, P. (2003). The experience of recovery from schizophrenia: towards an empirically validated stage model. *Australian and New Zealand Journal of Psychiatry, 37,* 586–594.

Anglin, D. M., Alberti, P. M., Link, B. G., & Phelan, J. C. (2008). Racial differences in beliefs about the effectiveness and necessity of mental health treatment. *American Journal of Community Psychology, 42,* 17–24.

Anthony, W. (1993). Recovery from mental illness: The guiding vision of the mental health service system in the 1990s. *Psychosocial Rehabilitation Journal, 16*(4), 11–23.

Bachrach, L. (1988). Defining chronic mental illness: A Concept Paper. *Hospital & Community Psychiatry, 39,* 383–388.

Barrio, C., Yamada, A. M., Hough, R. I., Hawthorne, W., Garcia, P., & Jeste, D. V. (2003). Ethnic disparities in use of public mental health case management services among patients with schizophrenia. *Psychiatric Services, 54*(9), 1264–1270.

Bass, J. K., Bolton, P. A., & Murray, L. K. (2007). Do not forget culture when studying mental health. *The Lancet, 370*(9591), 918–919.

Bassuk, E., Dawson, R., Perloff, J., & Weinreb, L. (2001). Post-traumatic stress disorder in extremely poor women: Implications for health care clinicians. *JAMWA, 56*(2), 79–85.

Bauldry, S., & McClanahan, W. (2008). Ready4Work: Final Research Report. Department of Labor Washington, DC: Department of Labor.

Bellack, A. S. (2006). Scientific and consumer models of recovery in schizophrenia: Concordance, contrasts, and implications. *Schizophrenia Bulletin, 32*(3), 432–442.

Berkman, L. F., Glass, T., Brissette, I., & Seeman, T. (2000). From social integration to health: Durkheim in the new millennium. *Social Science and Medicine, 51,* 843–857.

Black, D. W., Warrack, G., & Winokur, G. (1985). The Iowa Record-Linkage Study: I. Suicides and accidental deaths among psychiatric patients. *Archives of General Psychiatry, 42*(1), 71–75.

Blau, J. (2003). *The dynamics of social welfare policy.* NY: Oxford University Press.

Bolton, J., Cox, B., Clara, I., & Sareen, J. (2006). Use of alcohol and drugs to self-medicate anxiety disorders in a nationally representative sample. *Journal of Nervous and Mental Disease, 194*(11), 818–825.

Bogdan, R., & Taylor, S. J. (1989). Relationships with severely disabled people: The social construction of humanness. *Social Problems, 36*(2), 135–148.

Bolton, J. M., Robinson, J., & Sareen, J. (2009). Self-medication of mood disorders with alcohol and drugs in the National Epidemiologic Survey on Alcohol and Related Conditions. *Journal of Affective Disorders, 115*(3), 367–375.

Bond, G. R., Drake, R. E., & Becker, D. R. (2008). An update on randomized controlled trials of evidence-based supported employment. *Psychiatric Rehabilitation Journal, 31*(4), 280–289.

Braithwaite, R. L., Treadwell, H. M., & Arriola, K. R. J. (2005). Health disparities and incarcerated women: A population ignored. *American Journal of Public Health, 95,* 1679–1681.

Brown, L. D., Shepherd, M. D., Merkle, E. C., Wituk, S. A., & Meissen, G. (2008). Understanding how participation in a consumer-run organization relates to recovery. *American Journal of Community Psychology, 42,* 167–178.

Brown, L. D., Shepherd, M. D., Wituk, S. A., & Meissen, G. (2007). How settings change people: Applying behavior setting theory to consumer-run organizations. *Journal of Community Psychology, 35,* 399–416.

Burt, M. R., Aron, L. Y., Douglas, T., Valente, J., Lee, R., & Iwen, B. (1999). *Homelessness: Programs and the people they serve. Summary report: Findings of the National Survey of Homeless Assistance Providers and Clients.* Washington, DC: U.S. Housing and Urban Development and Urban Institute.

Bureau of Justice Statistics. (2006). *Mental health problems of prison and jail inmates* (NCJ 213600). Washington, DC: Department of Justice.

Campbell, J. (1992). The Well-Being Project: Mental health clients speak for themselves. In Third Annual conference proceedings on state mental health agency research. Alexandria, VA: National Association for State Mental Health Program Directors Research Institute.

Center for Substance Abuse Treatment (2007). The Epidemiology of Co-Occurring Substance Use and Mental Disorders. COCE Overview Paper 8. (DHHS Publication No. (SMA) 07–4308). Rockville, MD: Substance Abuse and Mental Health Services Administration, and Center for Mental Health Services.

Chamberlin, J. (1990). The Ex-patients' movement: Where we've been and where we're going. *The Journal of Mind and Behavior, 11*(3), 323–336.

Chamberlin, J., & Rogers, J. (1990). Planning a community-based mental health system: Perspective of service recipients. *American Psychologist, 45*(11), 1241–1244.

Chinman, M. J., Rosenheck, R., Lam, J. A., & Davidson, L. (2000). Comparing consumer and nonconsumer provided case management services for homeless persons with serious mental illness. *Journal of Nervous & Mental Disease, 188,* 446–453.

Chinman, M., Weingarten, R., Stayner, D., & Davidson, L. (2001). Chronicity reconsidered: Improving person–environment fit through a consumer-run service. *Community Mental Health Journal, 37*(3), 215–229.

Choe, J. Y., Teplin, L. A., & Abram, K. M. (2008). Perpetration of violence, violent victimization, and severe mental illness: Balancing public health concerns. *Psychiatric Services, 59*(2), 153–164.

Compton, W., Kevin, P., Conway, K. P., Stinson, F. S., & Grant, B. F. (2006). Changes in the prevalence of Major Depression and comorbid substance use disorders in the United States between 1991–1992 and 2001–2002. *American Journal of Psychiatry, 163,* 2141–2147.

Cook, B. I., McGuire, T., & Miranda, J. (2007). Measuring trends in mental health care disparities. *Psychiatric Services, 58*(12), 1533–1540.

Cook, J., Blyler, C., Burke-Miller, J., McFarlane, W., Leff, H., Mueser, K., et al. (2008). Effectiveness of supported employment for individuals with schizophrenia: Results of a multi-site, randomized trial. *Clinical Schizophrenia & Related Psychoses, 2*(1), 37–46.

Cooper, L., Beach, M. C., Johnson, R. L., & Inue, T. S. (2006). Delving below the surface: Understanding how race and ethnicity influence relationships in health care. *Journal of General Internal Medicine, 21,* S21–S27.

Corrigan, P. W. (2006). Impact of consumer-operated services on empowerment and recovery of people with psychiatric disabilities. *Psychiatric Services, 57*(10), 1493–1496.

Corrigan, P. W., & McCracken, S. G. (2005). Place first, then train: An alternative to the medical model of psychiatric rehabilitation. *Social Work, 50,* 31–39.

Corrigan, P., Mueser, K., Bond, G., Drake, R., & Solomon, P. (2008). Principles and practice of psychiatric rehabilitation: An empirical approach. New York, NY: Guilford Press.

Coyne, J. C., & Marcus, S. C. (2006). Health disparities in care for depression possibly obscured by the clinical significance criterion. *American Journal of Psychiatry, 163,* 1577–1579.

Delahanty, J., Ram, R., Postrado, L., Balis, T., Green-Paden, L., & Dixon, L. (2001). Differences in rates of depression in schizophrenia by race. *Schizophrenia Bulletin, 27*(1), 29–38.

Dadíc-Hero, E., Torić, I., Ruzík, K., Medved, P., & Graovac, M. (2009). Comorbidity—a troublesome factor in PTSD treatment. *Psychiatric Danubina, 21*(3), 420–424.

Davidson, L., O'Connell, M., Tondora, J., Styron, T., & Kangas, K. (2006). The top ten concerns about recovery encountered in mental health system transformation. *Psychiatric Services, 57*(5), 640–645.

Davidson, L., Shahar, G., Stayner, D. A., Chinman, M. J., Rakfeldt, J., & Tebes, J. K. (2004). Supported socialization for people with psychiatric disabilities: Lessons from a randomized controlled trial. *Journal of Community Psychology, 32,* 453–477.

Dickerson, F. B., Brown, C. H., Daumit, G. L., LiJuan, F., Goldberg, R. W., Wohlheiter, K., et al. (2006). Health status of individuals with serious mental illness. *Schizophrenia Bulletin, 32*(3), 584–589.

Dixon, L. (2002). Assertive Community Treatment: Twenty-five years of gold. *Psychiatric Services, 51*(6), 759–765.

Dixon, L., Hackman, A., & Lehman, A. (1997). Consumers as staff in Assertive Community Treatment Programs. *Administration and Policy in Mental Health, 25*(2), 199–208.

Dixon, L., McFarlane, W. R., Lefley, H., Lucksted, A., Cohen, M., Falloon, I., et al. (2001). Evidence-based practices for services to families of people with psychiatric disabilities. *Psychiatric Services, 52*, 903–910.

Doescher, M. P., Saver, B. G., Franks, P., & Fiscella, K. (2000). Racial and ethnic disparities in perception of physician style and trust. *Archives of Family Medicine, 9*, 1156–1163.

Doornbos, M. M. (1996). The strengths of families coping with mental illness. *Archives of Psychiatric Nursing, 5*(4), 214–220.

Drake, R. E., & Bond, G. R. (2008). Editorial: Supported employment 1998–2008. *Psychiatric Rehabilitation Journal, 31*(4), 274–276.

Drake, R. E., Essock, S. M., Shaner, A., Carey, K. B., Minkoff, K., Kola, L., et al. (2001). Implementing dual diagnosis services for clients with a severe mental illness. *Psychiatric Services, 52*(4), 469–476.

Drake, R. E., Mueser, K. T., Brunette, M. F., & McHugo, G. J. (2004). A review of treatments for people with severe mental illness and co-occurring substance use disorders. *Psychiatric Rehabilitation Journal, 27*(4), 360–374.

Drapalski, A. L., Marshall, T., Seybolt, D., Medoff, D., Peer, J., Leith, J., et al. (2008). Unmet needs of families of adults with mental illness and preferences regarding family services. *Psychiatric Services, 59*(6), 655–662.

Drury, L. (2003). Community care for people who are homeless and mentally ill. *Journal of Health Care for the Poor and Underserved, 14*(2), 194–207.

Druss, B. G., Wang, P. S., Sampson, N. A., Olfson, M., Pincus, M. A., Wells, K. B., et al. (2007). Understanding mental health treatment in persons without mental diagnoses: Results from the National Comorbidity Survey Replication. *Archives of General Psychiatry, 64*(10), 1196–1203.

Druss, B. G., Hwang, I., Sampson, N. A., Petukhova, M., Wang, P. S., & Kessler, R. C. (2009). Impairment in role functioning in mental and chronic medical disorders in the United States: Results from the National Comorbidity Survey Replication. *Molecular Psychiatry, 14*(7), 728–737.

Ellison, M. L., & Dunn, E. (2006). Empowering and demedicalized case management practices: Perspectives of mental health consumer leaders and professionals. *Journal of Social Work in Disability and Rehabilitation, 5*(2), 1–17.

Elway, A. R., Ranganathan, G., & Eisen, S.V. (2008). Race-ethnicity and diagnosis as predictors of outpatient service use among treatment initiators. Psychiatric Services, *59*(11), 1285–1291.

Felker, B., Yazel, J. J., & Short, D. (1996). Mortality and medical comorbidity among psychiatric patients: A review. *Psychiatric Services, 47*(12), 1356–1363.

Fisher, G. (2009). *The empowerment model of recovery: Finding our voice and having a say.* Retrieved from http://www.power2u.org/articles/recovery/model_recovery. html

Fisher, G., & Ahern, L. (2002). Evidence based practices and recovery [Letters]. *Psychiatric Services, 53*(5), 632–633.

Fisher, G., Benson, P., & Tessler, R. (1990). Family response to mental illness: Developments since deinstitutionalization. In J. R. Greenley (Ed.), *Research in community and mental health: Mental disorder in social context* (pp. 273–294). Greenwich, CT: JAI.

Fisher, D. B., & Chamberlin, J. (2004). Consumer-directed transformation to a recovery-based mental health system. SAMHSA/USDHHS: National Empowerment Center, Inc.

Forquer, S., & Knight, E. (2001). Managed care: Recovery enhancer or inhibitor? *Psychiatric Services, 52*(1), 25–26.

Frese, F. J., & Davis, W. W. (1997). The consumer–survivor movement, recovery, and consumer professionals. *Professional Psychiatry, Research and Practice, 28*(3), 243–245.

Gaines, A. D. (1992). Ethnopsychiatry: The cultural construction of psychiatries. In A. D. Gaines (Ed.), *Ethnopsychiatry: The cultural construction of professional and folk psychiatries* (pp. 3–50). Albany, NY: State University of New York Press.

Gijsen, R., Hoeymans, N., Schellevis, F. G., Ruwaard, D., Satariano, W. A., & van den Bos, G. A. (2001). Causes and consequences of comorbidity: A review. *Journal of Clinical Epidemiology, 54*(7), 661–674.

Goldberg, R. W., Lucksted, A., McNaty, S., Gold, J. M., Dixon, L., & Lehman, A. (2001). Correlates of long-term unemployment among inner-city adults with serious and persistent mental illness. *Psychiatric Services, 52*(1), 101–103.

Goldman, H. H., & Grob, N. (2006). Defining 'mental illness' in mental health policy. *Health Affairs, 25*(3), 737–749.

Goldman, H. H., & Morrissey, J. P. (1985). The alchemy of mental health policy: Homelessness and the fourth cycle of reform. *American Journal of Public Health, 75*(7), 727–731.

Goldman, H. H., Morrissey, J. P., Rosenheck, R. A., Cocozza, J., Blasinsky, M., Randolph, F., & the ACCESS National Evaluation Team. (2002). Lessons from the evaluation of the ACCESS Program. *Psychiatric Services, 53*(8), 967–970.

Gonzalez, G., & Rosenheck, R. A. (2002). Outcomes and service use among homeless persons with serious mental illness and substance abuse. *Psychiatric Services, 53*(8), 437–446.

Gould, R. A., & Clum, G. A. (1993). A meta-analysis of self-help treatment approaches. *Clinical Psychology Review, 13*, 169–186.

Granfield, R., & Cloud, W. (2001). Social context and "natural recovery": The role of social capital in the resolution of drug-associated problems. *Substance Use and Misuse, 36*, 1543–1570.

Grob, G. (2008). Mental health policy in the United States. *International Journal of Law and Psychiatry, 31*, 89–100.

Grossman, C. I. (2004). Labels and language: Implications for prevention of the DSM definition of mental disorder. *The Journal of Primary Prevention, 24*(4), 513–522.

Guarnaccia, P. J. (1998). Multicultural experiences of family caregiving: A study of African American, European American, and Hispanic American families. *New Directions for Mental Health Services, 77,* 45–61.

Harris, K. M., & Edlund, M. J. (2005). Use of mental health care and substance abuse treatment among adults with co-occurring disorders. *Psychiatric Services, 56*(8), 954–959.

Hopper, K. (1988). More than passing strange. Homelessness and mental illness in New York City. *American Ethnologist, 15*(1), 155–167.

Hopper, K., Jost, J., Hay, T., Welber, S., & Haughland, G. (1997). Homelessness, severe mental illness and the institutional circuit. *Psychiatric Services, 48*(5), 659–665.

Horvitz-Lennon, M., Kilbourne, A. M., & Pincus, H. A. (2006). From silos to bridges: Meeting the general health care needs of adults with severe mental illnesses. *Health Affairs, 25,* 659–669.

Hsiao, C., & Van Riper, M. (2010). Research on caregiving in Chinese families living with mental illness: A critical review. *Journal of Family Nursing, 16*(1), 68–100.

Interian, A., Martinez, I. E., Guarnaccia, P. J., Vega, W. A., & Escobar, J. I. (2007). A qualitative analysis of the perception of stigma among Latinos receiving antidepressants. *Psychiatric Services, 58*(12), 1591–1594.

Jacobson, N., & Greenley, D. (2001). What is recovery? A conceptual model and explication. *Psychiatric Services, 52*(4), 482–485.

Johnson, R. L., Roter, D., Powe, N. R., & Cooper, L. A. (2004). Patient race/ethnicity and quality of patient–physician communication during medical visits. *American Journal of Public Health, 94,* 2084–2090.

Kane, C. F., & Blank, M. B. (2004). NPACT: Enhancing programs of Assertive Community Treatment for the seriously mentally ill. *Community Mental Health, 40*(6), 549–559.

Kerker, B., Bainbridge, J., Li, W., Kennedy, J., Bennani, Y., Agerton, et al. (2005). *The health of homeless adults in New York City.* A report from the New York City Departments of Health and Mental Hygiene and Homeless Services.

Kessler, R. C., Chiu, W., Demler, O., & Walters, E. (2005). Prevalence, severity, and comorbidity of 12-month DSM-IV disorders in the National Comorbidity Survey Replication. *Archives of General Psychiatry, 62,* 617–627.

Kessler, R., Berglund, P. W., Demler, O., Jin, O., Merikangas, K., & Walters, E. (2005). Lifetime prevalence and age-of-onset distributions of DSM-IV disorders in the National Comorbidity Survey Replication. *Archives of General Psychiatry, 62,* 593–602.

Kessler, R. C., Heeringa, S., Lakoma, M. D., Petukhova, M., Rupp, A. E., Schoenbaum, M., Wang, P. S., & Zaslavsky, A. M. (2008). Individual and societal effects of mental disorders on earning in the United States: Results from the National Comorbidity Survey Replication. *American Journal of Psychiatry, 165*(6), 703–711.

Kessler, R., Merikangas, K., Berglund, P. E., Koretz, D., & Walters, E. (2003). Mild disorders should not be eliminated from the DSM-V. *Archives of General Psychiatry, 60,* 1117–1122.

Keyes, K. M., Hatzenbuehler, M. I., Alberti, P., Narrow, W. E., Grant, B. F., & Hasin, D. S. (2008). Service utilization differences for Axis I psychiatric and substance use disorders between white and Black adults. *Psychiatric Services, 59*(8), 893–901.

Kim, H., & Salyers, M. P. (2008). Attitudes and perceived barriers to working with families of persons with severe mental illness: Mental health professionals' perspectives. *Community Mental Health Journal, 44,* 337–345.

Klein, A. R., Cnaan, R. A., & Whitecraft, J. (1998). Significance of peer social support with dually diagnosed clients: Findings from a pilot study. *Research on Social Work Practice, 8,* 529–551.

Kleinman, A. (1988). *Rethinking psychiatry: From cultural category to personal experience.* New York, NY: The Free Press.

Kleinman, A., Eisenberg, L., & Good, B. (2006). Culture, illness, and care: Clinical lessons from anthropologic and cross-cultural research. *Focus, 4*(1), 140–149. (Reprinted from the *Annals of Internal Medicine, 88,* 251–258, 1978.)

Knudsen, H. K., Ducharme, L. J., & Roman, P. M. (2007). Racial and ethnic disparities in SSRI availability in substance abuse treatment. *Psychiatric Services, 58*(1), 55–62.

Koegel, P., Burnam, M. A., & Baumohl, J. (1996). The causes of homelessness. In *The National Coalition for the Homeless Homelessness in America* (pp. 24–33). Washington, DC: Oryx Press.

Koegel, P., Burnam, M. A., & Farr, R. K. (1998). The prevalence of specific psychiatric disorders among homeless individuals in the inner city of Los Angeles. *Archives of General Psychiatry, 45,* 1085–1092.

Koyangi, C. (2007). *Learning from history: Deinstitutionalization of people with mental illness as precursor to long-term care reform.* Washington, DC: The Kaiser Commission on Medicaid and the Uninsured.

Kurtzweil, P. L., Scogin, F., & Rosen, G. M. (1996). A test of the fail-safe for self-help programs. *Professional Psychology: Research and Practice, 27,* 629–630.

Lamb, H. R., & Weinberger, L. E. (2001). Persons with severe mental illness in jails and prisons: A review. *Psychiatric Services, 49,* 483–492.

Lamb, H. R., & Weinberger, L. E. (2004). Mentally ill persons in the criminal justice system: Some perspectives. *Psychiatric Quarterly, 75*(2), 107–126.

Lam, J. A., & Rosenheck, R. (1998). The effect of victimization on clinical outcomes of homeless persons with serious mental illness. *Psychiatric Services, 49,* 678–683.

Laudet, A. B., Morgen, K., & White, W. L. (2006). The role of social supports, spirituality, religiousness, life meaning, and affiliation with 12-step fellowships in life satisfaction among individuals in recovery from alcohol and drug use. *Alcohol Treatment Quarterly, 24*(1–2), 33–73.

Lawn, S., Battersby, M. W., Pols, R. G., Lawrence, J., Parry, T., & Urukalo, M. (2007). The mental health expert patient: Findings from a pilot study of a generic chronic condition self-management programme for people with mental illness. *International Journal of Social Psychiatry, 53*(1), 63–74.

Le Fauve, C. E., Lowman, C., Litten, R. Z. I., & Mattson, M. E. (2003). Introduction: National Institute on Alcohol Abuse and Alcoholism workshop on treatment research priorities and health disparities. *Alcoholism: Clinical & Experimental Research, 27,* 1318–1320.

Leeies, M., Pagura, J., Sareen, J., & Bolton, J. M. (2010). The use of alcohol and drugs to self-medicate symptoms of posttraumatic stress disorder. *Depression and Anxiety, 27*(4), 731–736.

Lidz, C. W., Banks, S., Simon, L., Schubert, C., & Mulvey, E. P. (2007). Violence and mental illness: A new analytic approach. *Law and Human Behavior, 33*(1), 23–31.

Link, B. G., Cullen, F. T., Struening, E., Shrout, P., & Dohrenwend, B. P. (1989). A modified labeling theory approach in the area of mental disorders: An empirical assessment. *American Sociological Review, 54,* 100–123.

Link, B. G., Struening, E. L., Rahav, M., Phelan, J. C., & Nuttbrock, L. (1997). On stigma and its consequences: Evidence from a longitudinal study on men with dual diagnoses of mental illness and substance abuse. *Journal of Health and Social Behavior, 38,* 177–190.

Link, B. G., & Phelan, J. C. (2001). Conceptualizing stigma. *Annual Review of Sociology, 27,* 363–385.

Lopez, S. R., & Guarnaccia, P. J. (2000). Cultural psychopathology: Uncovering the social world of mental illness. *Annual Review of Psychology, 51,* 571–598.

Loveland, D., & Boyle, M. (2007). Intensive case management as a jail diversion program for people with a serious mental illness: A review of the literature. *International Journal of Offender Therapy and Comparative Criminology, 51*(2), 130–150.

Lovell, D., Gagliardi, G., & Peterson, P. (2002). Recidivism and use of services among persons with mental illness after release from prison. *Psychiatric Services, 53,* 1290–1296.

Luoma, J. B., Twohig, M. P., Waltz, T., Hayes, S. C., Roget, N., Padilla, M., & Fisher, G. (2007). An investigation of stigma in individuals receiving treatment for substance abuse. *Addictive Behaviors, 32,* 1331–1334.

Lurigio, A., & Swartz, J. (2006). Mental illness in correctional populations: The use of standardized screening tools for further evaluation or treatment. *Federal Probation, 70*(2), 29–35.

Lutterman, T., Berhane, A., Phelan, B., Shaw, R., & Rana, V. (2009). *Funding and characteristics of state mental health agencies, 2007.* HHS Pub. No. (SMA) 09-4424. Rockville, MD: Center for Mental Health Services, Substance Abuse and Mental Health Services Administration.

McGurk, S. R., Mueser, K. T., Harvey, P. D., LaPuglia, R., & Marder, J. (2003). Cognitive and symptom predictors of work outcomes for clients with schizophrenia in supported employment. *Psychiatric Services, 54*(8), 1129–1135.

Mancini, M., & Lawson, H. (2009). Facilitating positive emotional labor in peer-providers of mental health services. *Administration in Social Work, 33,* 3–22.

Mancini, M. A. (2005). An evaluation of a peer-operated case management program: Lessons learned. Technical report presented to the Executive Director, St. Louis Empowerment Center.

Mancini, M., & Rogers, R. (2007). Narratives of recovery from serious psychiatric disabilities: A critical discourse analysis. *Critical Approaches to Discourse Analysis across Disciplines, 1*(2), 35–50.

Mechanic, D. (1989). *Mental health and social policy.* Englewood Cliff, NJ: Prentice-Hall.

Mechanic, D., & Tanner, J. (2007). Vulnerable people, groups, and populations: Societal view. *Health Affairs, 26*(5), 1220–1230.

Mitton, C. R., Adair, C. E., McDougall, G. M., & Marcoux, G. (2005). *Psychiatric Services, 56*(9), 1070–1076.

Mizrahi, T., Lopez-Humphries, M., & Torres, D. (2009). The social construction of client participation: The evolution and transformation of the role of service recipients in child welfare and mental disabilities. *Journal of Sociology & Social Welfare, 36*(2), 35–61.

National Coalition on Disability [NCD]. (2000). *From privileges to rights: People labeled with psychiatric disabilities speak for themselves.* Washington, DC: National Council on Disability.

National Council on Disability. (2004a). *Livable communities for adults with disabilities.* Washington, DC: National Council on Disability.

National Council on Disability. (2004b). *Consumer directed health care.* Washington, DC: National Council on Disability.

National Council on Disability. (2006). *Creating livable communities.* Washington, DC: National Council on Disability.

National Council on Disability. (2007). *Issues in creating livable communities for adults with disabilities: Proceedings of the Panel.* Washington, DC: National Council on Disability.

National Council on Disability. (2008). *Inclusive livable communities for adults with disabilities.* Washington, DC: National Council on Disability.

Najavits, L. M., Weiss, R. D., & Shaw, S. R. (1997). The link between post-traumatic stress disorder and substance abuse in women: A research review. *American Journal on Addictions, 6*(4), 273–283.

National Advisory Mental Health Council. (1993). Health care reform for Americans with severe mental illnesses. *American Journal of Psychiatry, 150*(10), 1447–1465.

Neale, J. (1997). Homelessness and theory reconsidered. *Housing Studies, 12*(1), 47.

Neibacher, S. (December, 1990). *Homeless people and health care: An unrelenting challenge. Paper Series 14.* New York, NY: United Hospital Fund of New York.

Neighbors, H. W., Caldwell, C., Williams, D. R., Nesse, R., Taylor, R. J., McKeever Bullard, K., et al. (2007). Race, ethnicity, and the use of services for mental disorders. *Archives of General Psychiatry, 64*, 485–494.

New York State Office of Mental Health. (2010). *Patient Characteristics Survey (PCS): Important notes.* Retrieved from http://bi.omh.state.ny.us/pcs/index?p_tab=notes

Norcross, J. (2000). Here comes the self-help revolution in mental health. *Psychotherapy: Theory, Research, Practice, Training, 37*(4), 370–377.

Ohayoon, M. M., & Schatzberg, A. F. (2010). Social phobia and depression: Prevalence and comorbidity. *Journal of Psychosomatic Research, 68*(3), 235–243.

Organista, K. C. (2007). *Solving Latino psychosocial and health problems: Theory, practice and populations*. Hoboken, NJ: John Wiley & Sons.

Padgett, D. K. (2007). There's no place like (a) home: Ontological security among persons with serious mental illness in the United States. *Social Science & Medicine, 64*, 1925–1936.

Parabiaghi, A., Bonetto, C., Ruggeri, M., Lasalvia, A., & Leese, M. (2006). Severe and persistent mental illness: A useful definition for prioritizing community-based mental health service interventions. *Social Psychiatry and Psychiatric Epidemiology, 41*, 457–463.

Parks, J., Svendsen, D., Singer, P., & Foti, M. E. (2006). *Morbidity and mortality in people with serious mental illness*. Alexandria, VA: National Association of State Mental Health Program Directors. Retrieved from www.nasmhpd.org

Peterson, N. A., & Zimmerman, M. A. (2004). Beyond the individual: Toward a nomological network of organizational empowerment. *American Journal of Community Psychology, 34*, 129–145.

Pharoah, F., Rathbone, J., Mari, J., & Streiner, D. (2004). Family intervention for schizophrenia. The Cochrane Library (Issue 2). Oxford, UK: Wiley.

Quarantin, L. C., Netto, L. R., Andrade-Nascimento, M., Galva'o-de Almeida, A., Sampaio, A. S., Miranda-Scippa, A., et al. (2009). Co-morbid mood and anxiety disorders in victims of violence with posttraumatic stress disorder. *Revista Brasileira de Psiquiatria, 31*(Suppl II), S66–S76.

Resnick, S. G., & Rosenheck, R. A. (2008). Integrating peer-provided services: A quasi-experimental study of recovery orientation, confidence, and empowerment. *Psychiatric Services, 59*, 1307–1314.

Ridgway, P. (2001). ReStorying psychiatric disability: Learning from first person narratives. *Psychiatric Rehabilitation Journal, 24*(4), 335–343.

Roberts, G., & Wolfson, P. (2004). The rediscovery of recovery: Open to all. *Advances in Psychiatric Treatment, 10*, 37–49.

Rogers, J. A., Vegare, M. J., Baron, R. C., & Salzer, M. S. (2007). Barriers to recovery and recommendations for change: The Pennsylvania Consensus Conference on Psychiatry's Role. *Psychiatric Services, 58*(8), 1119–1123.

Rogers, E. S., Teague, G. B., Lichenstein, C., Campbell, J., Lyass, A., Chen, R., et al. (2007). Effects of participation in consumer-operated service programs on both personal and organizationally mediated empowerment: Results of multisite study. *Journal of Rehabilitation Research & Development, 44*(6), 785–800.

Rosenheck, R. (2000). Cost-effectiveness of services for mentally ill homeless people: The application of research to policy and practice. *American Journal of Psychiatry, 157*, 1563–1570.

Rosenheck, R., Leslie, D., Keefe, R., McEvoy, J., Swartz, M., Perkins, D., et al. (2006). Barriers to employment for people with schizophrenia. *The American Journal of Psychiatry, 163*(3), 411–417.

Rothbard, A., Kuno, E., Schinaar, A., Hadley, T., & Turk, R. (1999). Service utilization and cost of community care for discharged safe hospital patients: A 3-year follow-up study. *American Journal of Psychiatry, 156*(6), 920–927.

Rowe, M., Bellamy, C., Baranoski, M., Wieland, M., O'Connell, M. J., Benedict, P., et al. (2007). A peer-support, group intervention to reduce substance use and criminality among persons with severe mental illness. *Psychiatric Service, 58,* 955–961.

Ruggeri, M., Leese, M., Thornicroft, G., Bisoffie, G., & Tansella, M. (2000). Definition and prevalence of severe and persistent mental illnes. *British Journal of Psychiatry, 177,* 149–155.

Rüsch, N., Corrigan, P. W., Wassel, A., Michaels, P., Larson, J. E., Olschewski, M., Wilkniss, S., & Batia, K. (2009). Self-stigma, group identification, perceived legitimacy of discrimination and mental health service use. *The British Journal of Psychiatry, 195,* 551–552.

Saha, S., Arbaelez, J. J., & Cooper, L. A. (2003). Patient physician relationship and racial disparities in the quality of health care. *American Journal of Public Health, 93*(10), 1713–1719.

Salzer, M. (2002). Consumer-Delivered Services as a best practice in mental health Care Delivery and the development of practice guidelines. *Psychiatric Rehabilitation Skills, 6*(3), 355–383.

SAMHSA. (2005). National consensus statement on mental health recovery. Retrieved from http://www.mentalhealth.samhsa.gov/publications/allpubs/sma05-4129

SAMHSA (May 20, 1993). Final notice establishing definitions for (1) children with a serious emotional disturbance, and (2) adults with a serious mental illness. *Federal Register, 58*(96), 29422–29425.

SAMHSA. (2006). *Results from the 2005 National Survey on Drug Use and Health: National Findings* (Office of Applied Studies, NSDUH Series H-30, DHHS Publication No. SMA 06-4194). Rockville, MD.

SAMHSA. (2010). *Uniform reporting data definitions.* Retrieved from http://mentalhealth.samhsa.gov/funding/pilotstudy/datadefinitions.asp

SAMHSA. (2001) *Cultural competence standards in managed care mental health services: Four underserved/underrepresented racial/ethnic groups.* Retrieved from http://mentalhealth.samhsa.gov/publications/allpubs/SMA00-3457/preface.asp

Scheid, T. L. (1999). Employment of individuals with mental disabilities: Business response to the ADA's challenge. *Behavioral Science Law, 17,* 73–91.

Schiff, A. C. (2004). Recovery and mental illness: Analysis and personal reflections. *Psychiatric Rehabilitation Journal, 27*(3), 212–218.

Schinnar, A., Rothbard, A., & Kanter, R. (1991). Adding state counts of the severely and persistently mentally ill. *Administration and Policy in Mental Health, 19*(1), 3–12.

Schinnar, A., Rothbard, A., Kanter, R., & Jung, Y. (1990). An empirical literature review of definitions of severe and persistent mental illness. *The American Journal of Psychiatry, 147*(12), 1602–1608.

Scogin, F., Bynum, J., Stephens, G., & Calhoun, S. (1990). Efficacy of self-administered treatment programs: Meta-analytic review. *Professional Psychology: Research and Practice, 21,* 42–47.

Scott, C. K., Dennis, M. L., & Foss, M. A. (2005). Utilizing recovery management checkups to shorten the cycle of relapse, treatment reentry, and recovery. *Drug and Alcohol Dependence, 78,* 325–338.

Semple, S. J., Grant, I., & Patterson, T. L. (2005). Utilization of drug treatment programs by methamphetamine users: The role of social stigma. *The American Journal on Addictions, 14*, 367–380.

Shea, J. M. (2010). Coming Back Normal: The process of self-recovery in those with schizophrenia. *Journal of American Psychiatric Nurses Association, 16*(1), 43–51.

Slade, M., Powell, R., & Strathdee, G. (1997). Current approaches to identifying the severely mentally ill. *Social Psychiatry & Psychiatric Epidemiology, 32*, 177–184.

Smedley, B. D., Stith, A. Y., & Nelson, A. R. (Eds.). (2002). *Unequal treatment: Confronting racial and ethnic disparities in health care.* Washington, DC: National Academy Press/Institute of Medicine.

Smith, J. E., Meyers, R. J., & Delaney, H. D. (1998). The community reinforcement approach with homeless alcohol-dependent individuals. *Journal of Consulting Clinical Psychology, 66*, 541–548.

Solomon, P., & Draine, J. (1995). The efficacy of a consumer case management team: Two-year outcomes of a randomized trial. *Journal of Mental Health Administration, 22*, 135–146.

Snow, D. A., Baker, S. G., Anderson, L., & Martin, M. (1986). The myth of pervasive mental illness among the homeless. *Social Problems, 33*(5), 407–423.

Steadman, H. J., Deane, M. W., Morrissey, J. P., Westcott, M. L., Salasin, S., & Shapiro, S. (1999). A SAMHSA research initiative assessing the effectiveness of jail diversion programs for mentally ill persons. *Psychiatric Services, 50*(12), 1620–1623.

Stuart, H. (2006). Mental illness and employment discrimination. *Current Opinions in Psychiatry, 19*(5), 522–526.

Sullivan, G., Burnam, A., Koegel, P., & Hollenberg, J. (2000). Quality of Life of homeless persons with mental illness: Results from the Course-of-Homelessness Study. *Psychiatric Services, 51*(9), 1135–1141.

Talbott, J. A. (2000). The past and future of mental health services: An interview with Leona Bachrach. *Psychiatric Services, 51*(12), 1511–1512.

Teplin, L. A., McClellan, G. M., Abram, K. M., & Weiner, D. A. (2005). Crime victimization in adults with severe mental illness. *Archives of General Psychiatry, 62*, 911–921.

The President's New Freedom Commission on Mental Health. (2003). *Achieving the promise: Transforming mental health care in America.* Rockville, MD: SAMHSA (SMA03-3831).

Trainor, J., Shepherd, M., Boydell, K., Leff, A., & Crawford, E. (1997). Beyond the services paradigm: The impact of consumer/survivor initiatives. *Psychiatric Rehabilitation Journal, 21*(2), 132–140.

Tsemberis, S. J., Gulur, L., & Nakae, M. (2004). Housing First, consumer choice, and harm reduction for homeless individuals with dual diagnosis. *American Journal of Public Health, 94*, 651–656.

Tsemberis, S., & Eisenberg, R. F. (2000). Pathways to housing: Supported housing for street dwelling homeless individuals with psychiatric disabilities. *Psychiatric Services, 51*, 487–493.

Tsemberis, S. J., Moran, L., Shinn, M., Asmussen, S. M., & Shern, D. L. (2003). Consumer preference programs for individuals who are homeless and have psychiatric disabilities: A drop-in center and a supported housing program. *American Journal of Community Psychology, 32*(3/4), 305–317.

Turner, R. J., & Avison, W. R. (2003). Status variations in stress exposure: Implications for the interpretation of research on race, socioeconomic status, and gender. *Journal of Health and Social Behavior, 44*(4), 488–505.

USDHHS. (2001). *Mental health: Culture, race, and ethnicity—A supplement to mental health: A report of the Surgeon General.* Rockville, MD: U.S. Department of Health and Human Services, Substance Abuse and Mental Health Services Administration, Center for Mental Health Services.

USDOJ. (2009). *Briefs filed in three states to enforce Supreme Court's Olmstead Decision.* Retrieved from http://blogs.usdoj.gov/blog/archives/451

Van Tosh, L., Ralph, R. O., & Campbell, J. (2000). The rise of consumerism. *Psychiatric Rehabilitation Skills, 4*(3), 383–409.

Van Tosh, L., & del Vecchio, P. (2000). *Consumer-operated self-help programs: A technical teport.* Rockville, MD: U.S. Center for Mental Health Services.

Venner, K. L., Matzger, H., Forcehimes, A. A., Moos, R. H., Feldstein, S. W., Willenbring, M. L., et al. (2006). Course of recovery from alcoholism. *Alcoholism, Clinical and Experimental Research, 30,* 1079–1090.

Vogel, H. S., Knight, E., Laudet, A., & Magura, A. S. (1998). Double Trouble in recovery: Self-help for people with dual diagnoses. *Psychiatric Rehabilitation Journal, 21*(4), 356–364.

Wahl, O. F. (2006). *Media madness: Public images of mental illness.* New Brunswick, NJ: Rutgers University Press.

Wagner, D., & Cohen, M. B. (1991). The power of the people: Homeless protestors in the aftermath of social movement participation. *Social Problems, 38*(4), 543–561.

Walter, U., & Petr, C. (2004). *Report #10: Best practices in children's mental health: Attendant care for children and youth.* Kansas: State of Kansas Department of Social and Rehabilitation Services.

Wang, P. S., Lane, M., Olfson, M., Pincus, H. A., Wells, K. B., & Kessler, R. C. (2005). Twelve-month use of mental health services in the United States: Results from the National Comorbidity Survey Replication. *Archives of General Psychiatry, 62,* 629–640.

Ware, N. C., Hopper, K., Tugenberg, T., Dickey, B., & Fisher, D. (2007). Connectedness and citizenship: Redefining social integration. *Psychiatric Services, 58*(4), 469–474.

Wellman, B., & Gulia, M. (1999). The network basis of social support. In Barry Wellman (Ed.) *Networks in the global village: Life in contemporary communities* (pp. 83–118). Boulder, CO: Westview Press.

Wells, K., Klap, R., Koike, A., & Sherbourne, C. (2001). Ethnic disparities in unmet need for alcoholism, drug abuse, and mental health care. *American Journal of Psychiatry, 158,* 2027–2032.

White, W. L. (2008). *Toward recovery management and recovery oriented systems of care: Scientific rationale and promising practices.* SAMHSA/CSAT: Northeast Addiction Technology Transfer Center, the Great Lakes Addiction Technology

Transfer Center, and the Philadelphia Department of Behavioral Health & Mental Retardation Services (DBH/MRS).

White, W. L. (2005). Recovery: Its history and renaissance as an organizing construct. *Alcoholism Treatment Quarterly, 23*(1), 3–15.

White, W. L. (2006). *Let's go make some history: Chronicles of the new addiction recovery advocacy movement.* Washington, DC: Johnson Institute and Faces and Voices of Recovery.

White, W., & Kurtz, E. (2006). *The varieties of recovery experience: A primer for addiction treatment professionals and recovery advocates.* Chicago, IL: Great Lakes Addiction Technology Transfer Center.

Wolf, J., Burnam, A., Koegel, P., Sullivan, G., & Morton, S. (2001). Changes in subjective quality of life among homeless adults who obtain housing: A prospective examination. *Social Psychiatry and Psychiatric Epidemiology, 36,* 391–398.

Woodward, A., Taylor, R., Bullard, K., Neighbors, H., Chatters, L., & Jackson, J. (2008). Use of professional and informal support by African Americans and Caribbean Blacks with mental disorders. *PsychiatricServices, 59*(11), 1292–1298.

Young, S. L., & Ensing, D. S. (1999). Exploring recovery from the perspective of people with psychiatric disabilities. *Psychiatric Rehabilitation Journal, 22*(3), 219–232.

Legal and Legislative Citations

ADAMHA Reorganization Act of 1992, Pub. L. No. 102-321, 106 Stat. 323 (1992).

Americans with Disabilities Act of 1990, Pub. L. No. 101-336, § 2, 104 Stat. 328 (1991).

Executive Order No. 13217 66 FR 31373 (2001).

Mental Health Amendments of 1990, Pub. L. No. 101-639, 104 Stat. 4600 (1990).

Mental Health Systems Act. Public Law 96-398, Oct. 7, 1980, S. 1177, S. Rept. 96–712, H.R. 7299, H. Rept. 96–977, H. Conf. Rept. 96–1367.

Mental Retardation Facilities and Community Mental Health Centers Construction Act of 1963 P.L. No.88-164, 77 Stat. 282 (1963).

National Mental Health Act of 1946, Pub. L. No. 79-487 § 538, 60 Stat. 421 (1946).

Olmstead v. L.C., 527 U.S. 581, 119 S.Ct. 2176 (1999).

Omnibus Budget Reconciliation Act of 1981, Pub. L. No. 97-35, 95 Stat. 357 (1982).

Omnibus Budget Reconciliation Act of 1990, Pub. L. No. 101-508, 104 Stat. 1388 (1990).

Presidential Proclamation No. 6158 (1990) http://www.loc.gov/loc/brain/proclaim.html

State Comprehensive Mental Health Services Plan Act of 1986, Pub. L. No. 99-660, 100 Stat. 3794 (1986).

CHAPTER TWO

Innovative Programs for Consumers with Psychiatric Disabilities

Phyllis Solomon, Lisa Schmidt, Peggy Swarbrick, and Edie Mannion

INTRODUCTION

With the recent issuance of two major reports on the state and future directions of mental health services and treatment by the U.S. federal government, there has been escalating promotion of evidence-based practices and a recovery orientation for adults with psychiatric disabilities (Department of Health and Human Services, 1999, 2003). The evidence-based and emerging best practices to be discussed in this chapter fall within the domain of psychiatric rehabilitation that began in the 1940s with the establishment of Fountain House psychosocial rehabilitation center in New York City.

Psychiatric Rehabilitation

Psychiatric rehabilitation involves systematic processes and interventions by which adults with severe psychiatric disorders are assisted in achieving full integration into communities of their choosing through environmental supports and modifications and personal skills and resource acquisition. Due to functional impairments across primary life domains of living, learning, working, and socializing that result from psychiatric disabilities, psychiatric rehabilitation services cover a broad spectrum of interventions, such as intensive case management, employment programs, and self-management skill training, to name a few. These services are designed to include the principles, values, and practices of being person centered and strengths based, ensuring self determination, respect and dignity, and collaborative engagement in the delivery of services.

Recovery-Oriented Services

As apparent from the values and orientation of psychiatric rehabilitation services, an orientation that focuses on recovery has always been inherent in the approaches, practices, and goals of psychiatric rehabilitation. While there are many definitions of recovery, the most widely accepted description is by Anthony (1993): "a deeply personal, unique process of changing one's attitudes, values, feelings, goals, skills and/or roles. It is a way of living a satisfying, hopeful, and contributing life even with limitations caused by the illnesses. Recovery involves the development of new meaning and purpose in one's life as one grows beyond the catastrophic effects of mental illness" (p. 15). Thus, recovery in this context differs from the traditional medical model orientation of service delivery focused on maintenance, compliance, and stabilization. In contrast to the conventional use of the term recovery, the concept of recovery being promoted focuses on the process of how adults with severe mental illness live their lives, given their illness rather than focusing on an absence of symptoms related to the illnesses. This definition, as does the recovery orientation, emerged from the perspectives of mental health consumers and is very much about hope, choice, self determination, and shared decision making.

 This chapter describes each of the currently accepted evidence-based practices and emerging best practices for adults with severe mental illness. Two case examples of innovative programs are presented. The chapter concludes with future directions with regard to funding, services, and approaches.

EVIDENCE-BASED PSYCHIATRIC REHABILITATION PRACTICES

Assertive Community Treatment

Assertive Community Treatment (ACT) is now widely accepted as an evidence-based practice for adults with severe mental illnesses. Developed in the 1970s by Marx, Test, and Stein (1973) as a community-based alternative to psychiatric hospitalization, this program was originally called Training in Community Living before it was renamed ACT.

ACT is a comprehensive self-contained total system of care for individuals with severe psychiatric disorders. It was designed to transfer many of the functions, services, and supports of public psychiatric hospitals into the community, and consequently, is sometimes called "the hospital without walls." The program is comprised of a multidisciplinary team that includes a psychiatrist, nurse, and social workers; specialists such as employment and substance abuse providers, contingent on the target population served; and case managers who serve the coordinating function of the team (Corrigan, Mueser, Bond, Drake, & Solomon, 2008). Some teams include peer providers and/or family members (Dixon, Kraus, & Lehman, 1994; Dixon et al., 1998). The team is available 24/7, 365 days a year and has a staff to client ratio of 1 to 10 or 12. An ACT team generally serves no more than 120 clients at any given time.

The goal of ACT is to reduce the need for psychiatric hospitalizations and increase the clients' independence and integration into the community. This is an extremely intensive service and is generally reserved for individuals who have spent extensive time in the hospital or on the streets, and those who are difficult to manage, for example, those with co-occurring disorders and/or involvement with the criminal justice system (Department of Health and Human Services, 2003).

One of the central features of the program model is continuous care, personalized to meet the specific needs of a given individual. Care is flexible and accommodates to the needs of the consumers served. The ACT team is responsible for all the treatment, rehabilitation, and social services that their consumers require. Team services include medication, supportive treatment, skill training, crisis intervention, as well as assistance with employment and housing. Services are provided *in vivo*, wherever clients live, learn, work, and socialize. The team also engages in assertive outreach to clients, which is provided for as long as ACT services are needed. The team meets on a daily basis to review the status of each of the clients so that all members are up to date on their knowledge regarding those being served by the team.

It is important to note that there have been a number of variants of ACT. Some have been developed to serve specialized populations, for example, forensic clients (Solomon, 2003; Solomon & Draine, 1995; Wilson, Tien, & Eaves, 1995). Furthermore, ACT has served as a foundation on which to offer a diversity of particular programs for adults with psychiatric disabilities (Solomon, 1999). Supported employment programs to be discussed below have been incorporated within ACT teams. Standard skill training as well as cognitive adaptation training have also been included into ACT programs (Bellack, 2004; Glynn et al., 2002; Velligan et al., 2000).

Extensive research on ACT programs has concluded that ACT teams are more likely to maintain persons with severe psychiatric illnesses in treatment, increase housing stability, decrease psychiatric hospitalizations, reduce lengths of hospital stay, and improve client and family satisfaction with services when compared to standard case management services. ACT teams work collaboratively with hospitals, and emergency services, to reduce the most intensive services and minimize disruptions in community stays. Due to reduced hospitalizations, ACT is often a cost-effective service (Corrigan et al., 2008). Research has found that increased fidelity to the ACT model results in better outcomes for clients (Bond, Drake, Mueser, & Latimer, 2001; Scott & Dixon, 1995). Based on the research, ACT is promoted as an evidence-based practice and the federal agency, Substance Abuse Mental Health Services Administration (SAMHSA), has a toolkit for implementing this program model.

Cognitive-Behavioral Strategies

Interventions adapted from services first conceived for other populations hold promise both for improving cognitive functioning, and compensating for cognitive deficits associated with serious mental illness. These interventions employ two primary strategies, behavioral modification and cognitive remediation. Behavior modification services include social skills training (Bellack, Mueser, Gingerich, & Agresta, 2004; Liberman, 2008), and environmental accommodations (Maples & Velligan, 2008). Cognitive change strategies involving talk therapies include Cognitive Behavioral Therapy (CBT) (Beck, Rector, Stolar, & Grant, 2009; Kingdon & Turkington, 1994) and mindfulness-based approaches adapted from Kabat-Zinn (1990), such as trauma informed therapy (e.g., Najavits, 2007), as well as dialectical behavioral therapy (Linehan, 1993). The most widely implemented of these strategies for persons with severe mental illness, social skills training, and CBT are discussed.

Much attention has been paid to social skills training (Liberman, 2008), particularly for people with schizophrenia, who often exhibit poor interpersonal skills due to neuro-cognitive impairments. These impairments lead to inadequate perception and responsiveness to social cues and social expectations. Impoverished, isolated living situations and active symptoms also present barriers to effective social engagement. Social skills training offers a systematic approach to (1) identifying skills the person wants and needs, (2) describing the behavioral steps required to perform the skill, and (3) establishing practice opportunities for skill acquisition. Just a few of the many skill areas targeted for training include conversational skills, assertiveness, conflict management, medication management, work-related skills, and substance use refusal skills. The practitioner creates a teaching plan based on the specific motivation and practical needs of the learner. The training is usually conducted in small groups with people who have similar skill deficits. The group is often co-led so that initial participation includes observation of competent role models performing each step of the skill. Then the group members are given opportunities to learn each component step using role-playing scenarios of commonly encountered social situations. To compensate for cognitive deficits, the "students" repeatedly perform each component and then begin to sequence these behaviors until the performance becomes rote, with positive reinforcement provided for successive approximations of skill performance. Homework involving skill practice outside the training situation is used to improve the transfer of skill performance to the needed "real life" environment. The group reviews and discusses homework experiences to further refine performance and subsequent homework assignments. Friends and supporters are actively recruited to guide and reinforce skill performance in the applicable community situation, reflecting the concern that skills learned in a treatment setting do not always transfer to community-based social situations. Some research suggests that case management follow-up also increases the probability that skills are performed when needed (Liberman et al., 1998).

Skills training curricula suited to the most common social situations are available through various sources including the UCLA-affiliated Psychiatric Rehabilitation Consultants or through textbooks including Bellack et al. (2004). Research on the effectiveness of social skills training suggests it is an evidence-based best practice for specific targeted skills, but the generalizability of its *in vivo* application is yet to be determined, which is essential for its effectiveness (Bellack, 2004). Improvements have been reported in the behavioral performance of skills, and social role functioning, which in turn may improve the person's sense of self-efficacy. However, social skills training "is best conceptualized as a targeted treatment that can achieve important outcomes when applied in conjunction with other critical interventions, including pharmacotherapy, case management, and substance abuse treatment, as well as environmental supports such as housing" (Bellack, 2004, p. 381).

CBT is a short-term treatment intervention originally conceived to help people struggling with neuroses related to anxiety and depression (Beck, Rush, Shaw, & Emery, 1979). It has since been widely adapted to the treatment of substance use disorders (Beck, Wright, Newman, &

Liese, 1993) and is expected to be as effective as a complementary tool for the treatment of psychotic disorders. It is typically provided through individual sessions over several months by a licensed clinician. CBT for schizophrenia helps clients understand symptoms such as hallucinations and delusions within the context of normal human reactions to stress. After building a strong affiliation with the client, the therapist begins to gently examine dysfunctional thoughts and beliefs. Alternate views and explanations for experiences are explored through collaborative dialogue and Socratic reasoning. Over time, the person's understanding of the cause and effect of symptoms changes, and sometimes these symptoms disappear altogether or at least become less intrusive with regard to functioning. A competing cognitive therapy model, Acceptance and Commitment Therapy, shifts the focus from modifying the content or veracity of hallucinations and delusions to learning to accept them as uncontrollable internal experiences that do not have to dominate one's attention. The client learns to be mindful of the present moment and to engage in goal-directed behavior, thus, altering his/her response to persistent symptoms (Pankey & Hayes, 2003).

Research has demonstrated that various forms of CBT, when applied consistently over an extended period of time, lead to significant reductions in the presence and intensity of psychotic symptoms (Bellack, 2004), and less hospitalizations (Bach & Hayes, 2002). This service is recommended in combination with pharmacological intervention for the treatment of serious mental illness (SMI).

Family Psycho-Education and Support

Families of persons with SMI shoulder much responsibility for their relatives, often functioning as *de facto* case managers, which results in emotional and financial stress and burden whether or not their relative resides with them. However, families frequently do not have the requisite knowledge, information, and skills necessary to undertake these responsibilities. Consequently, there has been, increasing recognition of the importance of providing information and support to these families. This recognition has resulted in a proliferation of family educational interventions, which primarily fall within two domains, family psycho-education interventions and family education. It is also important to note that the term "family" is broader than the traditional notion of families related by blood or marriage, but recognizes that many persons with psychiatric disabilities have primary supporters who are not necessarily family members in the traditional sense. Therefore, the term family in the present context is extended to traditional family members as well as other supporters identified by the consumer.

Originally, family psycho-educational interventions were developed in response to research that found that discharged psychiatric patients who returned to their families with high expressed emotion (EE), that is, highly critical, hostile, and over-involved, quickly had an exacerbation of their symptoms and were rehospitalized (Brown, Carstairs, & Topping 1958; Brown, Monck, Carstairs, & Wing, 1962). In response to these findings, a diversity of family psycho-educational interventions was developed by professionals, such as psychiatrists and psychologists as adjuncts to treatment. These interventions differ with regard to their theoretical orientation, format, duration, and location. The frameworks vary, from behavioral management, cognitive behavioral, family systems theory, to social support. Some of the interventions employ more than one of these orientations. Usually, these interventions last at least 2 years and may be delivered to an individual family member, but are frequently delivered to the family unit. Some are multifamily group interventions and generally, the client participates to some degree. Currently, most of these interventions are conducted in a clinic setting, but they may also take place in another location, such as in the family's home. These interventions usually include two or more mental health professionals (e.g., a psychiatrist, psychologist, and social workers). Initially designed for families of individuals with schizophrenia spectrum disorders, these interventions have been modified for families whose relatives have been diagnosed with bipolar, major depression, and substance abuse as well as other disorders (McFarlane, Dixon, Lukens, & Lucksted, 2003). The orientation of these interventions is a strengths perspective centered on the belief that families are competent therapeutic agents who can work collaboratively with providers to affect positive outcomes for their relatives (Corrigan et al., 2008).

Numerous randomized controlled trials of psycho-educational interventions have resulted in many narrative reviews and meta-analyses (e.g., Corrigan et al., 2008; Pharoah, Rathbone, Mari, & Streiner, 2004). They have found that regardless of the specific intervention, family psycho-education is effective in reducing rates of rehospitalization, as long as the intervention lasts a minimum of 9 months. Based on this research, family psycho-education is now considered an evidence-based practice.

As a result, SAMHSA has developed a toolkit to assist in the promotion and implementation of the McFarlane model (McFarlane, 2002) of family psycho-education. This model is considered a second-generation treatment model as it combines aspects of two different interventions, family behavioral management and multifamily approaches. In the initial stage of the model, the practitioner meets individually with the families of five to six consumers and forms a relationship. The practitioners then meet with the families twice a month. Family members in these structured groups assist each other in learning skills to cope with the illness of their relative. These families are provided education about the illness, taught problem-solving techniques, and gain support and suggestions from other family members. Consumers participate in these groups as well. These interventions were originally developed for families whose relatives were being discharged from psychiatric inpatient facilities. Now family psycho-education is offered to those residing in the community and not necessarily living with the family, and the emphasis has moved toward social and vocational rehabilitation.

There have been a number of difficulties with the implementation and uptake of family psycho-education in the mental health system including a lack of reimbursement, limited time, resources, and skills of providers as well as families' unwillingness to commit to such a time-consuming intervention. Consequently, the Veterans' Administration as well as some states (e.g., New York) now promotes a family consultation approach. In family consultation, the provider functions as an advisor, collaborating with an individual family member or a family unit on an as needed basis to clarify a situation, obtain resources, to problem solve, or to accomplish an agreed upon objective (Bernheim, 1982; Bernheim & Lehman, 1985; Mannion, Draine, Solomon, & Meisel, 1997). This intervention may be conducted in person or over the phone (see case example: Innovations in Family Inclusion).

INNOVATIONS IN FAMILY INCLUSION: "THE PHILADELPHIA STORY"

Edie Mannion, MFT

Family consultation is increasingly utilized to engage family members of individuals receiving a variety of behavioral health treatment and recovery services. In this approach, staff members negotiate with program participants about the people in their lives who are significantly affecting their recovery positively and/or negatively, such as biological relatives, spouses, romantic partners, friends, roommates, clergy and personal care home providers, and whose involvement with their services will not jeopardize their safety or legal proceedings such as divorce or child custody issues. Once a specialized family release form is signed, staff then call the designated persons to offer them a phone appointment or meeting and engage in the following activities, usually without the program participant (at least initially) to improve honesty and improve manageability of the session: (1) Sharing clinical information approved by the participant; (2) Eliciting and addressing their questions or concerns (within the constraints of the release form); and (3) Asking for other information they deem relevant to helping the participant (with the understanding that any information provided can be shared with the participant). This family consultation approach allows the provider to assess the needs of the family so that they can make appropriate referrals to other supportive, educational family services available in the community, such as family support groups and workshops. They are given packets which summarize these resources and other helpful information.

Implementation of this approach is part of Philadelphia's transformation to a more recovery-oriented system. Recently, the City of Philadelphia Department of Behavioral Health/Mental Retardation Services (DBH/MRS) made "family inclusion and leadership" one of the four pillars of its transformation and the 2009–2010 Annual Plan of DBH/MRS states: "Renewed emphasis on family inclusion is perceived as a key element required for the success of system-wide recovery transformation efforts." Case management and day programs were the first to respond to the challenge of improving family inclusion in their programs. Medicaid billing regulations are less of a problem in these types of programs because collateral contacts are billable, and day program rates can be bundled to include time spent with family members.

The Community Treatment Team and the Targeted Case Management Program of Horizon House, Inc. are undergoing a multi-phase process for using family consultation to structure time spent with their participants' significant people. They began with administrative approval in adapting standards for family inclusion developed by the Family Resource Network (FRN), a coalition of family education and support providers, including affiliates of the National Alliance on Mental Illness and the Mental Health Association of Southeastern PA. FRN developed "model standards" to clarify the types of family-friendly policies and procedures necessary for including participants' "significant people" in services systematically and proactively. The four components of the training for case managers included: (1) Clarifying procedures for handling various types of family–provider communication that do not violate federal and state confidentiality laws; (2) An algorithm for helping their participants identify which family members are appropriate for family inclusion; (3) Skill-based training in family consultation for engagement and trust-building, using role plays based on actual cases; and (4) Ongoing case conferences to continue reinforcing the skills taught and trouble-shoot challenging cases.

The day programs have used a different approach. The pilot programs sent their "recovery coaches" and certified peer specialists to a committee to brainstorm ways to better include family members. They did a field study of family inclusion kicked off by training in negotiating with participants about family inclusion and family consultation skills. They invited program participants and their family members who agreed to be in the field study to speak about their experiences at a conference attended by staff of the next tier of transforming programs. The positive testimonies inspired motivation for forming a "Family Inclusion Learning Collaborative." Monthly meetings attended by staff, participants, and family members of six-day programs are used to share ideas, resources, and events that promote family-inclusive activities. The collaborative is currently considering sponsoring evening monthly "family group consultation" meetings, in which selected staff will be trained in family consultation adapted for family groups (Mannion et al., 1997). Group participants are helped to define their top priority question or concern, and then taught a problem solving process in which the group participates in addressing the priorities. Both individual and group family consultation strategies can improve staff confidence that their conversations with family members and other significant people can be constructive and productive, whether they occur in an individual or group setting.

Family education is an emerging best practice with increasing research evidence. It was originally developed by family members themselves to respond to their own needs for practical advice and information (Hatfield, 1994). These educational programs provide knowledge about the causes, consequences, and treatment of the illness as well as teach problem-solving techniques, illness management skills, and ways to cope with the illness of a relative. These are often freestanding programs, not necessarily provided by the mental health system, and are delivered in libraries, churches, or other locations that are not stigmatizing. These are generally brief interventions that range from a couple of hours to 10 or 12 weekly sessions of about 1–2 hours. Currently, the most widely delivered program is Family-to-Family sponsored by the National Alliance on Mental Illness. Other family educational programs are facilitated by professionals or a combination of professionals and family members. Randomized clinical trials in this area are increasing and are demonstrating the effectiveness of these interventions (Dixon et al., 2004; Pickett-Schenk, Lippincott, Bennett, & Steigman, 2008).

Illness Management and Recovery

Nonpharmacological illness management strategies have grown as psychiatric rehabilitation practice develops and the experiential knowledge of people with a mental illness is disseminated. The strategies born of these developments are often based on the observation that people who progress in their recovery learn ways to manage stress and cope with risks for relapse. Services that help people to accomplish their personal recovery are becoming widely available. Psycho-education regarding the etiology and impact of mental illness (SAMHSA, 2010a) and 'Wellness Recovery Action Planning (WRAP) are two important strategies.'

The Illness Management and Recovery (IMR) Evidence-Based Practice Toolkit (SAMHSA, 2010a) is a teaching curriculum developed by a panel of experts. It includes several empirically based practices associated with psycho-education, skills teaching, and relapse prevention (Mueser et al., 2002). IMR is designed to help consumers of mental health services self-manage their mental illness and make progress toward recovery. IMR employs teaching strategies known to be effective in helping people with cognitive deficits. These include shaping and reinforcement techniques, role modeling, and role playing. Strategies are incorporated to enhance motivation by connecting personal goals to learning objectives and increasing the person's hope for recovery. The program consists of nine modules that practitioners use to run group or individual sessions that are conducted over 3–6 months. Topics include basic facts about serious mental illness; strategies for treatment, relapse prevention and recovery, and the development of coping skills and social supports. Each module follows a structured format and offers discussion topics, informational handouts, and suggestions for homework. Recent research has demonstrated its effectiveness (Hasson-Ohayon, Roe, & Kravetz, 2007; Mueser et al., 2006; Roe, Hasson-Ohayon, Salyers, & Kravetz, 2009).

WRAP is a self-help method of illness management developed by Copeland (1997) in response to her personal struggle with bipolar disorder. She surveyed many people with serious mental illness from around the United States and learned what people have done to successfully cope with their symptoms and restore a sense of wellness. Based on this qualitative research, she developed a system that has been taught to consumers of mental health services as well as providers who sometimes facilitate the process. A WRAP consists of several components, written and revised periodically by the person in recovery. The plan includes a personal description of what the person is like when well, what she/he needs to do every day to stay well, what things (people, feelings, events, etc.) trigger a return of symptoms, and strategies the consumer can use to respond to the various stages of decompensation that may arise. An emergency plan is developed and shared with trusted supporters who are responsible for communicating the person's treatment preferences in the event she/he is not competent to do so. The emergency plan is patterned after the medical advanced directive and may include preferences for or against specific medications and other treatment procedures. The plan may specify preferred treatment providers and settings, and provide the name of the person who can be included in confidential sharing of information. Twenty-five states now recognize the psychiatric advance directive as a binding legal document (National Resource Center on Psychiatric Advanced Directives, 2009).

Inclusion of Health and Wellness in Interventions

In addition to control of symptoms and the course of illness, illness management has expanded to consider the overall promotion of health. A recent epidemiological study has indicated that people with SMI die 25 years sooner on average than the rest of the population (Parks, Svendsen, Singer, & Foti, 2006). There are various contributors to this alarming statistic. People with SMI have poor access to medical care, and psychiatric symptoms may interfere with the ability to effectively seek medical treatment. Additionally, newer antipsychotic medications are associated with disease-provoking metabolic changes. Consequently, health problems such as high blood pressure, heart disease, diabetes, and obesity are increasing in prevalence. The lack of integration and coordination of the physical and behavioral health-care systems further aggravate these conditions.

Services tailored to the needs of people with psychiatric disabilities that promote physical health are sorely needed. To that end, it is recommended that all clients receive a comprehensive physical assessment and link with a primary care physician. When medical services are required, providers of both physical and behavioral health care must work in an integrated fashion to insure that a full range of bio-psychosocial supports are available to adequately address the problem. This may include home visits to monitor medication adherence, transportation to appointments, information and support for caregivers, and other case management-oriented activities as required.

In order to maintain wellness, programs in manual format, such as "Solutions for Wellness" (Eli, n.d.) offer practitioners psycho-educational materials and activities they can use to support healthy eating, and exercise as well as illness management and recovery applications. The "Facing us Clubhouse" is a free, interactive online wellness tool sponsored by Depression Bi-polar Support Alliance (DBSA). It is easy to use and introduces people to the methods of journaling, health charting, wellness recovery action planning, relaxation, and creative expression. This website also offers videos, music, workshops, and online courses to further the process of recovery.

Integrated Treatment For Co-Occurring Disorders

Many people with serious mental illnesses also have substance use disorders. By some estimates as many as 50% of those with psychiatric disabilities will experience problems with addictions during their lifetime (Regier et al., 1990). Treatment resources for substance use and mental illness are frequently offered by different organizations, with separate funding streams, and disparate treatment philosophies. Services may be offered sequentially, whereby one disorder is considered primary and treated first and the other disorder is treated later; or in parallel, both disorders are treated simultaneously by different unaffiliated agencies or providers. These approaches inadvertently create barriers to recovery and relapse prevention. Consumers receiving treatment from multiple, segregated service sectors tend to drop out of treatment prematurely, resulting in high rates of relapse, and poor health outcomes (Drake, Mueser, Brunette, & McHugo, 2004). However, integration of services alone does not necessarily improve outcomes (Donald, Dower, & Kavanagh, 2005).

One approach to solving this dilemma is Integrated Treatment for Co-occurring Disorders (Mueser, Noordsy, Drake, & Fox, 2003; SAMHSA, 2010b) which establishes a multidisciplinary treatment team with expertise to manage both disorders and provide a coordinated, "whole person" approach to assessment, planning, and intervention within a "stages of change" framework (Miller & Rollnick, 2002; Prochaska & Diclemente, 1984). The essential ingredients of this service model are varied and evidence based. Psycho-education is offered to explain the actions of common substances of abuse and how their effects interact with symptoms of mental illness. An assessment of the client's status with respect to making a change in their behavior is conducted to ensure that a meaningful intervention is offered when the client is most receptive. These stages of change include (1) precontemplation, (2) contemplation, (3) preparation, (4) action, and (5) maintenance/relapse prevention. Clients learn to use positive coping skills to manage symptoms and stressors as well as strategies to respond to lapses in behavior that might normally lead to relapse. If the person is not yet ready to abstain from substance use, harm reduction strategies become the focus of coping skills training. Harm reduction services include teaching people how to avoid infectious diseases, securing safe housing and clean needles, and managing finances among other areas. The aim of motivational counseling is to increase the likelihood that the consumer will prepare for, and then engage, in active treatment. Linkage to social supports such as 12-step meetings, day programs, and other prosocial groups are developed to promote abstinence, well-being, and long-term recovery.

These strategies are particularly helpful for people with high levels of impairment related to the interaction of both disorders (Drake et al., 2001). For instance, someone with a diagnosis of a bipolar disorder who is at high risk for relapsing into cocaine use during a manic episode needs support from a team that can assess level of service needs based on the status of each disorder, monitor psychotropic medication, and teach coping skills to effectively respond to high-risk situations that may provoke a mood swing as well as a lapse in abstinence.

Supported Employment ˌ

Much of one's personal identity and social mobility is associated with employment. In the United States, unemployment rates rarely exceed 10%, yet for people with serious mental illnesses, that rate often exceeds 70% (Pratt, Gill, Barrett, & Roberts, 2007). Supportive interventions that help people achieve competitive employment success have been a primary focus of psychiatric rehabilitation (Drake & Bond, 2008).

Supported employment services are provided by a bachelor's degree level specialist who develops the client's employment readiness through work assessment, supportive counseling, and information gathering. The specialist analyzes the costs and rewards of working and links the client with resources that limit the negative impact of income on entitlements. Once a type of employment is chosen, job search and development activities are started. Job development may include visiting potential workplaces and marketing employees to potential employers. Job search assistance may include help in completing job applications and arranging or preparing for the interview. The employment specialist provides ongoing support or "coaching" once the person is employed. Coaching services include assistance with on-the-job skills such as personal hygiene, appropriate dress, requesting feedback, getting along with others, communicating needs, and making reasonable accommodations in the workplace. These accommodations help to compensate for disability by modifying the work space or how the job is performed. Examples include flexible scheduling, job task modification or restructuring, adapting employee training or supervision, making policy changes, modifying the physical environment or providing special equipment. Reasonable accommodations are a guaranteed right under the Americans with Disabilities Act of 1990.

The most recognized supported employment model is "Individual Placement and Support" (IPS) which Becker and Drake (2003) describe in detail. The IPS model is a "place first and then train" approach that stresses rapid job placement followed by the provision of needed support to acclimate to the specific demands of the chosen work setting (SAMHSA, 2009). The IPS model also stresses the importance of the coordination and integration of mental health services and employment services. The IPS employment specialist provides ongoing support throughout the process of acquiring and maintaining a job, providing assistance as needed.

Competitive employment rates of up to 75% have been achieved by people involved with supported employment services (Bond, Drake, & Becker, 2008). This is a significant improvement over usual services such as those offered by state vocational rehabilitation offices (Bond et al., 2001). Additionally, service recipients' use of other mental health treatment is reduced, resulting in significant cost saving to mental health-care systems (Bush, Drake, Xie, McHugo, & Haslett, 2009). However, there is still a considerably high unemployment rate among this population and the challenge to remove disincentives to working such as employer stigma, the loss of SSI and Medicaid benefits and concern about the stress of working is ongoing.

EMERGING BEST PSYCHIATRIC REHABILITATION PRACTICES

Peer-Provided Services

Peer-provided services are delivered by individuals who identify as having a severe psychiatric diagnosis and are, or have been, a recipient of mental health services, for the primary purpose of helping others with a psychiatric diagnosis. Peer-provided services are recovery oriented and empowerment enhancing and emphasize self-determination. Their premise is that individuals who have shared common experiences are in a better position to provide support to others like themselves than those who themselves have not had mental illness. These programs include a diversity of service models from the delivery of case management, crisis intervention services, community outreach to offering drop-in services. With the recent New Freedom Commission Report identifying peer-provided services as an emerging best practice and promoting recovery oriented services, there has been a renewed interest in these services (see case example: Wellness and Recovery Education Project).

WELLNESS AND RECOVERY EDUCATION PROJECT: A PEER-DELIVERED INNOVATION

Margaret Swarbrick, PhD, OTR, CPRP

Individuals with psychiatric disability living in institutional settings often have limited awareness of recovery resources and natural supports that would help them succeed in the community. They also have limited exposure to people who role model their own recovery. "Recovery Network" was developed to communicate a message of recovery and wellness, delivered by peer educators, to patients and staff of the five state psychiatric hospitals in New Jersey (Swarbrick & Brice, 2006). The program was designed by Collaborative Support Program of New Jersey, a peer-run organization that has a long history of developing and implementing innovative services for people living with mental illness (Swarbrick, 2009).

Peer educators (persons in recovery and living with mental illness) are trained to share their personal recovery experiences, teach healthy coping skills, and offer other information for the purpose of instilling hope and preparing patients for reintegration into the community. Recovery and wellness principles are stressed in an effort to get patients and staff to think more holistically about mental health. These principles include maintaining healthy eating habits, getting adequate rest and sleep, developing positive personal relationships, engaging in recreation and intellectually stimulating activities, and nurturing a sense of spiritual well-being. Peer educators help to introduce and connect people at the hospital to a wide variety of natural community supports and resources including self-help.

Peer educators facilitate structured group experiences for patients once a week with group size ranging from 8 to 15 participants. Each session consists of an introduction to a recovery concept followed by a relevant personal story by the peer educator. These stories create hope, purpose, and inspiration by showing that a person with a mental illness can and has resumed valued social roles such as neighbor, friend, worker, student, parent, sibling, family member, and community citizen (Swarbrick & Brice, 2006). Then each group member has an opportunity to discuss the designated topic and identify personally relevant goals. The peer educator is responsible for creating a safe, open, trusting, and supportive environment for all group members; guiding the group activity and discussion; keeping the channels of communication open; sensing moods and feelings within the group; keeping the group focused on the task; and most importantly inspiring hope for recovery.

Peer educators also offer wellness and recovery training within the hospital's new employee orientation program. This is especially powerful when the peer is also an ex-patient of a psychiatric institution. Hospital and project staffs have even collaborated on ways to incorporate recovery principles into hospital-run therapeutic services. The Recovery Network represents an effort to transition the mental health system toward a recovery-oriented service environment. The project has been running since 2005 and has been well received by participants and the hospital staff.

Solomon (2004) has categorized peer-provided services into four domains: mutual support or self-help groups, peer-operated services, peer-professional partnership services, and peers as employees, or more recently designated as peer specialists. Mutual support or self-help groups are small voluntary groups that offer mutual assistance for achieving a particular purpose. A diversity of groups serve people with specific problems and diagnoses. Traditionally, these groups met in person, but with the proliferation of Internet access online groups are now common. Peer-operated services or peer-run services are those that are designed, managed, operated, and delivered by individuals with a psychiatric illness. Partnerships are those in which peers partner with nonpeers, but more than half of those involved in administering and delivering the services are peers. For the most part, these various types of peer-support services are adjunctive to traditional mental health services rather than replacement. Peers as employees are individuals who identify as a recipient of mental health services and are hired by nonpeer agencies, such as community mental health centers, to fill either designated peer positions or existing agency positions. Peer specialists help other peers to regain control over their lives and their own process of recovery by demonstrating competence and offering role models of recovery (Sabin & Daniels, 2003). The number of peer specialists has greatly expanded, with mental health agencies now receiving reimbursement for this service through the Medicaid mental health rehabilitation option, which was initially pioneered by the State of Georgia and has now expanded to a number of states (Sabin & Daniels, 2003). Currently, 13 states use this Medicaid waiver option (states can apply for a waiver, which is approval for a variation from the standardized Medicaid benefit/service array) and 30 states have criteria required for employment and training of peer specialists (Davidson & Rowe, 2008). To be eligible for reimbursement, peers are required to meet certain qualifications which vary by location, but frequently include current or past recipient of mental health services and a high-school diploma or GED. Generally, the person must also be certified through successful completion of a peer training program. There are a number of organizations that provide peer specialist certification training, both nationally and locally. The National Association of Peer Specialists, Inc. (NAPS), which was founded in 2004, is dedicated to the promotion of peer specialists throughout the United States.

Peer-provided services are considered an emerging best practice as the evidence to date has been relatively limited. The research has found that these services can be feasibly implemented and that outcomes of the service are at least as effective as those provided by nonpeer providers (Solomon, 2004).

Supported Education

Serious mental illness often first appears at the time young adults are finishing high school or attending college. Early in the onset of illness, symptoms can be frightening, confusing, and disruptive, often derailing continued education. Supported education (SEd) services help students with psychiatric disabilities successfully pursue their educational goals (Mowbray, Brown, Furlong-Norman, & Sullivan-Soydan, 2002), which in turn may lead to improved employment opportunities (Murphy, Mullen, & Spagnolo, 2005; Nuechterlein et al., 2008). Indeed, the core components of this service mirror those offered by supported employment. The SEd specialist acts as a case manager and provides a broad range of services that support students with psychiatric disabilities through each stage of academic pursuit, from career exploration, to admission/enrollment, through course selection and academic achievement (Mowbray et al., 2005).

The core services of supported education typically include career counseling, assistance with applications for admission and financial aid, facilitation of academic services and supports within the school, and ongoing support as needed throughout the student's academic experience. The supported education specialist may also help the student develop a social support network, link with tutoring or other mentoring resources, and acquire academic survival skills such as time management. If symptoms appear to be presenting barriers to success, SEd services may assist the student in linking with the school's disability services office or with faculty. The specialist may help with developing reasonable accommodations that modify the classroom environment or the way in which information is presented. Support accommodations may also include help with note taking, such as the use of a tape recorder, or extended deadlines and alternate formats (e.g., verbal vs. written) for projects and exams. When required, the SEd specialist provides supportive counseling and referral to other behavioral health services. Together these services, supports, and accommodations are designed to "empower adults with SMI to choose their own educational goals, and acquire the tools necessary for achievement in post secondary educational settings attain their highest potential and succeed in their efforts" (Mowbray et al., 2005, p. 10).

There are a variety of approaches to offering supported education (Unger, 1990). The self-contained classroom provides a protected learning environment exclusively for students with psychiatric diagnoses. It typically prepares participants for regular college classes, but may also offer studies leading to certification programs for peer specialists (Ratzlaff, McDiarmid, Marty, & Rapp, 2006) or technical careers not typically needing a college degree (Best, Still, & Cameron, 2008). On-site support is the second approach to SEd. A trained rehabilitation specialist, perhaps employed by the school's disability office or contracted through a behavioral health agency (e.g., Hain & Gioia, 2004), is available at the school. Mobile support programs are offered directly by community-based mental health agencies that provide both health and education support services to their clients who are enrolled in regular college classes.

The evidence for the effectiveness of supported education generally demonstrates that students with psychiatric disabilities can successfully participate in and complete college level courses (Unger & Pardee, 2002). Furthermore, students are generally satisfied with the support they receive and subsequent employment reflects a good fit between the level of education and the kind of job secured (Mowbray et al., 2005).

Supported Housing/Housing Models

Since the era of deinstitutionalization in the 1960s and 1970s, people with serious mental illnesses have often lacked safe, affordable housing. Over 20% of people who are homeless at any point of time have serious mental illnesses (National Coalition for the Homeless, 2008). These individuals often lack the skills and resources needed to maintain themselves in independent residential settings. They do not have adequate income to afford rent, food, and transportation. They may be barred or evicted from subsidized housing due to criminal conviction, substance use, treatment noncompliance, or bizarre behavior that disturbs the neighbors. These situations diminish a person's quality of life and present significant barriers to recovery and community integration.

Yet, there is a debate about how best to help people with mental illness reintegrate into residential communities (Yanos, Barrow, & Tsemberis, 2004). The "continuum paradigm" matches individuals to housing based on their level of functioning. This model requires residents to make transitions from more to less intensively supervised settings before independent living is attempted. Thus, a person might initially live in a congregate setting such as a group home operated by a mental health agency, attend a day treatment program, and receive 24-hour on-site supervision and support by trained residential staff. These staffs monitor medication, teach independent living skills, and facilitate social/recreational activities. As the resident learns to manage household chores, demonstrates adherence to treatment and gains confidence to live more independently, she/he "graduates" to less supervised housing, ultimately leaving mental health-sponsored housing altogether for an independent apartment. The transition(s) to more independent housing has often been difficult to achieve for a variety of reasons. Residents tend to get comfortable in one place: making friends, establishing routines, building a "place called home." Also, the environmental demands of congregate living do not always match the demands of a more independent living situation; so, for example, skills that have been learned in a group home are not always transferable to living alone in an apartment. And finally, the stock of affordable apartments is inadequate for many people living on fixed income benefits, making it difficult to find a new place to live (O'Hara, Cooper, Zovistoski, & Buttrick, 2007).

The supported housing model has emerged to address some of the difficulties discussed above and to also better reflect the principles of choice, respect, and normalization associated with the philosophy of psychiatric rehabilitation (Rog, 2004). The supported housing approach suggests that people with mental illness choose a place to live that is independent of treatment. Thus, they typically become normalized tenants, bound to the requirements of a standard lease. Behavioral health support is brought to the setting as needed (and accepted by the resident), thus eliminating the need to make transitional moves to more independent settings over time. Another unique feature of this model is that continued stay is not predicated on adherence to treatment, which tests the sensibilities of some treatment providers, but honors the philosophy of separation of housing and treatment. The menu of services offered by a supported housing program are similar overall to the transitional housing model, with the primary distinction that services are chosen to meet the current needs of the client wherever they live, rather than remain fixed to a particular level of housing. "Housing First" is an application of the supported housing model. It incorporates harm reduction strategies, such as not requiring abstinence, with supported housing principles and has been shown to be well suited to help people who are chronically homeless and have substance use disorders (Tsemberis, Gulur, & Nakae, 2004).

The systematic review of research regarding the outcomes of the various housing programs discussed above suggests that housing stability, and psychiatric symptoms improved and hospitalizations declined with each model of housing (Leff et al., 2009). Leff however, reported that supported housing received higher user satisfaction ratings than other models of housing.

Mental Health Criminal Justice Diversion and Reentry Programs

Both mental health and criminal justice providers have become increasingly concerned about the growing numbers of adults with severe mental illness involved with the criminal justice system. Individuals with psychiatric disorders have long been incarcerated, but today they are over-represented in the criminal justice system (Loveland & Boyle, 2007) and have a far greater likelihood of being confined in jails than in psychiatric hospitals (Morrissey & Cuddeback, 2008). There is also economic pressure in many states to reduce the cost of their prison programs, by reducing their prison populations, thus, contributing to many individuals with behavioral health disorders being released without adequate planning. Since the safety net of state psychiatric hospitals is no longer available on a wide scale, individuals with SMI often do not receive the intensive community-based treatment they may need. Therefore, the involvement of those with mental illness in the criminal justice system has precipitated the development of jail diversion programs and jail/prison re-entry programs.

Jail diversion is eliminating or reducing the time that an individual with SMI spends in jail by diverting that individual with an encounter with the criminal justice system to a mental health treatment alternative. There are two types of diversion, prebooking and postbooking diversion. Prebooking occurs prior to arrest and before charges are filed, and involves police discretion, whereas postbooking occurs after the formal charges are filed by the police officer and may involve "judges, district attorneys, jail administrators, public defenders, and possibly probation officers" (Morrissey & Cuddeback, 2008, p. 528).

A number of prebooking, police-mental health clinician collaborations have been developed with some involving police bringing individuals to mental health programs for assessment and treatment, while in others, mental health clinicians are hired by a law enforcement agency to work alongside police officers. The most widely known and implemented of police-based diversion programs is Crisis Intervention Teams (CIT), which was initially developed in Memphis, Tennessee in response to a highly publicized incident in which police shot a person with mental illness (Compton, Bahora, Watson, & Oliva, 2008; Watson, Morabito, Draine, & Ottati, 2008). The program involves 40 hours of didactic and experiential training to self-selected police officers in the basics of mental illness, de-escalation techniques when managing crises, and methods of transporting individuals in crises. These trained police officers function as frontline responders who are equipped to transport individuals with mental illness to the mental health treatment program and away from the criminal justice system by means of a "no refusal" policy for such cases (Compton et al., 2008; Morressey & Cuddeback, 2008). This model has been endorsed by the National Alliance on Mental Illness (NAMI).

Research to date on the effectiveness of this intervention seems to indicate that CIT has promise, but the studies have a number of methodological and conceptual limitations, including small sample sizes and lack of multivariate statistical procedures. Further research is needed to determine the essential elements for an effective program, such as whether a single drop-off point is required or a partnership between stakeholders is sufficient to redirect individuals from criminal justice involvement to mental health treatment (Compton et al., 2008).

Relatively recently there has been an increasing proliferation of Mental Health Courts as a post booking diversion mechanism. This emergence is due in large part to federal legislation that provided initial funding for these courts. These are specialized courts that evolved from the success of drug courts and are consistent with other specialized courts like family or juvenile courts. They are basically designed to divert nonviolent persons with mental illnesses (who are usually charged with misdemeanors) away from criminal justice and into the mental health system through collaborative efforts between mental health clinicians and court personnel to develop a therapeutic intervention. Although courts vary as to eligibility criteria, such as charges, diagnoses, and history of mental health treatment involvement, all require voluntary participation in the court program, a willingness to accept and follow their treatment plan as well as monitoring by the court. In return, charges and/or sentences are reduced. Research to date shows promise for these mental health courts in reducing recidivism and subsequent violence (Corrigan et al., 2008; McNiel & Binder, 2007).

Individuals leaving prison and jails receive little in the way of planning, other than possible supervision by a parole officer, if they have not maxed out of their sentence, which is commonly the case for persons with severe mental illnesses. Re-entry planning in actual practice, if done at all, consists of nothing more than referrals to treatment and resource supports (Draine & Herman, 2007). Community re-entry programming has to respond to the needs and risks of the individual being released as well as the public safety concerns of the community and the availability and receptivity of the community's resources (Draine, Wolff, Jacoby, Hartwell, & Duclos, 2005). These authors note that current models must "focus on conceptualizing the process of service delivery—describing what should be done for an individual" (p. 692).

Draine and colleagues have put forth a Shared Responsibility and Interdependent Model of Reentry for prisoners with mental illness that involves four domains of support: housing, jobs, services, and treatment. Consequently, Forensic Assertive Community Treatment (FACT) and Intensive Case Management have been used for persons being released from jails and prisons, as well as for jail diversion, but there is need for further research as to the effectiveness of FACT for criminal justice involved clients (Loveland & Boyle, 2007; Morrissey, Meyer, & Cuddeback, 2007; Solomon, 2003). Currently, Critical Time Intervention (CTI) is being tested as a possible reentry program for persons with mental illness who are leaving prisons. CTI is a time-limited intervention that has been shown to be effective for individuals being discharged from institutions by assisting them in making connections to needed community resources. It further tries "to enhance engagement with treatment and community supports through building problem-solving skills, motivational coaching, and advocacy with community agencies" (Draine & Herman, 2007, p. 1577).

FUTURE DIRECTIONS

The absence of an integrated funding stream has challenged the implementation and delivery of innovative services for people with co-occurring disorders and with long-term support needs, as well as family caregivers. Failing an increase in funding, offering consumers control over how healthcare dollars are spent might shakeout ineffective and nonessential services. A number of self-directed care models (Cook, Russell, Grey, & Jonikas, 2008) where participants have control over a set amount of dollars for purchasing services they desire, are receiving attention, particularly given that the New Freedom Commission (Department of Health and Human Service, 2003) strongly endorsed such an approach. Widespread dissemination of evidence-based practices will also have an impact on the nature of services for this population. Although implementing these services has been somewhat problematic, a growing emphasis on translational research and implementation science may increase success in this arena. Greater focus on recovery services seems to be increasing employment opportunities for peer specialists and family providers, and hopefully this may result in more innovative and effective services with a reallocation of funding priorities.

Another challenge is the failure of education and training programs to fully prepare the behavioral health-care workforce to work in partnership with consumers of service and to teach skills that facilitate a personal path to recovery. Most direct care positions are held by workers with a generalist background in psychology or social work who have been trained to apply a medical model and employ an authoritarian orientation. Many academic programs do not know of, understand, nor support and agree with less than very traditional approaches such as one-to-one therapy. In-service training, when it occurs, tends to reinforce conventional, reimbursable service approaches, and does not necessarily lead to improved clinical competencies. Furthermore, a great proportion of those in the public sector working with people with the most severe cases of mental illness have a bachelor's degree at best. Many lack a recovery orientation that promotes collaboration and shared decision making rather than the traditional authoritative model of medicine.

As recognized in the New Freedom Commission, the mental health system requires a total transformation, not simply another reform effort. The federal government, particularly SAMHSA, is taking the lead in this system transformation. There is an emphasis on the inclusion of people of diverse racial and ethnic backgrounds to eliminate disparities in access to mental health care and in the overall quality of mental health. People in recovery and their family members have also been actively recruited to help shape a new philosophy and methodology for ensuring that individuals with serious mental illness recover a rich quality of life with all the privileges and responsibilities of people living in all communities across the country.

REFERENCES

Anthony, W. A. (1993). Recovery from mental illness: The guiding vision of the mental health service system in the 1990s. *Psychosocial Rehabilitation Journal, 16,* 12–23.

Bach, P., & Hayes, S. C. (2002). The use of Acceptance and Commitment Therapy to prevent the rehospitalization of psychotic patients: A randomized controlled trial. *Journal of Consulting and Clinical Psychology, 70,* 1129–1139.

Beck, A. T., Rector, N. A., Stolar, N., & Grant, P. (2009). *Schizophrenia: Cognitive theory, research, and therapy.* New York, NY: Guilford Press.

Beck, A. T., Rush, A. J., Shaw, B. F., & Emery, G. (1979). *Cognitive therapy of depression.* New York, NY: Guilford Press.

Beck, A. T., Wright, F. D., Newman, C. F., & Liese, B. S. (1993). *Cognitive therapy for substance abuse.* New York, NY: Guilford Press.

Becker, D. R., & Drake, R. E. (2003). *A working life for people with severe mental illness.* New York, NY: Oxford Press.

Bellack, A. S. (2004). Skills training for people with severe mental illness. *Psychiatric Rehabilitation Journal, 27*(4), 375–391.

Bellack, A. S., Mueser, K. T., Gingerich, S., & Agresta, J. (2004). *Social skills training for schizophrenia: A step-by-step guide* (2nd ed.). New York, NY: Guilford Press.

Bernheim, K. (1982). Supportive family counseling. *Schizophrenia Bulletin, 8,* 634–648.

Bernheim, K., & Lehman, A. (1985). *Working with families of the mentally ill.* New York, NY: Norton.

Best, L. J., Still, M., & Cameron, G. (2008). Supported education: Enabling course completion for people experiencing mental illness. *Australian Occupational Therapy Journal, 55*, 65–68.

Bond, G. R., Drake, R. E., & Becker, D. R. (2008). An update on randomized controlled trials of evidence-based supported employment. *Psychiatric Rehabilitation Journal, 31*(4), 280–289.

Bond, G. R., Drake, R. E., Mueser, K., & Latimer, E. (2001). Assertive Community Treatment for people with severe mental illness: Critical ingredients and impact on patients. *Disease Management and Health Outcomes, 9*, 141–159.

Brown, G., Carstairs, G., & Topping, G. (1958). The post-hospital adjustment of chronic mental patients. *Lancet, 2*, 685–689.

Brown, G., Monck, E., Carstairs, G., & Wing, J. (1962). The influence of family life on the course of schizophrenic illness. *British Journal of Preventive and Social Medicine, 16*, 55–68.

Bush, P. W., Drake, R. E., Xie, H., McHugo, G. J., & Haslett, W. R. (2009). The long-term impact of employment on mental health service use and costs for persons with severe mental illness. *Psychiatric Services, 60*(8), 1026–1031.

Compton, M., Bahora, M., Watson, A., & Oliva, J. (2008). A comprehensive review of extant research on Crisis Intervention Team (CIT) Programs. *Journal of American Academy of Psychiatry Law, 26*, 47–55.

Cook, J., Russell, C., Grey, D., & Jonikas, J. (2008). A self-directed care model for mental health recovery. *Psychiatric Services, 59*, 600–602.

Copeland, M. E. (1997). *Wellness recovery action plan*. Dummerston, VT: Peach Press.

Corrigan, P., Mueser, K., Bond, G., Drake, R., & Solomon, P. (2008). *Principles and practice of psychiatric rehabilitation: An empirical approach*. New York, NY: Guilford Press.

Davidson, L., & Rowe, M. (2008). *Peer support with criminal justice settings: The role of forensic peer specialists*. Retrieved July 30, 2009, from http://www.gainscenter.samhsa.gov

Department of Health and Human Services. (1999). *Mental health: A report of the Surgeon General*. Rockville, MD: U.S. Department of Health and Human Services, Substance Abuse and Mental Health Services Administration, Center for Mental Health Services, National Institutes of Health, National Institute of Mental Health.

Department of Health and Human Services. (2003). *New Freedom Commission on Mental Health: Achieving the promise: Transforming mental health care in America. Final report*. (No. DHHS pub no SMA-03–3832). Rockville, MD: Author.

Dixon, L., Kraus, N., & Lehman, A. (1994). Consumers as service providers. The promise and challenge. *Community Mental Health Journal, 30*, 615–625.

Dixon, L., Lucksted, A., Stewart, B., Burland, J., Brown, C., Postrado, L., et al. (2004). Outcomes of the peer-taught 12-week Family-to-Family education program for severe mental illness. *Acta Psychiatrica Scandinavica, 109*, 207–215.

Dixon, L., Stewart, B., Kraus, N., Robbins, J., Heckman, A., & Lehman, A. (1998). The participation of families of homeless persons with severe mental illness in an outreach intervention. *Community Mental Health Journal, 34*, 251–259.

Donald, M., Dower, J., & Kavanagh, K. (2005). Integrated versus non-integrated management and care for clients with co-occurring mental health and substance use disorders: A qualitative systematic review of randomized controlled trials. *Social Science & Medicine, 60,* 1371–1383.

Draine, J., & Herman, D. (2007). Critical Time Intervention for reentry from prison for persons with mental illness. *Psychiatric Services, 58,* 1577–1581.

Draine, J., Wolff, N., Jacoby, J., Hartwell, S., & Duclos, C. (2005). Understanding community re-entry of former prisoners with mental illness: A conceptual model to guide new research. *Behavioral Sciences and the Law, 23,* 689–707.

Drake, R. E., & Bond, G. R. (Eds.). (2008). Special 10th anniversary issue on supported employment. *Psychiatric Rehabilitation Journal.*

Drake, R. E., Essock, S. M., Shaner, A., Carey, K. B., Minkoff, K., Kola, L., et al. (2001). Implementing dual diagnosis services for clients with a severe mental illness. *Psychiatric Services, 52*(4), 469–476.

Drake, R. E., Mueser, K. T., Brunette, M. F., & McHugo, G. J. (2004). A review of treatments for people with severe mental illness and co-occurring substance use disorders. *Psychiatric Rehabilitation Journal, 27*(4), 360–374.

Eli, L. (n.d.). *Solutions for wellness.* Retrieved October 7, 2010 from http://www.solutionsforwellness.info/index.aspx

Glynn, S., Marder, S., Liberman, R., Blair, K., Wirshing, W., Wirshing, D., et al. (2002). Supplementing clinic-based skills training with manual-based community support sessions: Effects on social adjustment of patients with schizophrenia. *American Journal of Psychiatry, 159,* 829–837.

Hain, R., & Gioia, D. (2004). Supported Education Enhancing Rehabilitation (SEER): A community mental health and community college partnership for access and retention. *American Journal of Psychiatric Rehabilitation, 7*(3), 315–328.

Hasson-Ohaon, I., Roe, D., & Kravetz, S. (2007). A randomized controlled trial of the effectiveness of the illness management and recovery program. *Psychiatric Services, 58,* 1461–1466.

Hatfield, A. (1994). Family education theory and practice. In A. Hatfield (Ed.), *Family interventions in mental illness. New Directions for mental health services* (Vol. 62, pp. 3–11). San Francisco: Jossey-Bass.

Kabat-Zinn, J. (1990). *Full catastrophe living: Using the wisdom of your mind to face stress, pain and illness.* New York, NY: Dell Publishing.

Kingdon, D. G., & Turkington, D. (1994). *Cognitive–behavioral therapy of schizophrenia.* New York, NY: Guilford Press.

Leff, H. S., Chow, C. M., Pepin, R., Conley, J., Allen, I. E., & Seaman, C. A. (2009). Does one size fit all? What we can and can't learn from a meta-analysis of housing models for persons with mental illness. *Psychiatric Services, 60*(4), 473–482.

Liberman, R. P. (2008). *Recovery from disability: Manual of psychiatric rehabilitation.* Arlington, VA: American Psychiatric Publishing Incorporated.

Liberman, R. P., Wallace, C. J., Blackwell, G., Kopelowicz, A., Vaccaro, J. V., & Mintz, J. (1998). Skills training vs. psychosocial occupational therapy for persons with persistent schizophrenia. *American Journal of Psychiatry, 155,* 1087–1091.

Linehan, M. M. (1993). *Cognitive behavioral treatment of borderline personality disorder.* New York, NY: Guilford Press.

Loveland, D., & Boyle, M. (2007). Intensive case management as a jail diversion program for people with a serious mental illness. *International Journal of Offender Therapy and Comparative Criminology, 51*, 130–150.

Mannion, E., Draine, J., Solomon, P., & Meisel, M. (1997). Applying research on family education about mental illness to development of a relatives' group consultation model. *Community Mental Health Journal, 20*, 43–50.

Maples, N. J., & Velligan, D. I. (2008). Cognitive adaptation training: Establishing environmental supports to bypass cognitive deficits and improve functional outcomes. *American Journal of Psychiatric Rehabilitation, 11*(2), 164–180.

Marx, A., Test, M. A., & Stein, L. (1973). Extra-hospital management of severe mental illness. *Archives of General Psychiatry, 29*, 505–511.

McFarlane, W. (2002). *Multifamily groups in the treatment of severe psychiatric disorders.* New York, NY: Guilford Press.

McFarlane, W., Dixon, L., Lukens, E., & Lucksted, A. (2003). Family psychoeducation and schizophrenia: A review of the literature. *Journal of Marital and Family Therapy, 29*, 223–245.

McNiel, D., & Binder, R. (2007). Effectiveness of a mental health court in reducing criminal recidivism and violence. *American Journal of Psychiatry, 164*, 1395–1403.

Miller, W. R., & Rollnick, S. (2002). *Motivational interviewing: Preparing people to change addictive behavior* (2nd ed.). New York, NY: Guilford Press.

Morrissey, J. P., & Cuddeback, G. S. (2008). Jail diversion. In K. T. Mueser & D. V. Jeste (Eds.), *Clinical handbook of schizophrenia.* New York, NY: Guilford Press.

Morrissey, J., Meyer, P., & Cuddeback, G. (2007). Extending Assertive Community Treatment to criminal justice settings: Origins, current evidence, and future directions. *Community Mental Health Journal, 43*, 527–544.

Mowbray, C. T., Brown, K. S., Furlong-Norman, K., & Sullivan-Soydan, A. (2002). *Supported education and psychiatric rehabilitation: Models and methods.* Columbia, MD: IAPSRS.

Mowbray, C. T., Collins, M. E., Bellamy, C. D., Megivern, D. A., Bybee, D., & Svilvagyi, S. (2005). Supported education for adults with severe mental illness: An innovation for social work and psychiatric rehabilitation practice. *Social Work, 1*(50), 7–20.

Mueser, K. T., Corrigan, P. W., Hilton, D., Tanzman, B., Schaub, A., & Gingerich, S. (2002). Illness management and recovery for severe mental illness: A review of the research. *Psychiatric Services, 53*(10), 1272–1284.

Mueser, K., Meyer, P., Penn, D., Clancy, R., Clancy, D. M., & Salyers, M. P. (2006). The Illness Management and Recovery program: Rationale, development, and preliminary findings. *Schizophrenia Bulletin, 32*(Suppl 1) S32–S43.

Mueser, K. T., Noordsy, D. L., Drake, R. E., & Fox, L. (2003). *Integrated treatment for dual disorders: A guide to effective practice.* New York, NY: Guilford Press.

Murphy, A. A., Mullen, M., & Spagnolo, A. (2005). Enhancing individual placement and support: Promoting job tenure by integrating natural supports and supported education. *American Journal of Psychiatric Rehabilitation, 8*, 37–61.

Najavits, L. M. (2007). Seeking safety: An evidence-based model for substance abuse and trauma/PTSD. In K. Witkiewitz & G. A. Marlatt (Eds.), *Therapist's guide to evidence-based relapse prevention* (pp. 141–167). New York, NY: Academic Press.

National Coalition for the Homeless. (2008). *Mental illness and homelessness.* Retrieved August 7, 2009 from http://www.nationalhomeless.org/factsheets/Mental_Illness.html

National Resource Center on Psychiatric Advance Directives. (2009). *State by state information.* Retrieved July 30, 2009 from http://www.nrc-pad.org/

Nuechterlein, K. H., Subotnik, K. L., Turner, L. R., Ventura, J., Becker, D. R., & Drake, R. E. (2008). Individual placement and support for individuals with recent-onset schizophrenia: Integrating supported education and supported employment. *Psychiatric Rehabilitation Journal, 31*(4), 340–349.

O'Hara, A., Cooper, E., Zovistoski, A., & Buttrick, J. (2007). *Priced out in 2006. The housing crisis for people with disabilities.* Boston, MA: Technical Assistance Collaborative, Inc.

Pankey, J., & Hayes, S. C. (2003). Acceptance and commitment therapy for psychosis. *International Journal of Psychology and Psychological Therapy, 3*(2), 311–328.

Parks, J., Svendsen, D., Singer, P., & Foti, M. E. (Eds.). (2006). *Morbidity and mortality in people with serious mental illness* [Technical Report]. Retrieved July 28, 2009, from http://www.nasmhpd.org/general_files/publications/med_directors_pubs/Technical%20Report%20on%20Morbidity%20and%20Mortaility%20-%20-Final%2011-06.pdf

Pharoah, F., Rathbone, J., Mari, J., & Streiner, D. (2004). *Family Intervention for schizophrenia.* The Cochrane Library (Issue 2). Oxford, UK: Wiley.

Pickett-Schenk, S., Lippincott, R., Bennett, C., & Steigman, P. (2008). Improving knowledge through family-led education: The Journey of Hope. *Psychiatric Services, 59*, 46–56.

Pratt, C. W., Gill, K. J., Barrett, N. M., & Roberts, M. M. (2007). *Psychiatric rehabilitation* (2nd ed.). San Diego: Academic Press.

Prochaska, J. O., & Diclemente, C. C. (1984). *The transtheoretical approach: Crossing traditional boundaries of therapy.* Homewood, IL: Dow Jones-Irwin.

Ratzlaff, S., McDiarmid, D., Marty, D., & Rapp, C. (2006). The Kansas Consumer as Provider program: Measuring the effects of a supported education initiative. *Psychiatric Rehabilitation Journal, 29*(3), 174–182.

Regier, D. A., Farmer, M. E., Rae, D. S., Locke, B. Z., Keith, S. J., Judd, L. L., et al. (1990). Co-morbidity of mental disorders with alcohol and other drug abuse: Results from the epidemiologic catchment area (ECA) study. *Journal of the American Medical Association, 264*, 2511–2518.

Roe, D., Hasson-Ohayan, I., Salyers, M., & Kravetz, S. (2009). A one year follow-up of Illness Management and Recovery: Participants' accounts of its impact and uniqueness. *Psychiatric Rehabilitation Journal, 32*, 285–291.

Rog, D. J. (2004). The evidence on supported housing. *Psychiatric Rehabilitation Journal, 27*(4), 334–344.

Sabin, J., & Daniels, N. (2003). Strengthening the consumer voice in managed care: VII. The Georgia Peer Specialist Program. *Psychiatric Services, 54,* 497–498.

SAMHSA. (2009). *Supported employment. Implementation resource kit.* Retrieved October, 24 2008, from http://store.samhsa.gov/shin/content/SMA08-4365/SMA08-4365-01.pdf://store.samhsa.gov/shin/content/SMA08-4365/SMA08-4365-01.pdf

SAMHSA. (2010a). *Illness management and recovery evidence-based practice.* Retrieved October 7, 2010, from http://store.samhsa.gov/product/SMA09-4463

SAMHSA. (2010b). *Integrated treatment for co-occurring disorders.* Retrieved October 7, 2010, from http://store.samhsa.gov/product/SMA08-4367

Scott, J., & Dixon, L. (1995). Assertive Community Treatment and case management of schizophrenia. *Schizophrenia Bulletin, 21,* 657–668.

Solomon, P. (1999). Evolution of service innovation for adults with severe mental illness. In D. Biegel & A. Blum (Eds.), *Innovation in practices and service delivery across the life span* (pp. 147–168). New York, NY: Oxford University Press.

Solomon, P. (2003). Case management and the forensic client. In W. Fisher (Ed.), *Community-based interventions for criminal offenders with severe mental illness.* New York, NY: JAI.

Solomon, P. (2004). Peer support/peer provider services: Underlying processes, benefits, and critical ingredients. *Psychiatric Rehabilitation Journal, 27,* 392–401.

Solomon, P., & Draine, J. (1995). One year outcomes of a randomized trial of case management with seriously mentally ill clients leaving jail. *Evaluation Review, 19,* 256–273.

Swarbrick, M. (2009). Collaborative Support Programs of New Jersey. *Occupational Therapy in Mental Health.* Taylor & Francis, 25(3,4), 224–238.

Swarbrick, M., & Brice, G. (2006). Sharing the message of hope, wellness and recovery with consumers and staff at psychiatric hospitals. *American Journal of Psychiatric Rehabilitation, 9,* 101–109.

Tsemberis, S., Gulur, L., & Nakae, M. (2004). Housing first, consumer choice, and harm reduction for homeless individuals with dual diagnosis. *American Journal of Public Health, 94,* 651–656.

Unger, K. (1990). Supported postsecondary education for people with mental illness. *American Rehabilitation, 16,* 10–14.

Unger, K., & Pardee, R. (2002). Outcomes measure across program sites for postsecondary supported education programs. *Psychiatric Rehabilitation Journal, 25(1),* 300–304.

Velligan, D. I., Bow-Thomas, C. C., Huntzinger, C., Ritch, J., Ledbetter, N., Prihoda, T. J., et al. (2000). Randomized controlled trial of the use of compensatory strategies to enhance adaptive functioning in outpatients with schizophrenia. *American Journal of Psychiatry, 157(8),* 1317–1323.

Watson, A., Morabito, M., Draine, J., & Ottati, V. (2008). Improving police response to persons with mental illness: A multi-level conceptualization of CIT. *International Journal of Law and Psychiatry, 31,* 359–368.

Wilson, D., Tien, G., & Eaves, D. (1995). Increasing the community tenure of mentally disordered offenders: An assertive case management program. *International Journal of Law and Psychiatry, 18,* 61–69.

Yanos, P. T., Barrow, S. M., & Tsemberis, S. (2004). Community integration in the early phase of housing among homeless persons diagnosed with severe mental illness. *Community Mental Health Journal, 40*(2), 133–150.

CHAPTER THREE

Children, Youth, and Families

Needs and Issues

Heidi Arthur, Susan Bowler, and Nina Rose Fisher

INTRODUCTION

Federal and state agencies, advocates, and private service providers agree that children and youth arrive at the doors of existing mental health, substance abuse, juvenile justice, and child welfare service systems with co-occurring needs, which require highly coordinated services from multiple agencies. They must overcome pervasive stigma to seek treatment, only to encounter a fragmented maze of providers with bewildering and sometimes contradictory eligibility, funding, and service requirements. The door at which children and youth arrive is often dictated by what happens to be available, rather than which services would meet their specific needs. At the community level, services are too often unevenly distributed, substantial gaps are common, and measures of service quality are evolving.

The system is heavily weighted toward care for those with a high level of acuity. For example, children are unlikely to receive service as soon as they begin skipping school, but may find themselves in a detention center a couple of years later for shoplifting. Often, services are organized around the needs and values of providers—from hours and locations to the cultural values and assumptions sensitivity of professionals. Children and their families need treatment options and providers that are aligned with real needs rather than bureaucratic necessity.

Culture is the lens through which each individual understands the world—including health, illness, and recovery. Yet, the service system is disproportionately drawn from the ranks of white, middle-class people

71

serving diverse ethnic, racial, and linguistic communities. As well, the service system is not organized to deal with the full range of challenges children, youth, and families face in the process of recovery. While family needs may include housing, food, and employment, as well as parental behavioral health and medical care there is very limited infrastructure in the service system for joint and integrated planning.

This chapter explores these issues as they affect children and youth with mental health and substance abuse challenges needs within the juvenile justice and child welfare systems. Chapter 5, *Programming Approaches for Children, Youth, and Families*, explores recommended models and interventions.

CO-OCCURRING NEEDS

As I was growing up, it became obvious that I had some big issues. My temper tantrums were especially bad. I would go on kicking and screaming for hours as a child. I was easily distracted, and I never listened to my mother . . . I also struggled with an eating disorder, and I became a frequent cutter . . . As a teenager I was sick of treatment, refused medications, and was often out of control. In these bad times I was raped, so now I'm dealing with PTSD and other problems related to a really traumatic experience. (Kayla Paulson, Reflections of a Youth 'N Action! Member.) (Matarese et al., 2008, p. 293)

Despite the manner in which service systems are typically organized and funded, most children, youth, and families present multiple needs that require help from an array of systems and providers. A National Co-Morbidity Study found that 8–11 million people in the United States have a mental health or substance abuse diagnosis and identified the median age of onset for mental health issues to be 11—*one half of these consumers developed their problem before age 11* and half developed it afterward. For 85% of these people, the mental health problem preceded the substance abuse issues, meaning that they handled their mental health issues by self-medication with drugs and alcohol (Kessler, 1994). Close to half of all youth receiving mental health services in the United States also have a co-occurring disorder (US HHS, 2002).

Mental health disorders frequently begin in childhood and the complications of co-occurring substance use disorders, as well as serious impairment, may be avoidable with early detection and effective treatment. According to SAMHSA's National Survey on Drug Use and Health in 2008, 12.4% of adolescent females and 4.3% of adolescent males experienced a major depressive episode (MDE); 9.2% of females and 2.9% of males experienced severe impairment and 37.4% had used illicit drugs during the same period. Drug use was 17.2% among youth who did not report an MDE in the past year. Similarly, the rates of past month daily cigarette use and heavy alcohol use were higher for youth with MDE (3.6% and 3.4%, respectively) than for youth who did not have MDE (1.8% and 1.8%, respectively) (SAMHSA, 2009).

Too often, co-occurring needs go unidentified. Although one out of every eight adolescents with a mental illness has a co-occurring substance abuse problem, less than 60% are appropriately diagnosed (King, Gaines, Lambert, Summerfelt, & Bickman, 2000). In 2008, 37.7% of youth aged 12–17 with past year MDE received treatment for depression (i.e., saw or talked to a medical doctor or other professional or used prescription medication). Among youth with past year MDE, 21.7% saw or talked to a medical doctor or other professional only, 2.9% used prescription medication only, and 13.1% received treatment from both sources for depression. In 2008, 3.1 million youth aged 12–17 (12.7%) received treatment or counseling for problems with behavior or emotions in a specialty mental health setting (inpatient or outpatient care). Additionally, 11.8% of youth received services in the education setting, and 2.9% received mental health services in a general medical setting in the past 12 months. Mental health services were received in both a specialty setting and either the education or general medical settings (i.e., care from multiple settings) by 5.3% of youth (SAMHSA, 2009).

Youth whose functioning is impaired by behavioral problems like conduct disorder or attention deficit disorder are more likely to develop substance abuse disorders than youth with mood disorders like anxiety or depression, yet even those youth are two to four times more likely to develop substance abuse disorders than youth without mental disorders (US HHS, 2000).

When children and youth do not receive appropriate treatment, poor school performance, truancy, family and peer conflicts, medical problems, later unemployment and homelessness, incarceration, and high rates of suicide too often result (US HHS, New Freedom Commission, 2003). The majority of adults with multiple mental health and substance abuse disorders (80%) report that their problems began in their youth too often result (US HHS, 2000). Of the one million youth in formal contact with the justice system (i.e., charges and/or court appearance), two thirds have one or more alcohol, drug, and mental disorders and one quarter have serious mental illnesses (US HHS, 2007).

STIGMA

Our children are dying. The schools, court counselors, and social workers try. They have the knowledge but they have not lived what we have lived. They have not lived with a child who cries all night and does not know why. They have not lived with the school calling every day saying, "Come and get your child." We truly feel that professionals only see our children as "behaviors"—our children are more than that. They are beautiful, loving children who are hurting inside where no one can see.
(Jones, 2005)

Stigma has been widely identified as a barrier to effective intervention for children and families, among other affected populations. The Surgeon General's Report on Mental Health, which was prepared by the Substance Abuse Mental Health Service Administration's (SAMHSA) Center for Mental Health Services in partnership with the National Institute of Mental Health (NIMH) of the National Institutes of Health, indicated that stigma is "manifested by bias, distrust, stereotyping, fear, embarrassment, anger, and/or avoidance." Because stigma leads others to avoid people with mental disorders (Corrigan & Penn, 1999; Penn & Martin, 1998), people are understandably reluctant to self-identify as having mental problems or seek services and assistance.

Stigma also occurs treatment, when parents are blamed for their children's problems, told they will outgrow their challenges, or labeled as "anxious parents."

This stigma is compounded when families have other needs, including poverty or when youth and family culture is not understood by the service system. Mental illness may manifest in behavioral issues and social skill deficits (Ostman & Kjellin, 2002) and in social isolation that compounds self-esteem problems and increases feelings of hopelessness experienced by children and families (Prince & Prince, 2002). Stigma may lead to social adjustment problems that further perpetrate this cycle (Perlick et al., 2001).

CULTURAL FACTORS

Many factors influence a family's willingness to seek services, including varying rates of insurance, mistrust and fear of treatment providers; different cultural perceptions of illnesses, health, ways of seeking help, language, and communication patterns; racism; and discrimination by individuals and institutions. Highly individualized care that is consumer driven and includes staff representative of the targeted population and trained to understand and address cultural differences is critical. For instance, parenting approaches may differ based on immigration history (level of acculturation) and/or responses to community forces. For example, parents living in areas where children may be at risk due to community threats such as violence or prevalence of gangs often focus on reducing the chances that their children will engage in high-risk behaviors. Treatment professionals may perceive a low level of parental warmth when these parents emphasize control and monitoring to keep children safe and out of the criminal justice system (Hopkins, Huici, & Bermudez, 2005). In fact science may ratify these parents' approach: a positive association exists between parental monitoring and youth avoidance of risk-taking behavior in urban areas where such risks lead to well-known negative outcomes, especially among Black adolescents (Miller, McKay, & Baptiste, 2007). Clinicians without a strong cultural lens could inappropriately assess this style. Culture may also impact treatment participation. Studies of treatment engagement have noted that treatment dropouts are linked to lower parental education, the belief that mental health distress should be handled by children independently, and the belief that emotional and behavioral problems require increased discipline (McKay et al., 2004). When treatment professionals do not understand underlying cultural values, they cannot work effectively with families to engage them in treatment and build an effective treatment alliance.

Disproportionality, a primary consequence of stigma has been the focus of many state and federal efforts in recent years. Due to assessments based on racial prototypes by well-meaning clinicians, Black children are more readily placed in foster care than White children (Stehno, 1982; Whaley, 1998). According to research compiled by the Child Welfare League of America (CWLA), no significant or even marginal race differences exist in the incidence of maltreatment and yet, abuse or neglect substantiation rates among white children are half the rate nationally reported among African American/black and American Indian/Alaska Native children (CWLA, 2005).

From the research it is clear that youth of color are treated more harshly than White youth at every stage of the juvenile justice process, even when they present the same histories and are accused of the same crimes. Black adolescents are more often referred to secure correctional facilities, while White youth with the same violent behavior and psychopathology are more often referred to mental health services as outpatients (Stehno, 1982). Youth of color are markedly over represented in the juvenile justice system, as a result of racially disparate treatment at various stages of decision-making processes. Black youth are more likely than White youth—with the same offenses—to be referred to juvenile court, to be detained prior to trial in secure facilities, to be formally charged in juvenile court, to be waived for disposition in adult courts, and to be committed to a juvenile or adult correctional institution (National Council on Crime and Delinquency, 2007) While government data reveal that White youth use and sell more drugs than Black youth, Blacks are more likely to be charged with drug offenses than Whites—at each stage of criminal processing (Hill, 1999; Snyder, Sickmund, & Bilchik, 1999).

FAMILY AND YOUTH INVOLVEMENT

He was patient with me and didn't force me to go on medications, but he didn't let me rule them out either. After one more stupid mistake, it was obvious to me that I needed to be on medication. I feel like a partner in my treatment team. (Matarese et al., 2008, p. 293)

The gap between providers and consumers often creates a system in which consumers are planned *for* not planned *with*. Plans and treatment may not motivate or even have relevance for the family and are often static, created at the point of intake and then not routinely or truly reassessed again.

Working in partnership with youth and families may cause professionals to fear that they will lose power and control, have responsibility without authority, lose their personal and professional identity and value, or develop interventions that hurt the child (Adams, Biss, Muhammad, Myers, & Slayton, 1998). Yet families are a permanent part of a child's life, while providers may come and go. Families have a vested interest in their child's wellness that cannot be underestimated. It is increasingly understood that providers need to focus on strengths when addressing challenges and treat every family and youth with dignity and respect—allowing them to make their own decisions about medications, where to go for treatment, who to talk with, and how long treatment should last. To do otherwise may engender distrust and resistance. Families may feel pressured and resort to "false cooperation" - completing the specified treatment program without really making needed changes.

The President's New Freedom Commission on Mental Health (US HHS, 2003) called for "family and consumer driven care" (p. 35), which has been further defined by the Federation for Families for Children's Mental Health in partnership with SAMHSA. The Federation conducted a two-year development process, which led to the determination that families must have a primary decision-making role in the care of their children and in the policies and procedures governing the care for all children in the community. "Family driven" services are those in which families are "choosing supports and providers, setting goals, designing and implementing programs, monitoring outcomes, partnering in funding decisions, and determining effectiveness of program interventions." Definition developed at the 16th Annual Federation of Families for Children's Mental Health Conference, 2004.)

Children and youth have traditionally been left out of planning discussions, but their participation is now considered essential to effective service delivery, particularly in their Individualized Education Program (IEP), the educational program mandated in the United States by the Individuals with Disabilities Act (IDEA) for each child with a disability. As providers come to respect that families and youth are the experts on their lives, true needs and priorities can come to light for creative problem solving that is responsive and individualized.

The New Freedom Commission also prodded the system to offer a range of effective, community-based treatment options in order to ensure family choices and engage a comprehensive community response to children's and youth's needs. In addition to greatly improving the service system, expanding options to community-based alternatives to inpatient treatment improves engagement in community-based treatment and reduces unnecessary institutionalization. Without community-based support and treatment options, troubled children and youth are too often placed in out-of-state treatment facilities, hours away from their families and communities, which impedes their effective treatment.

DEVELOPMENTAL ISSUES

Our typically developing children usually have a voice; those with disabilities often do not. They often have services available to them; those with disabilities often do not. And our social workers know how to interact with typically developing children—but they often don't have a clue how to support children with disabilities. (Foster and adoptive parent National Council on Disability, 2008, p. 115)

While developmental disabilities are pervasive within most children's treatment settings, very often mental health and substance abuse treatment services are based on adult models and fail to accommodate even the standard developmental needs presented by children and youth. Children and youth require family involvement in all stages of treatment and family support to follow-through. In addition, the differences between young children, latency age children, preadolescents, and teens are vast. Interventions have to be gauged to the developmental strengths and needs appropriate to each age group.

Brain studies and social science research show conclusively that adolescents are less mature than adults. In addition, emotional maturation is often disrupted among youth with mental health and substance abuse disorders. Youth with Serious Emotional Disturbance frequently exhibit problems coping with frustration and retaining focus and persisting when gratification is delayed. They may experience complicated dependency and resentment, black and white thinking (in which things/people are all good or all bad), and may only live in the present, unable to plan ahead or avoid repeating mistakes. They may lie to avoid consequences, test limits well into adolescence, and be unable to effectively communicate feelings, which can lead to cutting behavior and suicidal gestures (Federation of Families for Children's Mental Health, 2001).

Youth with learning disabilities or an emotional disturbance are arrested at higher rates than their nondisabled peers (Chesapeake Institute, 1994; SRI International, 1997) and studies of incarcerated youth reveal that as many as 70% suffer from disabling conditions (Leone, Rutherford, & Nelson, 1995). The juvenile justice system is overflowing with youth whose behavior problems related to mental health and substance use disorders have led to incarceration. Nonetheless, an estimated 200,000 youthful offenders are tried in adult courts every year, many of whom are punished in adult prisons or probation/parole systems. Studies consistently find that young people prosecuted and punished in the adult justice system are more likely to reoffend than similar youth retained in the juvenile system. Some live in states that define the age of juvenile jurisdiction at 16 or 17, rather than 18, and many others are transferred to adult courts through ill-considered transfer and waiver laws passed in the 1990s.

FRAGMENTED SYSTEMS

We were told we'd have to enroll our son in one program, finish that, and then send him away to treatment. Our son was away for two years and he did not come home recovered from mental illness or substance abuse. He was a stranger to us. (Federation of Families for Children's Mental Health, 2001, p. 2)

Youth with co-occurring mental health and substance abuse disorders and their families seldom receive the help they need. Instead, they are served by an uncoordinated array of service systems, including schools, primary care doctors, mental health providers, child welfare programs, probation offices, detention centers, etc. The adults who fill hospital emergency rooms, homeless shelters, substance abuse treatment programs, psychiatric hospitals, and prisons today very bounced from one system to another as children. The 2002 President's New Freedom Commission *Interim Report* highlighted system fragmentation as a primary concern for human services delivery: "... the mental health delivery system is fragmented and in disarray ... lead[ing] to unnecessary and costly disability, homelessness, school failure and incarceration." (p. 1) The report asserted that more individuals, including children and youth, could recover from even the most serious mental illnesses if they had access in their communities to treatment and supports that are tailored to their needs. Increasingly, multiple programs with disparate objectives and requirements finance services and supports for those with mental illnesses, including state and local general fund appropriations, Medicare, Social Security (Social Security Income/Social Security and Disability Income payments), vocational rehabilitation, education, Temporary Assistance for Needy Families (TANF), juvenile justice and criminal justice, child welfare, and federal block grants. While each program provides essential assistance, together they create a financing approach that is complex, fragmented, and inconsistent in its coverage.

Integrated care is difficult to achieve in a service environment where some services are public while others are privately operated. Different layers of government pay for different services (e.g., child welfare and mental health are county functions but juvenile justice is a state function), and there is an array of decision makers setting priorities (courts, juvenile justice, schools). Different funders are tied to different problems and eligibility criteria differ across systems for families increasing the potential for contradictory case plans. There is limited infrastructure to navigate and integrate planning when family members and caregivers also have challenges, since adult and children's systems are separate and parallel.

CONVERGING NEEDS WITHIN THE JUVENILE JUSTICE AND CHILD WELFARE SYSTEMS

The Juvenile Justice Division of the CWLA has noted that people who were abused or neglected as children are 59% more likely to have been arrested as a juvenile (CWLA, 2002). Disability among the juvenile justice population is 3–5 times that of the general juvenile population: learning disabilities and emotional disturbance are prevalent (National Council on Disability, 2003). Despite services from two systems charged with their well-being, these young people are rarely appropriately served. For five years, The National Center on Addiction and Substance Abuse (CASA) at Columbia University analyzed the impact of substance abuse and the juvenile justice system on juvenile offenders. The resulting report, *Criminal Neglect: Substance Abuse, Juvenile Justice and the Children Left Behind* (CASA, 2004), is the most comprehensive study ever undertaken of substance abuse and the state juvenile justice systems. Created for juvenile offenders who are generally 10–17 years old, the juvenile justice system today is largely serving children aged 15 and younger (57.7%). This study, currently being updated, was based on 2000 data, the latest available in sufficient detail to permit such an in-depth analysis.

Among its key findings are the following:

▪ Four of every five children and teens (78.4%) in juvenile justice systems—1.9 of 2.4 million arrests of 10–17-year-olds—are under the influence of alcohol or drugs while committing their crime, test positive for drugs, are arrested for committing an alcohol or drug offense, admit having substance abuse and addiction problems, or share some combination of these characteristics.
▪ Of the 1.9 million arrests of juvenile offenders with substance abuse and addiction problems, only about 68,600 juveniles—3.6%—receive any form of substance abuse treatment.
▪ Mental health services are rare for incarcerated youth and most of the education programs offered to detained youth do not meet minimum state educational criteria.

The report describes the juvenile justice system as "colleges of criminality" rather than institutions for rehabilitation and notes that at least 30% of adults in prison for felony crimes were incarcerated as juveniles. This system failure compounds the impact of the first-order concern: juvenile courts and corrections systems have become a dumping ground for youth with mental health problems, abuse and neglect histories, and learning disabilities who should be served by public systems with specialized expertise. Many youth are detained or placed in the juvenile justice system for minor offenses and end up in the system simply because of a lack of community-based service options (Anglin & Knorth, 2004, p. 141; Child Welfare League of America, 2002; Mears, Yaffe, & Harris, 2009).

According to the New Freedom Report (2003), there are more than 106,000 teens in juvenile justice facilities. The Northwestern Juvenile Project (Teplin, Abram, McClelland, Dulcan, & Mericle, 2002), a large-scale, four-year study in Chicago, found that 66% of boys and nearly 57% of girls in juvenile detention have at least one psychiatric disorder. More than 40% were diagnosed with oppositional defiant or conduct disorders, and depression and dysthymia were diagnosed in 17% of boys and 26% of detained girls. Fifty percent of these youth have a history of child abuse addiction to drugs. Notably, 46% of youth on probation met criteria for a serious emotional disorder compared to 67% of youth in a correctional setting. In contrast, 20% of children in the general American population have a diagnosable psychiatric disorder (SAMHSA, 1999; U.S. Department of Health and Human Services, 1999).

As noted, childhood victimization is a risk factor for subsequent delinquency. Children who are abused and neglected are more likely to experience a range of mental health, substance abuse, occupational, and educational deficiencies during adolescence and adulthood and more likely than other children to commit delinquent acts as adolescents and crimes as adults (OJJDP, 2009).

A report on Child Maltreatment and Juvenile Delinquency from the The Child Welfare League of America compiled the following statistics:

1. Child abuse and neglect increase the likelihood of children's future delinquency and criminality, including a 59% higher chance of juvenile arrest.
2. Children who have been maltreated have been shown to be younger at their time of arrest and arrested more frequently than children who were not maltreated.
3. Over 50% of youth offenders have been abused or neglected.
4. Maltreatment results in a high risk of a variety of negative outcomes for children.

These outcomes include a predisposition to later delinquency, serious and violent offending, placement in out-of-home residential facilities, the victimization of community members, and high rates of recidivism, school dropouts, teen pregnancy, and gang involvement (Tuell, 2002).

Too often, when a child or adolescent becomes involved with the juvenile justice system, other child-serving systems withdraw until the justice involvement ends. Outcome data on youth in the justice system indicate that youth with serious emotional disorders have the highest recidivism rates compared to other youth in the justice system and are often placed in residential settings designed to handle only one of their multiple issues or problems (Jones & Harris, 2000). In fact, the recidivism rates for juveniles receiving in-home and community-based interventions are equivalent if not better than those for high-risk juveniles placed in very expensive, restrictive residential programs (Jones, Harris, Fader, Burrell, & Fadeyi, 1999).

CONCLUSION

Fortunately, major foundations (e.g., Robert Wood Johnson, Annie E. Casey) and federal funders (e.g., Substance Abuse and Mental Health Services Administration, Administration for Children and Families) as well as many state and local jurisdictions are beginning to address these needs. Public education and community service delivery increasingly acknowledges and addresses stigma, and service mandates have evolved to require cross-system collaboration, community partnerships, and youth and family participation in program development, implementation, and evaluation. Models for comprehensive system change and for more targeted and population-specific interventions are being evaluated, refined, and disseminated. Within any program, addressing these issues in part or in whole can offer a valuable foundation for further enhancement and funding support. See the corresponding chapter, *Approaches to Child and Youth Mental Health Needs*, for a detailed description of the Systems of Care model and the Wraparound approach to service delivery, which exemplifies a comprehensive response to the needs described in this chapter.

REFERENCES

Adams, J., Biss, C., Muhammad, V. B., Meyers, J., & Slaton, E. (1998). *Learning from colleagues: Family/Professional partnerships moving forward together.* Alexandria, VA: National Peer Technical Assistance Network's Partnership for Children's Mental Health.

Anglin, J. P., & Knorth, E. J. (2004). Competing declarations on residential care for children and youth—Stockholm versus Malmö. *Child & Youth Care Forum, 33*(3), 141–149.

Chesapeake Institute. (1994). *National agenda for achieving better results for children and youth with serious emotional disturbance.* Washington, DC: Author.

Child Welfare League of America. (2003). *CWLA Statement: Children of Color in the Child Welfare System: Overview, vision, and proposed action steps.* Washington, DC: Author.

Corrigan, P. W., & Penn, D. L. (1999). Lessons from social psychology on discrediting psychiatric stigma. *American Psychologist, 54,* 765–776.

Federation of Families for Children's Mental Health. (2001). *Blamed and ashamed.* Alexandria, VA: Author.

Hill, B. (1999). *Institutional racism in child welfare. Race and society.* Rockville, MD: Elsevier.

Hopkins, S., Huici, V., & Bermudez, D. (2005). Therapeutic play with Hispanic clients. In E. Gil & A. A. Drewes (Eds.), *Cultural issues in play therapy* (pp. 148–167). New York, NY: The Guilford Press.

Jones, L. (2005). Another parent's perspective: Living with a child with Serious Emotional Disturbance. In M. Arbuckle & C. Herrick (Eds), *Child and adolescent mental health: Interdisciplinary systems of care* (p. 98). Sudbery, MA: Jones and Bartlett Publishers.

Jones, P. R., & Harris, P. W. (2000). *ProDes: System Trends 1999–2000*. Philadelphia, PA: Crime and Justice Research Institute.

Jones, P. R., Harris, P. W., Fader, J., Burrell, J. L., & Fadeyi, A. (1999). Identifying chronic juvenile offenders. *Corrections Compendium, 24*(8), 1–23.

Kessler, R. C. (1994). The National Comorbidity Survey: Preliminary results and future directions. *International Journal of Methods in Psychiatric Research, 4,* p114.1–114.13.

King, R. D., Gaines, L. S., Lambert, E. W., Summerfelt, W. T., & Bickman, L. (2000). The co-occurrence of psychiatric and substance abuse diagnoses in adolescents in different service systems: Frequency, recognition, cost, and outcomes. *The Journal of Behavioral Health Services & Research, 27,* 428.

Leone, P. E., Rutherford, R. B., Jr., & Nelson, C. M. (1995). *Special education in juvenile corrections*. Reston, VA: Council for Exceptional Children.

Matarese, M., Carpenter, M., Huffine, C., Lane, S., & Paulson, K. (2008). Partnerships with youth for youth-guided systems of care. In B. A. Stroul & G. M. Blau (Eds.), *The system of care handbook: Transforming mental health services for children, youth, and families* (pp. 275–300). Baltimore, MA: Brookes Publishing.

McKay, M. M., Hibbert, R., Hoagwood, K., Rodriguez, J., Murray, L., Legerski, J., et al. (2004). Integrating evidence-based engagement interventions into 'real world' child mental health settings. *Brief Treatment and Crisis Intervention, 4*(2), 177–186.

Mears, S. L., Yaffe, J., & Harris, N. J. (2009). Evaluation of Wraparound services for severely emotionally disturbed youths. *Research on Social Work Practice, 19,* 678–685.

Miller, S., McKay, M., & Baptiste, D. (2007). Social support for African American low-income parents: The influence of preadolescents' risk behavior and support role on parental monitoring and child outcomes. *Social Work in Mental Health, 5*(1&2), 121–145.

Morley, E., Rossman, S. B., Kopczynski, M., Buck, J., & Gouvis, C. (2000). Comprehensive responses to youth at risk: Interim findings from the safe-futures initiative. summary. Washington, DC: U.S. Department of Justice, Office of Justice Programs, Office of Juvenile Justice and Delinquency Prevention. NCJ 183841.

National Council on Crime and Delinquency. (2007). *And justice for some: Differential treatment of minority youth in the justice system*. Oakland, CA: Author.

National Council on Disability. (2003). *Addressing the needs of youth with disabilities in the Juvenile Justice System: The current state of evidence-based research*. Washington, DC: National Council on Disability.

National Council on Disability. (2008). Youth with disabilities in the foster care system: Barriers to success and proposed policy solutions, Washington, DC: Author. Retrieved 10/12/10 from: http://www.ncd.gov/newsroom/publications/2008/FosterCareSystem_Report.html.

National Federation of Families for Children's Mental Health. (2010). Citing Website. Retrieved 10/12/10 from: http://www.ffcmh.org/r2/publications2/family-driven-defined/.

National Center on Addiction and Substance Abuse (CASA). (2004). *Criminal neglect: Substance abuse, juvenile justice and the children left behind.* New York.

Office of Juvenile Justice Delinquency and Prevention. (2009). Juvenile Arrests 2008 Top Bulletin, December 2009. Summarizes 2008 juvenile crime and arrest data reported by local law enforcement agencies across the country and cited in the FBI report Crime in the United States 2008. 12 pages. NCJ 228479.

Ostman, M., & Kjellin, L. (2002). Stigma by association: Psychological factors in relatives of people with mental illness. *British Journal of Psychiatry, 181,* 494–498.

Penn, D. L., & Martin, J. (1998). The stigma of severe mental illness: Some potential solutions for a recalcitrant problem. *Psychiatric Quarterly, 69,* 235–247.

Perlick, D. A., Rosenheck, R. A., Clarkin, J. F., Sirey, J. A., Salahi, J., Struening, E. L., et al. (2001). Stigma as a barrier to recovery: Adverse effects of perceived stigma on social adaptation of persons diagnosed with bipolar affective disorder. *Psychiatric Services, 52*(12), 1627–1632.

Prince, P. N., & Prince, C. R. (2002). Perceived stigma and community integration among clients of assertive community treatment. *Psychiatric Rehabilitation Journal, 25*(4), 323–331.

SRI International, Center for Education and Human Services. (1997). *The National Longitudinal Transition Study: A summary of findings.* Washington, DC: U.S. Department of Education, Office of Special Education Programs.

Stehno, S. (1982). Differential treatment of minority children. *Social Work, 27*(1), 39–45.

Substance Abuse and Mental Health Services Administration. (2009). *Results from the 2008 National Survey on Drug Use and Health: National Findings.* Rockville, MD: (Office of Applied Studies, NSDUH Series H-36, HHS Publication No. SMA 09-4434.

Substance Abuse and Mental Health Services Administration. (1999). *The Relationship Between Mental Health and Substance Abuse Among Adolescents.* Rockville, MD: Office of Applied Studies, OAS Analytic Series #9, DHHS Publication No. (SMA) 99-3286.

Snyder, H. N., Sickmund, M., & Bilchik, S. (1999). National Center for Juvenile Justice Office of Juvenile Justice and Delinquency Prevention. Washington, DC.

Teplin, L., Abram, K., McClelland, G., Dulcan, M., & Mericle, A. (2002). Psychiatric disorders in youth in juvenile detention. *Archives of General Psychiatry, 59,* 1133–1143.

Tuell, J. A. (2002). *Child maltreatment and juvenile delinquency: Raising the level of awareness.* Department of Education, Office of Special Education and Rehabilitative Services, Office of Special Education Programs. Washington, DC: Child Welfare League of America.

U.S. Department of Health and Human Services. (1999). Mental Health: A Report of the Surgeon General. Rockville, MD: U.S. Department of Health and Human

Services, Substance Abuse and Mental Health Services Administration, Center for Mental Health Services, National Institutes of Health, National Institute of Mental Health, 1999, Chapter 2, 32–104.

U.S. Department of Health and Human Services. (2000, May). *Draft 3: Prevention of co-morbidity in children and adolescents: The nexus of mental health and substance abuse.* Washington, DC: U.S. Department of Health and Human Services, Substance Abuse and Mental Health Services Administration.

U.S. Department of Health and Human Services. (2002, November). *Report to Congress on the prevention and treatment of co-occurring substance abuse disorders and mental disorders.* Washington, DC: U.S. Department of Health and Human Services, Substance Abuse and Mental Health Services Administration.

U.S. Department of Health and Human Services. (2003). The President's New Freedom Commission on Mental Health. *Achieving the promise: Transforming mental health care in America.* Final Report (DHHS Publication No. SMA 03-3832). Washington, DC: U.S. Government Printing Office.

Whaley, A. L. (1998). Racism in the provision of mental health services. *American Journal of Orthopsychiatry, 68*(1), 47–57.

FURTHER READING

U.S. Department of Health and Human Services. (1999, April). *The relationship between mental health and substance abuse among adolescents.* Washington, DC: Department of Health and Human Services, Substance Abuse and Mental Health Services Administration.

U.S. Public Health Service. (2000). Report of the Surgeon General's Conference on Children's Mental Health: A National Action Agenda. Washington, DC: Department of Health and Human Services.

CHAPTER FOUR

Model Approaches for Children and Youth with Serious Emotional Disturbance

Systems of Care and Wraparound

Nina Rose Fischer

INTRODUCTION

The Systems of Care approach to service delivery has evolved over the past 20 years in response to children and families with multiple needs who face multiple systemic barriers to care. Every federal funding agency serving children and adolescents are funding Systems of Care programs, and most states and local jurisdictions are aligning their programming expectations to dovetail with this model of care. This chapter refers to approaches to youth with complex needs, as well as to overarching system reform that transforms service delivery to youth and families across systems. Wraparound is a service delivery system that supports a seamless System of Care.

HISTORY OF SYSTEMS OF CARE

Since the 1975 passage of the Individuals with Disabilities Education Act (Public Law (PL) 94-142), which ensures that all children with disabilities have access to a free and appropriate education in the least restrictive environment, there has been a growing movement to deliver services to children within their homes, schools, and communities. It has also become clear that no single child-serving agency, because of policy, programmatic, or financial limitations, has the ability to provide all the services and supports needed by families with children who have disabilities and/or are vulnerable to abuse and neglect. During the early 1980s, local educational authorities joined child welfare in supporting children with various disabilities, yet children with serious emotional disturbances often remained without service, underserved, or inappropriately served. In 1984, the National Institute of Mental Health, U.S. Department of Health and Human Services, initiated the Child and Adolescent Service System Program (CASSP) to help States plan for and design systems of care to address the mental health needs of children who were experiencing a serious emotional disturbance (Child Welfare Information Gateway, 2010).

The systems of care approach was originally created in response to concerns that:

▤   Children in need of mental health treatment were not getting the services they needed.
▤   Services were often provided in restrictive out-of-home settings.
▤   Few community-based services were available.
▤   Service providers did not work together.
▤   Families were not adequately involved in their child's care.
▤   Cultural differences were rarely taken into account (Stroul, 1996).

Adaptations of the systems of care approach are now being applied to other target populations who depend on public systems for services, including adults with substance use disorders (the SAMHSA Recovery Oriented System of Care program), the developmentally disabled, those with chronic health conditions, and individuals needing an array of social supports due to mental illness.

Historically, systems of care have focused on improving access to and availability of services, and on reducing service and funding fragmentation. In addition, systems of care aim to improve the skills, knowledge, and attitudes of frontline service providers. Increasingly, systems of care are concerned about "treatment efficacy," ensuring effective therapeutic interactions between practitioners and children in care and their families (Pires, 2002) and system reform.

A system of care offers a community partnership among families, youth, schools, and public and private organizations to provide coordinated mental health services and access to effective approaches to care. Partners include families, child welfare, education, mental health and substance abuse professionals, juvenile justice, primary health care, and other community organizations. The approach is fundamentally family driven and youth guided, culturally and linguistically competent, and community based (SAMSHA, 2010).

WRAPAROUND SERVICE

Wraparound service is an innovation that reflects the core principles of systems of care.

Wraparound's framework is highly individualized and allows for any service and intervention necessary to support a youth and family's stability and success. The Wraparound approach does not look at a family and force them to fit into systems. Wraparound demands that systems fit the needs of families. Thus, whatever is needed to support the stability of a youth and family in any system (child welfare, juvenile justice, substance use, mental health and mental retardation/developmental delays) can be implemented: therapy to address sexually aggressive behaviors, art therapy, a recreational program like martial arts, a special education school, or Aggression Replacement Therapy (OJJDP, 2009), one of the many Cognitive Behavioral therapies that are currently viewed as best practices.

Wraparound, also known by various terms, such as an individualized service planning, has become recognized as one of the most effective approaches to providing community-based comprehensive services to youth whose needs fall outside the boundaries of traditional mental health, child welfare, and juvenile probation services and span a variety of child-serving agencies (Blueprints, 2009; Potter & Mulkern, 2005; VanDenBerg, 2006). Wraparound has been described as a process, not a program, which maximizes the use of informal supports to create a comprehensive, integrated, and individualized treatment approach for youth, especially those who are transitioning home from residential care, juvenile detention, or foster care. The goals of Wraparound are parallel to systems of care as this process seeks to reduce the use of institutional care and replace fragmented approaches to youth with complex needs with more comprehensive service provision.

History of Wraparound

The Wraparound approach became more broadly known and adopted throughout the United States during the 1980s. In 1984, the Wraparound process became a cornerstone of the largest federal conceptualization of children's mental health care through its CASSP, which was designed to establish multilevel community-based systems to serve children with emotional, behavioral, and mental health needs. Both CASSP with Wraparound sought to address existing deficiencies in the mental health system including its fragmentation, overly professionalized service delivery, and use of restrictive out-of-home treatments (Potter & Mulkern, 2005).

One of the first of these CASSP programs, The Alaska Youth Initiative (AYI), is often cited as an example of Wraparound. The success of AYI led to many other community-based Wraparound initiatives, such as Milwaukee Wraparound and the North American Family Institute's Project Wraparound in Vermont (Netzel, 2004; Potter & Mulkern, 2005; VanDenBerg, 2006). In 1995, many of the 31 sites funded as demonstration grants by Children's Mental Health Services incorporated Wraparound as a foundation for their programs (Potter & Mulkern, 2005).

The effectiveness of the approach is well documented. The Milwaukee Wisconsin Child Welfare system established the Milwaukee Wraparound system in 1994 reducing the number of youth in Residential Treatment Centers by 90% (Cohen & Rae, 2002; Potter & Mulkern, 2005; VanDenBerg, 2006). Wraparound service provision significantly shortened their stays, reunited families, reduced the incidence of youth crime, and saved millions of dollars in treatment costs (Cohen & Rae, 2002). By reducing the number of children in Milwaukee institutions from 385 to 40 children, the program brought significant savings—a youth's average monthly expense in Wraparound was $3479 versus $7200 for institutional care. Institutional placements were reduced to an average of 3 months, down from 16 months. By 2002, Milwaukee Wraparound had served more than 800 children and their families, each an average of 16 months, with a $29 million annual budget—about the same that was being spent for the 385 children in institutions (Cohen & Rae, 2002).

Evaluation of Wraparound

The Wraparound Fidelity Index (WFI) was developed and peer reviewed by researchers from the University of Vermont and the University of Washington, and has been field tested with over 700 hundred families (Suter et al., 2005) proving the approach to be a recognized Best Practice (Blueprints, 2009; OJJDP, 2009). Comparative research studies of Wraparound and more traditional models of mental health service delivery to children and families showed significantly fewer placement changes for youths in the Wraparound program, fewer days on runaway, fewer days incarcerated, and older youth were significantly more likely to be in a permanency plan at follow-up (Clark et al., 1998; Pullman et al., 2006). Youths in the comparison group were three times more likely to commit a felony offense than youths in the Wraparound group. Of youth in Wraparound detained in juvenile facilities, their stays were less frequent than their peers. Wraparound youth showed significant improvement on standardized measures of behavioral and emotional problems, including increased behavioral and emotional strength and improved functioning at home at school, and in the community (Pullman et al., 2006).

Wraparound approaches differ widely in their implementation, process, structure, and underlying theories (Clark et al. 1998), but common in the various approaches is the push for less restrictive, more integrated, community-based, and coordinated services. Wraparound has produced positive outcomes for children who are experiencing multiple and complex challenges and for their families. Wraparound evaluation studies have used various research methods ranging from in-depth, qualitative interviews to quantitative designs with randomized subject selection and control groups. The strongest evidence for the effectiveness of the Wraparound approach has been produced by randomized controlled studies (Mears, Yaffe, & Harris, 2009).

Wraparound Principles

Programs that tout "Wraparound services" are becoming increasingly common though "high fidelity Wraparound services" must reflect the 11 core elements of Wraparound (Bruns et al. 2004; Suter et al., 2005). Each element is integral to successful Wraparound services. Case examples from two Wraparound programs in New York that serve youth with complex needs (histories of sexual aggression, developmental delays, severe emotional disturbance) through foster care to keep youth out of residential placement, and a preventive service program for relative caregivers, to keep youth out of foster care are used to exemplify the *11 core elements of Wraparound*:

1. *Family voice and choice:* family and youth/child perspectives are central during all phases of the Wraparound process. Planning is grounded in family members' perspectives, and the team provides options and choices that reflect the youth's and family's values and preferences.

Case Example

In the New York Wraparound program for foster children with complex developmental and emotional needs, the matching process between the foster parent, the child, and the birth family is based on giving the family and the youth voice and choice. Not only does the foster family receive access to all written documentation about the child, as well as meetings with the formal supports in the child's life (therapists, psychiatrists, doctors), the prospective foster parent meets with the natural support systems (birth family, neighbors, friends). The foster parent is required to decide after reading the written materials that they want to be a match. This prevents a feeling of abandonment when the foster parent actually meets the child. When the child and the foster parent meet, the child gets to decide if they are a match. The birth family specifically meets the foster parent to also have a voice in expressing to the foster parent about their child's likes, dislikes, and how they will all work together to provide necessary supports for the child.

2. *Team based:* the Wraparound team consists of individuals confirmed by the youth and family and committed to them through informal (extended family, neighbors, family friends, religious institution, and civic group members), formal (school, mental health, medical, and other professionals), and community support services (mentors, boys, and girls clubs, YMCA's, parks and recreation, youth vocational training programs, art's programs, etc.).

Case Example

In a New York Wraparound program for relative caregivers to prevent children from going into foster care, the Wraparound team is critical to the service delivery. When the referral is received from the Department of Social Services (DSS) all of the parties meet: the relative caregiver, birth family, DSS worker, program staff, and any other natural or formal supports that will be part of the plan. The team works together to develop a plan that will fit the individual needs of the children, relative caregivers, and birth families and to establish protocols for communication.

3. *Natural supports:* the team encourages full participation of members drawn from family members' networks of interpersonal and community relationships. The Wraparound plan reflects activities and interventions that draw on sources of natural support.

   The New York foster care Wraparound identifies all possible natural support systems in the foster family's community as well as the birth family's community to provide respite, recreational and educational supports, transportation, crisis counseling, and mentorship, to develop and support a tight network of support when the youth is out of the system. If there is a dearth of natural supports, the Wraparound team works diligently to cultivate relationships for the youth and families in the community that will support goal achievement. With the foster care program, a foster family used the Foster Mother's sister as respite in order to support a kinship support system.

4. *Collaboration:* team members work cooperatively and share responsibility for developing, implementing, monitoring, and evaluating a single Wraparound plan.

   In the Wraparound prevention program, the initial team that is identified continues to collaborate with formal and natural supports to enhance and expand the support network. Wraparound team meetings are planned on a monthly basis to ensure that collaboration is working effectively toward shared goals.

5. *Community based:* the team implements service and support strategies that take place in the most inclusive, most responsive, most accessible, and least restrictive settings possible; and that safely promote child and family integration into home and community life.

   In the foster care program, community services are identified during the matching process to ensure a network of support for the youth and families. The mainstream public schools are especially resistant to having youth with complex needs enrolled; thus, during the matching process, the Wraparound team works diligently to persuade the most appropriate community school setting that the team can provide the intensive daily supports to keep the child and community safe. The team was able to create a safety plan in a mainstream school setting for a young man with a history of sexual aggression, by working with the school community, the Principal, Guidance Counselor, and Security Guards, to establish everyone's role in the plan. Regular meetings were set up to evaluate the plan.

6. *Culturally competent:* the Wraparound process demonstrates respect for and builds on the values, preferences, beliefs, culture, and identity of the child/youth and family, and their community.

   An important example of cultural competence comes from the Wraparound foster care program. The Wraparound team identifies Lesbian/Gay/Bisexual/Trans families to be part of the foster parent pool. A young gay/trans man referred to the program requested that he wanted a Gay family in order to feel safe about his identity. His identity was a reason that he was not able to stay with his birth family. His ability to feel safe being his true self in his family was integral to his ability to believe he could achieve his goals.

7. *Individualized:* to achieve the goals laid out in the Wraparound plan, the team develops and implements a customized set of strategies, supports, and services.

    A young man in the foster care program with a history of sexual aggression was passionate about sound engineering. The program found him a mentor who worked in a recording studio. The young man was able to apprentice under the Sound Engineer, and then work at the studio. A young woman with severe psychiatric issues and a history of multiple hospitalizations from suicide attempts had a low tolerance for the intimacy of a family. Her behavior would start positive, and then she would become scared of rejection and sabotage the placement with aggressive behaviors. The Team was able to use two foster families to share time with her throughout the week, so that when her harmful behaviors began, she could start over with the other family to prevent further hospitalization.

8. *Strengths based:* the Wraparound process and the Wraparound plan identify, build on, and enhance the capabilities, knowledge, skills, and assets of the child and family, their community, and other team members. Being strengths based reduces the stigma that keeps youth stuck in negative self-perception.

    The foster care Wraparound team uses a youth's strengths to guide all aspects of service provision. When the foster care program meets with the youth, after reading all of the negative documentation that often precedes a youth in foster care, the team conducts an extensive strengths assessment to share with the foster parent: including likes, talents, positive characteristics, and how the youth likes to be helpful. A young woman with severe emotional disturbance was an amazing cook. She shared this with the team in the assessment. The team found a foster parent who also loved to cook. This shared love supported and enhanced their bond.

9. *Continuation of care:* services and supports must be provided unconditionally. In a crisis, services and supports should be added rather than placing the youth with a new provider.

    Both Wraparound programs have a no-reject policy. One of the youths in the foster care program was demonstrating compulsive aggressive behaviors and was not able to be kept safe in the community.

When he entered the hospital, the Wraparound team, the foster parent, and the birth family visited him weekly and were planning with the hospital how he would be transitioned back into the community.

10. *Flexible funding: Flexible funding and resources:* successful Wraparound teams are creative in their approach to service delivery and have access to flexible funds and resources to implement their ideas.

    Flexible funding is now available in New York through Bridges to Health that caps funding for foster children at $50,000/year to provide any service needed to support stability in the community and prevent residential care.

11. *Outcome based:* the team ties the goals and strategies of the Wraparound plan to observable or measurable indicators of success (Suter et al., 2005)

    The preventive service program conducts satisfaction surveys with children, families, and DSS workers to assess the success of the program. The Team meets monthly to discuss the feedback from the surveys and incorporates the improvements. The WFI is employed to measure the Team's fidelity to the Wraparound principles.

    Fidelity to the core principles is measured through the WFI, creating a solid foundation for policy makers and service providers to make positive changes in collaboration with youth and families. The challenges that tend to emerge from Wraparound include fidelity to four of the core elements: flexible funding and resources are hard to secure due to governmental funding restraints; cultural competency is difficult to ensure due to the complex issues in serving youth from diverse backgrounds; collaboration can be a challenge due to the obstacles faced in finding common ground among the youth, family, and natural and formal support members; and continuation of care can be hard to establish due to the difficulty in providing follow-up after discharge.

Wraparound Case Study

The following case study is taken from the New York Wraparound program for youth in foster care who have complex needs (2008). Tony was placed in a sex offender treatment facility when he was 11, completed the program when he was 14, and remained there until he was 16 because no other placements would take him, and he was not allowed to go home where he had molested his brothers. Having been in residential facility for five years, his understanding of how to socialize "normally" with his age group was negatively affected by his restrictive setting:

Tony, age 16

PHASE 1: Referral

Tony is a 16-year-old male who came to a New York Wraparound program from a secure sex offender treatment facility in out of state. He was placed there for sexually abusing his younger siblings, and had been there since he was 11 years old. Due to the geographic distance of his birth family from his out-of-state placement, he had rarely had visits and no family therapy or reunification attempts with his siblings had been made. Despite 5 years of treatment at the sex offender facility, he continued to have issues with sexual boundaries.

As a young child, Tony had taken the role of the "father" when his father had left the home, helping his mother take care of his siblings. Though only 11 years old when he was adjudicated, he had virtually all the freedom an adult would have, as his mother allowed him to come and go from home as he pleased and did not make sure whether he went to school. Upon Tony's entrance to the Wraparound program, Tony's early history was vague, though his mother reported that his father abused him for several years as a very young boy. She also reported having put him in a scalding hot tub to punish him when he was discovered abusing his siblings. In his initial interview, Tony was quiet though insightful and expressed understanding of his issues with sexual aggression. He indicated that he wanted to continue to do well and change his behavior. He was agreeable to Wraparound and requested a community-based foster home close to his family so that he could see his mother often and hopefully be reunified with his brothers shortly after his discharge. He expressed that he felt that the residential facility was suffocating him and said he needs to be allowed to go out when he is discharged to a foster home. Tony also hoped to be able to see his stepfather and get to know him, since his mother had remarried after Tony entered the facility. Tony had only met his stepfather twice. In addition to a Conduct Disorder diagnosis (due to his abuse of his siblings) Tony came to Wraparound with a diagnosis of Post Traumatic Stress Disorder (PTSD) (due to abuse he suffered as a child by his father (sexual) and mother (physical)), plus Mild Mental Retardation (IQ 65). He was prescribed psychotropic medications to treat the symptoms of these conditions.

Wraparound Team Meeting: February 1

When Tony came to the Wraparound program, the team met to discuss which clinical team (Social Worker and Case Manager) would work best with him and his family. A team was assigned based on case configuration, Tony and his family's needs, their proximity to the program, and foster home availability. Tony completed the five-child caseload for the assigned team, which also cared for two other boys from the same sex offender treatment facility. The Foster Parent Recruiter suggested a foster home that was proximal to the birth family, headed by a warm and affectionate single woman who works in the social service field and has strong boundaries, no other children in her home, and a willingness to work closely with Tony's mother and step father to facilitate reunification.

The Wraparound team discussed the services they thought Tony would need: a therapeutic school environment (within a regular high-school setting or in a specialized school); specialized therapy for sexually aggressive youth; after-school programming; summer camp; basketball program (basketball is a passion that Tony had shared he would play 24/7 if allowed); and art therapy, as that intervention seemed most effective during his residential care. The Team determined that he would benefit from services, and the Program Director called the Foster Parent to arrange for her to come in two days later to review Tony's chart.

PHASE 2: Transition Services Begin: February 2–February 22

After the Wraparound team met with the Medical Director to get his input on the plan, the Program Director introduced the Foster Mother to Tony via his chart and history and she agreed to take on his care. The Case Manager began contacting the school district and made plans for his admission to the local school District. A transitional school program was identified and assessed for Tony and the school gave a verbal consent for admission, telling the Team to follow-up when he is officially discharged from the facility.

PREPLACEMENT BEGINS: FEBRUARY 22–JUNE 1. The Program Director took the Foster Mother to meet Tony at the facility and learned that, due to Tony's defiant behavior (being disrespectful to staff, not following rules, and "throwing in their face" that he is leaving soon), Tony was not going to be discharged after all. The Wraparound team coordinated with the DSS to encourage the facility to reconsider and approve preplacement weekend visits. The Foster Mother visited Tony twice at the facility while awaiting approval for weekend visits, and Tony's Judge then ordered preplacement visits to occur. The Wraparound Case Manager began working on establishing community resources with the Foster Mother, including signing him up for camp and a basketball program that started at the end of August, as well as getting all needed approvals from the DSS. Case Manager visited the camp, speaking in person to the director to find out the level of supervision and confirm that no children under the age of 13 will be in the camp. The Social Worker coordinated with the community mental health clinic and arranged for his treatment to begin there upon discharge from the facility's care, including providing services to Tony's family. The Clinic agreed to provide sex offender-specific treatment while Wraparound provided family therapy. The Social Worker and the Case Manager met with the Foster Mother to go over upcoming appointments, and to arrange transportation to and from the camp and all his appointments, especially his therapy. Wraparound arranged for on-call coverage during each of Tony's preplacement visits.

The Social Worker, the Case Manager, and the Foster Parent worked out a supervision plan for Tony's first two weeks at home, during the times he would have been in school and a safety contract for his first 30 days. The Foster Mother identified a respite arrangement for him for during the day while she works and Tony is introduced to the summer camp he will be attending. Prior to his official Wraparound admission date, another team meeting was held to confirm that comprehensive plans were made in anticipation of his individualized needs. The Foster Mother began attending the biweekly Foster Parent support group and training meetings held at the Wraparound agency. The Wraparound Operations Manager made all appointments for Tony's initial psychiatric, physical and dental care.

PHASE 3: *Foster Home Admission to the Program: June 1 and forward*

Tony began home tutoring and summer camp. The Foster Mother contacted either the Social Worker or the Case Manager at least twice per week to keep the team informed and the Social Worker facilitate Service Plan Review meetings every 6 months. The Social Worker, the Case Manager, the Program Director, the Foster Parent, the Birth Mother, the Stepfather, and Tony discussed his 30-day Individual Service Plan, and completed an Individual Service Plan every 3 months thereafter. The Social Worker began individual sessions with Tony and with his parents, and family sessions were held together for at least 1 hour each per week (1 hour with Tony, 1 hour with his parents, and 1 hour for family sessions). The Case Manager met with Tony at least once per week, not including visiting and/or contacting his camp/school once per week. The Case Manager also visited the basketball program coach at least twice per month. The Foster Mother took Tony to all of his initial appointments and his ongoing mental health appointments ($\frac{1}{2}$ hour individual and 1 hour group per week, on different days). The Foster Mother also transported Tony for visits, once per weekend, with his mother who lived in another town. These visits occurred in a public location, as Tony was not yet allowed in the home due to his brothers being there. The Social Worker met monthly with the community mental health provider and talked to her weekly by phone to share information about Tony's progress. The Social Worker rented an office space in Tony's family's town for two weekly sessions—once with his parents individually and once for family therapy. Tony's Safety Contract was updated after 30 days.

Tony began exhibiting challenging behaviors after 1–2 months at home; so a new safety contract was put in place. He began leaving without permission to play basketball in the afternoons with his new friends from school; so the Foster Mother bought a basketball hoop for her backyard and allowed his friends to hang out at her house every afternoon.

Four Months After Admission

When Tony's behavior improved, his Foster Mother bought him a cell phone so that he could have some unsupervised time out and still be able to be in touch. A safety plan specific to the cell phone was developed with the team, Tony's sex offender therapist, his parents, and his school. A payment plan was arranged with Tony after he ran up a $400 phone bill the third month and he is placed on a prepaid cell plan. The cell phone worked for him: he called his Case Manager and/or Social Worker almost daily and his Foster Mother several times per day. He also began calling his Mother more often. Tony progressed in family, individual, and his sex offender work.

Six Months After Admission

Tony's parents had issues with their younger sons sexually acting out with one another and their visits and attendance at therapy was reduced severely. They saw Tony only about once per month. Tony began acting out again, leaving without permission almost daily for several hours, leading to several missing persons reports. Tony also took his Foster Mother's car one afternoon without permission and without a license. His Foster Mother called him when she realized the car was gone and told him to return it. The Social Worker and the Case Manager responded to the Foster Mother's call that day and held a meeting with her and Tony to discuss this behavior and consequences.

The Case Manager contacted the local police and got in touch with the youth officer who began meeting with Tony about his behavior and about possible criminal consequence after Tony admitted to hanging out with gang members. He denied being a part of a gang. A new safety contract was put in place, plus a behavior plan regarding his Absence Without Leave (AWOL) behavior. A mentor from the community was identified, a man who knew Tony's Foster Mother, and he began spending time with Tony each week. Tony resumed his progress in therapy.

Tony had a run in with a few guys at school after flirting with another boy's girlfriend. He was cornered in the bathroom and beaten up. The Social Worker, the Case Manager, and the Foster Mother responded to the school and the Foster Mother took Tony to meet up with his Mother before going to the hospital.

The Social Worker, the Case Manager, and the Foster Parent had a meeting at the school to discuss the incident, and planned for his future safety in school. Tony's Mother pressed charges against the boys. A team meeting was held to discuss more structure for Tony, including the possibility of a direct care person to shadow him during and after school to help with these behaviors, and the Social Worker began speaking to the DSS to negotiate this.

Four Years Later

Tony continues to live in a stable home, attends school regularly, plays on the baseball team, and now has regular visits with his entire birth family.

The above Case Study is an example of a youth that because of the stigma attached to his behaviors, many professionals believed he would be slotted for a residential placement until the age of 18. Wraparound was successfully able to stabilize Tony in the community using formal and natural supports with the consistent and creative intervention of a Wraparound team. Tony demonstrated warning signs of harmful behaviors during his adjustment, but the Wraparound team worked so closely with all parties involved in Tony's life. Safety plans were implemented to prevent escalation of harm and to maintain stability. This is a young man who was stigmatized by the label "sex offender" from 11 years old. The stigma would have haunted him throughout his adolescence, and research shows would have potentially intensified his harmful behaviors upon release at 18 because of his lack of socialization and alienation from his home and community. Fortunately he had the opportunity to function in the community with Wraparound services.

Wraparound and Evidence-Based Programs

Wraparound's motto is "whatever works"—individualizing services for youth and families and providing services across systems and departments. Wraparound is an overarching process that engages all involved people, including the child and their family, in identifying needs, problem solving to overcome obstacles and build on strengths, and improving service delivery by coordinating the appropriate services and programs for high needs youth and families (Clark et al., 1998; Pullman et al., 2006).

More and more "blueprint" evidence-based programs (EBPs) are funded by States to serve youth diagnosed with moderate to mild emotional disturbance and substance use within the juvenile justice and child welfare systems. Multisystemic therapy (MST), family functional therapy, and multidimensional treatment foster care (MTFC) are classified as EBPs based on randomized controlled studies that support their efficacy at providing diversion or aftercare from residential placement (Asscher et al., 2007; Breuck et al., 2006; Dembo, 2005).

MST is a home- and community-based intervention developed for adolescents that addresses conduct-related mental health needs by intervening in all the systems, institutions, and groups that affect the youth. These may include family, school, after-school programs, church, peer group, and community. MST often includes family therapy, structured family therapy, behavioral parent training, and other cognitive behavioral interventions. MST usually consists of about 60 hours of direct service over a 4-month period (Henggler, 1998; Schoenwald, Henggeler, Brondino, & Rowland, 2000).

Functional Family Therapy (FFT) is a home- and community-based intervention designed for 11–19-year-old youth who have disruptive behavior disorders, conduct disorder, oppositional defiant disorder, and delinquency. The intent of the intervention is to reduce risk factors and enhance protective factors. FFT is a short-term, high-quality intervention program with an average of 12 sessions over a 3–4-month period. Services are conducted in both clinic and home settings, and can also be provided in a variety of settings including schools, child welfare facilities, probation and parole offices/aftercare systems, and mental health facilities. FFT is a strength-based model. At its core is a focus and assessment of those risk and protective factors that impact the adolescent and his/her environment, with specific attention paid both to intrafamilial and extrafamilial factors, and how they present within and influence the therapeutic process.

In the MTFC program, foster parents are recruited, trained, and supported to become part of the treatment team and children are placed in a family setting for 6–9 months. Foster parents provide close supervision and implement a structured, individualized program for each child. The Program Supervisor designs the child's program with input from the treatment team. This intervention builds on the child's strengths while reinforcing clear rules, expectations, and limits to manage behavior. MTFC parents receive 12–14 hours of preservice training, participate in group support and assistance meetings weekly, and have access to program staff back-up and support 24 hours a day/7 days a week. In addition, MTFC parents are contacted daily (Monday through Friday) by telephone to provide the Parent Daily Report (PDR) information, which is used to relay information about the child's behavior over the last 24 hours to the treatment team and to provide quality assurance on program implementation. MTFC parents are paid a monthly salary and a small stipend to cover extra expenses.

The primary outcomes of evidence-based interventions include decrease in the rate and seriousness of antisocial behavior and prevention of juvenile justice recidivism (Asscher et al., 2007a). A longitudinal study on EBPs shows significant decreases in recidivism and harmful behaviors 6–18 months out, and the positive outcomes decrease significantly after 6 months out (Asscher et al., 2007b). None of the evidence-based interventions involves preplacement while children are in facilities or continuity of care after program completion, both elements which have proven to be effective in establishing stability and are routinely credited with the success of Wraparound.

While each has efficacy for children with mild-to-moderate emotional disturbances, these interventions are not intense or flexible enough to meet the needs of higher risk youth with fire setting, sexual aggression, and severe mental health and developmental delays. In fact, these EBPs typically restrict participation by youth with more severe behavioral needs (EBP, 2009).

"We should avoid 'a false dichotomy between the concepts of evidence-based interventions and systems of care—they go hand in glove'" (Pires, 2002). Research shows that although the evidence-based practices have positive outcomes in the short term, the more comprehensive and longer-term Wraparound plans that incorporate an evidence-based practice as part of a continuity of care plan are more effective than a sustaining long-term stability (Asscher et al., 2007).

Erie County, New York is an example of using Wraparound as an overarching philosophy of service provision including evidence-based practices. Erie County's System of Care uses Wraparound to provide a menu of individualized services to serve the needs of families and youth. Family Voices Network of Erie County represents the children's division within the Erie County Department of Mental Health and DSS.

This system of care provides support and services for children aged 5–17 to include children involved with Foster Care and Adoptive Services; Juvenile Justice, Probation, and Detention; DSS; Homeless Children; Children with Mental Health Needs and Children in Schools & Faith-based Communities.

The Wraparound philosophy purports the need to collapse departments that fragment services to needy families. Erie County is successful at providing individualized services across different needs. The network empowers children, youth, and families who are experiencing mental health issues by encouraging families to understand what they need to become independent in their communities. Each family is assigned a Care Coordinator who works with the family to assess the needs. The Care Coordinator works with a pool of providers who offer an array of services. The families choose the services that best match their needs. The Coordinator links the families to this service and monitors their progress, ensuring that all the principles of Wraparound, that is, voice and choice, continuity of care, and individualized service planning, are being addressed (www.familyvoicesnetwork.org/en/). Evidence-Based practices are included in the pool of services. If a youth has a juvenile justice issue and the family wants intensive therapy and monitoring, the family is referred to MST. The Care Coordinator then communicates with the MST provider throughout the treatment and develops an aftercare plan to sustain goal achievement.

CONCLUSION

Wraparound is an approach to service delivery that mends the cracks where high needs youth fall. Carl Dennis, a Chicago-based Wraparound originator wrote the seminal book *Everything is Normal Until Proven Otherwise*. He describes via compelling vignettes how resources are used creatively to keep youth with acute and challenging issues stabilized in the community. Initiatives like Bridges to Health in New York State allow

Departments of Social Services to apply flexible funding to support Wraparound services for families in need, to achieve Carl Dennis's vision to keep youth safe in the most normalizing and healthy ways. This flexible funding allows for the payment of any necessary services identified in a youth's Individual Service Plan. Milwaukee Wraparound prevents thousands of youth from entering institutions through collapsing systems, and by carving out a budget per youth and family, saving the State millions of dollars. Most importantly, Wraparound is able to reframe the needs of youth and families using culturally competent and strength-based principles to remove stigma and maximize stability in the community.

REFERENCES

Asscher, J., Deković, M., van der Laan, P., & Sander van Arum, P. (2007). Implementing randomized experiments in criminal justice settings: An evaluation of multi-systemic therapy in the Netherlands. *Criminology, 3*, 113–129.

Breuck, R., Sexton, T., Van Dam, A., Disse, C., Dorelijer, T., Slot, W., et al. (2006). The implementation and the cultural adjustment of functional family therapy in a Dutch psychiatric day treatment center. *Journal of Marital and Family Therapy, 32*(4), 515–529.

Bruns, E. J., Walker, J. S., Adams, J., Miles, P., Osher, T. W., Rast, J., et al. (2004). *Ten principles of the wraparound process.* Portland, OR: National Wraparound Initiative, Research and Training Center on Family Support and Children's Mental Health, Portland State University.

Child Welfare Information Gateway. (2010). System wide reform. www.childwelfare.gov/systemwide/reform/soc/history/history.cfm. Retrieved October 13, 2010.

Children and Families in the Child Welfare System. (2010). Systems of care. www.systemsofcare. samhsa.gov/2010. Retrieved October 11, 2010.

Clark, H., Boyd, A., Lee, B., Prange, M., Barrett, B., Stewart, E., et al. (1998). Individualized service strategies for children with emotional/behavioral disturbances in foster care: Summary of practice, findings, & systemic recommendations. *US Department of Education* (ERIC No. ED460488) Retrieved April 11, 2006, from ERIC database.

Cohen, S., & Rae, L. (2002). Wraparound plan delivers success at less cost. *Journal News*, December 15.

Dembo, R. (2005). Introduction. *Substance Use & Misuse, 40*, 879–885.

Henggeler, S. W. (1998). *Multisystemic treatment of antisocial behavior in children and adolescents.* New York: Guilford Press, xiii, 287 p.

Mears, S. L., Yaffe, J., & Harris, N. J. (2009). Evaluation of Wraparound services for severely emotionally disturbed youths. *Research on Social Work Practice, 19*, 678–685.

Netzel, A. (2004, January 22). John Bruchard. *Burlington Free Press.* Retrieved April 8, 2006, from http://depts.washington.edu/wrapeval/BFP_article.html.

Pires, S. A. (2002). *Building systems of care: A primer.* Human Service Collaborative. Washington, DC: National Technical Assistance Center for Children's Mental Health, Georgetown University.

Potter, D., & Mulkern, V. (2005). *Community living exchange: Wraparound services.* Retrieved April 17, 2006, from U.S. Department of Health and Human Services, Centers for Medicare & Medicaid Services Web site: http://72.14.203.104/search?q=cache:4anwp_hUiEMJ:www.cshp.rutgers.edu/

Pullman, M. D., Kerbs, J., Koroloff, N., Veach-White, E., Gaylor, R., & Sieler, D. (2006). Juvenile offenders with mental health needs: Reducing recidivism using wraparound. *Crime Delinquency, 52,* 375–397.

Schoenwald, S. K., Henggeler, S. W., Brondino, M. J., & Rowland, M. D. (2000). Multisystemic therapy: Monitoring treatment fidelity. *Family Process, 39,* 83–103.

Stroul, B. A. (Ed.). (1996). *Management and training innovations.* Baltimore, MD: Paul H. Brookes Publishing.

Substance Abuse & Mental Health Services Administration (SAMHSA). (2010). http://www.samhsa.gov/grants/2010/TI-10-007.aspx

Suter, J., Force, M., Bruns, E., Leverentz-Brady, K., Mehrtens, K., & Burchard, J. (2005, May). *Wraparound fidelity index 3.0.* Department of Psychiatry & Behavioral Sciences, Seattle: University of Washington.

VanDenBerg, V. (n.d.) *History of wraparound and systems of care.* Retrieved May 9, 2006, from http://www.vroonvdb.com/about_wraparound.html

Wraparound Fidelity Index. Retrieved March 3, 2006, from http://www.depts.washington.edu/wrapeval/WFI.html

CHAPTER FIVE

Sexual Minority and Gender-Variant Youth

The Heterogeneity of Health-Care Needs

Maria Messina, Sel J. Hwahng, and Anthony Vavasis

INTRODUCTION

The developmental processes and concerns of sexual minority youth (SMY) are similar to their heterosexual peers, but there is also enormous complexity and heterogeneity within this population (Ryan & Futterman, 1998). The first section introduces central concerns about SMY and access to health care, self-identification practices, resilience, and diversity. The next section addresses the impact of stigma, social isolation, and abuse on SMY's physical and mental health as well as HIV risk and substance use, while the final section concludes with a model health-care paradigm and describes in detail an innovative, cutting-edge youth health program called HOTT, "Health Outreach To Teens" at Callen–Lorde in New York City (NYC). Callen–Lorde Community Health Center provides sensitive, exceptional health care and related services primarily to diverse individuals from the lesbian, gay, bisexual, and trans/gender-variant communities, regardless of their ability to pay. To further this mission, Callen–Lorde promotes health education and wellness, and advocates for gay, lesbian, bisexual, and transgender health issues.

SMY face the same problems of adolescence as heterosexual youth in the United States, but have some unique concerns (Mallon, 1992). They care about puberty, friendships, family conflicts, peer pressure, and their future, and also face highly complex challenges learning how to manage stigma and discrimination (Owen, 1998; Ryan & Futterman, 1998).

In health care, the main relevance of disclosing sexual orientation and gender identities is to facilitate providers' accurate diagnoses and appropriate treatment, especially since heterosexuality is generally assumed when

107

(and if) a sexual history is taken (Eliason & Schope, 2001; Fish, 2006). However, obscuring the diversity and complexity of the human experience by locating an individual's identity "in their sex" (Whitlock & Kamel, 1989) may also reflect the nonholistic approach to health in Western societies where the medical model separates the body into discrete domains demonstrated by the specialties, for example, cardiac, obstetrics, ears, nose, throat, etc. (Fish, 2006).

Like their heterosexual counterparts, SMY require routine health care and are at risk for sexually transmitted diseases and HIV, pregnancy, substance abuse, and mental health problems. Many adolescents experiment with same-sex behaviors rendering themselves vulnerable to STDs and HIV, the second most common infectious disease diagnosed after upper respiratory viral infections (Ryan Futterman, 1998). However, because of their sexual orientations and gender identities, lesbian, gay, bisexual, transgender, or queer/questioning (LGBTQ) youth face the additional risk of increased stress, antigay violence including rape, and assault (Ryan Futterman, 1998).

Nomenclature

Following Savin-Williams (2001), SMY here refers to lesbian, gay, bisexual, trans/gender-variant,[1] unlabeled, sexually questioning, or youth who have same-sex attractions. Adolescent sexual identities are ever-evolving as they develop and may change multiple times over time. Youth may be attracted to or engage in same-sex activities or gender atypical behaviors but resist the labeling of LBGTQ, or may identify as gay or lesbian but are not exclusively involved with same-sex or same-gender relations. Some students use "faggot" and "queer" to denigrate and verbally abuse gay adolescents (Hunter and Schaecher, 1987; Smith, 1988; Yarbrough, 2003). In turn, some LGBT youth have adopted "queer" to confront the wounding use of this "epithet" by nongay individuals (Owen, 1998, p. 6). Many queer-identified youth may identify as genderqueer, gender-variant, queer women, or queer men.

Young people might consider the term "transgender" or "transsexual" to be "old school," used by an older generation that is trying to fit within a gender binary system (in which there are only two genders—men

---

[1]See pp. xx.

and women). Many youth, on the other hand, strive to complicate and break out of the gender binary system by creating social systems and worldviews that are comprised of multiple genders, or even sometimes *no* gender. Identifying terms used by the young "trans/gender-variant" person, for example, may not be understood by older members of the community, or by other ethnicities within the same generation: AG, aggressive, boi/gurl, butch queen, butch queen up in drags, fem aggressive, fem queen, femme boy, fourth-sex, gender bender, girl, liminal-gendered, lo-ho, no-ho, non-op, over, pass, queen, questioning, real, third-sex, third-gender, tranny boy, tranny fag, transbian, and transdyke (American Boyz, 2002; Barlow, 2002; Blumenstein & Hansbury, 2002; Boswell, 2002; Broadus 2003; Costain, 2002; Gino, 2001; Griffey, Giordano & Terry, 2002; Hwahng, 2002, 2003; Jessup/Beautiful Thunder, 2001; La Gaipa, Percival, Bell & Rosen, 2001; Lewis, 2002; Marshall, 2001, 2002; Mitchell, 2003; Nucitelli & McAdams, 2002; Nucitelli & Todd, 2002; Patton & Libman, 2003; Peddle, 2005; Rae, pers. comm., 2010; Sanchez, 2003; Solik & O'Malley, 2002).[2] The nomenclature is diverse, complicated, and ever changing, but possibly vital to the trans/gender-variant and other LGBT youth as they attempt to construct an understanding of their individual gender identities.

Less is known about "invisible" youth with same-sex attractions who do not identify as LGBTQ, and do not participate in research studies (Savin-Williams & Cohen, 2009). More is known about youth with problems who come to the attention of service-providing agencies than youth coming from supportive environments with self-esteem, resilience, and healthy developmental progressions. Initially, researchers focused on the most accessible—runaways, male sex workers, and delinquents— adolescents who were extremely vulnerable and at risk emotionally (Savin-Williams & Cohen, 2009). More research is needed on less vulnerable LGBTQ youth to balance the lack of representativeness of the sample.

Youth who resist "discrete identity labels" challenge HIV and other educational interventions to develop highly individualized approaches to

---

[2]"Transfeminine" is to "transwoman" what "MSM" is to "gay men." Both "transfeminine" and "MSM" are descriptive (versus identity) terms, and "transfeminine" connotes a much broader spectrum beyond the identity term "transwoman," which often assumes a binary sex/gender system where an individual crosses over from one gender to the other, often through hormone therapy and/or sexual reassignment surgery. In addition, transfeminine people of color rarely adopt the term "transwoman" as an identity term for themselves (Hwahng & Lin, 2009; Hwahng & Nuttbrock, 2007).

care for those who "don't fit into one box" (Welle, Fuller, Mauk & Clatts, 2006). Politically and personally, nonconformity and fluid partnering practices may be crucial expressions of self among these youth. In fact, "for queer-identified youth acutely aware of power hierarchies and role assignments, the doctor–patient or provider–patient relationship may need open negotiation and renegotiation" (Welle et al., 2006, p. 64).

Resilience

Although much of this chapter discusses risks and vulnerabilities among SMY, it is important to consider a balanced perspective that integrates resiliency, risk, and vulnerability. Brown and Colbourne (2005) explore resiliencies among queer youth involved in the LGB Youth Project, an independent, charitable organization society in Nova Scotia, Canada. This Project provides support, education, resource expansion, and community development to SMY and involves youth at all levels of the organization, including a youth board of directors. Patterns of queer youth resilience included having a sense of entitlement to express truth in their being (thus giving them the strength to "come out"), personal agency, autonomy, self-reliance, personal orientation toward rejecting the negativity and myths of heterosexism and homophobia, forming alternative family structures beyond families of origin, locating and securing the means to break social isolation, accessing gay and ally communities, and sharing identity.

Research indicates that sexual minorities and SMY often practice various forms of resiliencies; given the often enormous stressors, risk factors, and vulnerabilities that sexual minorities confront in their lives, there would be even greater health disparities and more negative health outcomes without these resiliencies. For instance, studies demonstrate that gay and lesbian adolescents use a wide variety of coping strategies and use these strategies at higher rates than heterosexual adolescents in the same schools (Lock & Steiner, 1999), lesbians use psychotherapy and counseling at higher rates than heterosexual women (Rothblum & Factor, 2001), and lesbian and bisexual women often create "families of choice" or strong support systems to combat the stressors of misogynist and homophobic victimization (Balsam, 2003). Indeed, social support is fundamental to sexual minority resiliency, since social support has been shown to be an important moderator of the impact of homophobic hate crimes (Otis & Skinner, 1996) and moderates the impact of traumatic experiences in childhood and adulthood (Carlson & Dalenberg, 2000; Goodenow et al., 2006).

Diversity

Poteat, Espelage, and Koenig (2009) maintain that racial minorities and questioning youth are underrepresented as are youth of multiple intersecting group identities (e.g., gender, sexual orientation, race) in research. Ethnic minorities' process of self-acceptance and "self-celebration" may be complicated by their ethnic, racial, or cultural identities that are not accepting of being LGBT-variant. Where there is religious conservatism, SMY may feel the conflict between acknowledging their sexual orientation and the message that this is against God and the community and risk losing the ethnic minority community's support, placing them, if they are female, in "triple jeopardy" (Owen, 1998). Owen (1998) maintains that racism in the lesbian, gay, and bisexual community may be as persistent as homophobia in some ethnic minority communities (see Familial Violence and Abuse section for more information). Some LGBTQ ethnic minority youth feel they must assimilate into the Euro-American LGBT communities. Gwadz, Clatts, Leonard, and Goldsamt (2004) state that youth of color are often highly vulnerable to a variety of risk factors and adverse effects, suggesting that ethnicity may be a useful indicator of vulnerability.

Studies on Native American populations have emphasized the importance of "identity attitudes" that provided protective mechanisms and accounted for changes of self-esteem, depression, anxiety, and interpersonal sensitivity (Duran & Walters, 2004; Walters, 1999). Identity attitudes are derived from enculturative beliefs and behaviors that arise from identification with, and recognition of resiliency within an individual's ethnic minority culture, often forged through resistant social movements. Another study suggests that enculturation can mitigate the negative effects of a risk factor or enhance the effects of another variable (e.g., identity attitudes) to decrease the probability of a negative health outcome (Zimmerman, Washienko, Walters, & Dyer, 1996).

Identity attitudes and enculturative behaviors appear to also be applicable to other LGBTQ people of color populations. One study of Asian-American youth revealed that Asian-American women who have sex with women (WSW) experienced greater discrimination from being Asian American than being a sexual minority compared to Asian American men who have sex with men (MSM) (Hahm, Wong, Huang, Ozonoff, & Lee, 2008). For young Asian-American WSW, then, greater participation in Asian-American communities would mitigate exposure to racial discrimination. Asian-American enculturative identification may therefore be a protective factor against the internalization of homophobia and other forms of internalized discrimination for Asian-American WSW (Hwahng & Lin, 2009).

Trans/Gender-Variant Youth

Much of this chapter discusses trans/gender-variant youth along with other SMY within various sections. However, some trans/gender-variant youth may have needs that extend beyond other SMY, particularly in relation to transitioning from one sex to another. Some approaches to the treatment of trans/gender-variant youth include a therapeutic intervention that is geared toward altering the youth's gender identity to be congruent with the biological sex, or supportive psychotherapy that strives to alleviate intrapsychic distress while allowing the youth to continue to mature into adulthood. Another intervention facilitates the cross-gender transition, addresses the manner in which society polarizes gender, draws attention to the ways gender dysphoric adolescents are marginalized and pathologized for not conforming to norms of Western culture, and actively determines the appropriateness for hormone therapy, and eventually sex reassignment surgery (Swann & Herbert, 2009).

In treating trans/gender-variant youth, many researchers and clinicians agree that a "one-size-fits-all" approach to the formulation of service-delivery policy is not adequate, and can actually harm youth by pressuring youth to fit the "needs" of service policy (Clatts, 1999). Clatts (1999) actually recommends more flexible service-delivery principles that can be used to guide a hierarchy of goals that serve to maximize the protection of health and well-being while minimizing intrusions to personal freedom and responsibility. It is important to view gender diversity among trans/gender-variant youth as an integral part of their identity and not pathology (Pazos, 2009).

STIGMA AND SOCIAL ISOLATION

Stigma derives from Greek and originally meant a mark or brand burned into the skin of a criminal, slave, or traitor to visibly identify them as blemished or morally polluted persons (Western Heritage Dictionary, 1976). Goffman (1963) refers to stigma as "spoiled identity," an attribute, behavior, or reputation which is socially discrediting in a particular way. Despite the increasing acceptance of nonheterosexual individuals and presence of adult role models in the United States, many SMY still grow up feeling shame and isolation in largely homophobic, heterosexist environments (Stone & Harvey, 2005). They may experience prejudice, discrimination, verbal insults, and violence from strangers, institutions (e.g., laws and statues), and even from known individuals (e.g., their parents) (National Gay and Lesbian Task Force Policy Institute, 1991; Pilkington & D'Augelli, 1995; Rosario, Hunter, & Gwadz, 1997). There are, however, strong regional differences in the United States, including, for example, the more conservative Bible belt areas in contrast to the Atlantic and Pacific Coasts which tend to be more tolerant though religious and political influences mediate as well as the geography (Sullivan, 2003).

Sullivan (2003) broadly defines homophobia as the dislike or hatred expressed toward sexual minorities including cultural and personal biases that are internalized or externalized. SMY may internalize society's antihomosexual sentiments and have negative feelings toward themselves because of their nonheterosexual orientation, whereas externalized homophobia is observable in critical and hostile behavior such as discrimination and violence. Citing social control theory, Sullivan (2003) characterizes externalized homophobia as a form of social control that serves to physically and psychologically intimidate sexual minorities and validate heterosexuality as the only normal sexual identity choice. Similarly, heterosexism is defined as the belief that heterosexuality is the only acceptable form of sexual orientation and that nonheterosexuals should be universally excluded from society's structures and institutions (Appleby & Anastas, 1995; Fassinger, 1991; Sears, 1997; Yarbrough, 2003). As such, heterosexism promotes and condones the individual expression of antigay prejudice (Herek, 1988; Krieglstein, 2003).

SUBSTANCE USE

Savin-Williams, Ritch, & Cohen, (1996) maintains that gay adolescents and their heterosexual counterparts misuse alcohol and/or other substances for different reasons. While heterosexual youth appear to engage in substance misuse due to peer pressure or thrill-seeking, gay adolescents are more likely muffling their growing awareness that they are not heterosexual, the distressing realization that a difficult road lies ahead, and taking "revenge" against parents and a society that rejects them (Savin-Williams, Ritch, & Cohen, 1996, p. 265).

Young WSW appear to be highly vulnerable to substance use and often initiate substance use even earlier than young men who have sex with men ("YMSM"). For instance, Hahm and colleagues (2008) found that young Asian-American women aged 18–27 who self-identified as nonheterosexual were more likely to initiate tobacco use, binge drinking, marijuana use, and other drug use than their heterosexual peers and young Asian-American sexual minority males. These findings suggest that special attention to young Asian-American WSW and substance use is needed.

In another study, young women who identified as lesbian or bisexual were significantly more likely than heterosexual women to report lifetime and recent use of alcohol, speed, marijuana, cocaine, heroin, and having injected drugs in a study measuring both sexual identity and sexual behavior (Scheer et al., 2003). Bisexual-identified women were more likely than lesbian-identified women to report lifetime use of amphetamines and cocaine, and heroin and cocaine use in the past 6 months.

African Americans were twice as likely to use substances daily, as were Latinos, although the latter was at a marginally statistically significant level in a study on young MSM, 17–28 years. Heterosexual-identified YMSM) were more than 4× as likely to use substances daily, and bisexual-identified YMSM were 1.69× more likely, but again, the latter was at a marginally statistically significant level. Overall, transfeminine[2] youth were less likely to use substances daily, unless they had been abused. For young MSM who had not experienced abuse, foster care increased their likelihood of daily substance use by a factor of 3.63 (Gwadz et al., 2004).

Epidemiological studies, however, rarely ask about sexual orientation (McCabe, Hughes, Bostwick, West, & Boyd, 2009). Whether or not gay men and lesbians do have a higher prevalence of alcohol and substance misuse, Cabaj (2000) suggests that internalized homophobia contributes toward a predisposition to substance use and abuse. Young LGBTQ children may learn to suppress and repress feelings of "difference" and find comfort in drinking alcohol or using drugs. Much less is known about men who have sex with men and women (MSMW), women who have sex with women and men (WSWM), and trans/gender-variant persons who also appear to be at "heightened" risk for substance abuse.

ABUSE AND VICTIMIZATION

Research demonstrates that school is one of the most influential environments critical to children's healthy development and well-being (Baker et al., 2001; Birkett, Espelage, & Koenig, 2009; Eccles et al., 1993; Ringeisen, Henderson, & Hoagwood, 2003). LGBTQ youth experience alarming rates of verbal and physical harassment, discrimination, bullying, and assault in schools across the United States (Birkett, Espelage, & Koenig, 2009; Bontempo & D'Augelli, 2002; D'Augelli, Pilkington, & Hershberger, 2002; Kosciw & Diaz, 2006). In the 2007 National School Climate Survey, 86% of LGBT students reported being verbally harassed; 44% reported being physically harassed; 61% felt unsafe at their school because of their sexual orientation; 33% reported skipping a day of school in the last month because of feeling unsafe; 44% had been physically harassed (e.g., pushed or shoved) in the last year at school because of their sexual orientation; 22% reported being physically assaulted (e.g., punched, kicked, injured with a weapon) because of their sexual orientation; and 14% because of their gender orientation (Kosciw, Diaz, & Greytak, 2008).

Recent exceptions are the Harvey Milk High School in NYC designed to be a safe space for students regardless of sexual orientations or gender identities as well as The School for Social Justice Pride Campus in Chicago also fostering a violence-free academic environment, particularly though not exclusively, catering to students targeted for their sexual orientations or gender identities. Kosciw, Greytak, and Diaz (2009) found that LGBTQ youth in rural communities and communities where the adult level of education is low face particularly hostile school environments. In an analysis of sexual minority adolescents, protective factors in six school-based surveys in Minnesota and British Columbia included family connectedness, school connectedness, and religious involvement.

A comparison of seven population-based high-school health surveys in the United Stated and Canada revealed that in all surveys except for one, adolescent girls were more likely to report sexual abuse than adolescent boys; however, gay and bisexual boys were nearly as likely to report sexual abuse as lesbian and bisexual girls. Lesbian and bisexual girls reported the highest prevalence of sexual abuse among girls, with 25–50% reporting a history of sexual abuse, compared to 10–25% of heterosexual girls reporting sexual abuse. Over 25% of bisexual boys and 20% of gay boys reported sexual abuse compared to fewer than 10% of heterosexual boys. Bisexual boys were up to 10 times as likely, and bisexual girls were at least twice as likely to report sexual abuse as their heterosexual peers (Saewyc et al., 2006).

With regard to physical abuse, girls of all orientations were more likely to experience physical abuse than boys, with lesbian and bisexual girls reporting a higher prevalence of physical abuse than heterosexual girls, and gay and bisexual boys (20–33%) reporting a higher prevalence of physical abuse than heterosexual boys (12.5%). Bisexual youth had at least twice the odds of physical abuse compared to their heterosexual peers, and in some surveys report sometimes higher and sometimes lower rates of physical abuse as compared to gay peers (Saewyc et al., 2006).

Several other studies also indicate that lesbian and bisexual female youth were more likely to experience a history of physical abuse and sexual abuse compared to heterosexual female youth (Austin et al., 2008; Balsam, Rothblum, & Beauchaine, 2005; Saewyc, Bearinger, Blum, & Resnick, 1999). It was also found that a vast majority of lesbian and bisexual female youths, 14–21 years, had experienced abuse and victimization due to their sexual orientation (sexual orientation victimization), often being threatened and/or attacked multiple times (D'Augelli, 2003). Female SMYs who had self-identified at younger ages reported more lifetime sexual orientation victimization as well as those who had disclosed to others at younger ages, and 14% of the overall sample had experienced sexual orientation victimization by mothers, fathers, or both parents. The National Lesbian Health Care Survey (NLHCS) specifically examined 1925 lesbian-identified women and revealed that 28.7% were sexually abused as children, with lesbians in the youngest age cohort (17–24 years) reporting the highest prevalence of childhood sexual abuse (CSA) while the oldest cohort (55 years and older) reporting the lowest prevalence (Descamps, Rothblum, Bradford, & Ryan, 2000). In addition, lesbians who had experienced CSA were slightly younger, had less education, and had lower income than lesbians who had not experienced CSA. Lesbians who had experienced CSA were significantly more likely to experience daily stress, depression, alcohol abuse, adult rape, intimate partner violence, and hate crimes compared to lesbians who had not experienced CSA. In another study of over 63,028 women, lesbian and bisexual women reported more physical abuse, sexual abuse, and forced sexual activity during childhood and adolescence, and greater chronicity of physical abuse in both childhood and adolescence. Lesbian and bisexual women who had been abused during childhood were also more likely to experience revictimization as adolescents compared to heterosexual women (Austin et al., 2008).

Another study examined low-income young women, 18–29 years, mostly women of color, and compared sexual self-identity with sexual behavior. Scheer and colleagues (2003) found that lesbian- and bisexual-identified young women were more likely to have experienced coerced sex than heterosexual-identified young women, and also found that WSWM reported significantly higher coerced sexual experiences, and higher rates of sexual victimization measured by having traded sex for drugs or money, threatened with force to engage in sex, and forced to engage in sexual activity compared to women who have sex with men only (WSMO).

Familial Violence and Abuse

Parents of LGBTQ youth who come out may respond with disappointment, shock, sadness, fear, or panic (D'Augelli, Hershberger, & Pilkington, 1998; Herdt & Koff, 2000). Some parents may distance themselves from their LBGTQ children (Saltzburg, 2004), or there may be familial emotional and/or physical abuse (Martin & Hetrick, 1988; Uribe & Harbeck, 1992). Parents may disown or expel them from home (Davis, Saltzburg, & Locke, 2009; Savin-Williams, 1994). Pilkington and D'Augelli (1995) found that among gay, lesbian, and bisexual adolescent and young adults, 22% of the female participants had been verbally assaulted and 18% had been physically assaulted by a family member because of their sexual orientation.

An interesting study by Balsam and colleagues (2005), compared lesbian, gay, bisexual, and heterosexual siblings (total $N = 1245$). Lesbians, gay men, bisexual women, and bisexual men reported higher levels of psychological, physical, and sexual abuse in childhood (as well as adulthood) compared to their heterosexual siblings and LGB children and youth may be singled out by their parents for maltreatment. In a study of ethnic minorities, lesbians of color (African American at 45.4%, and Latinas at 40%) had experienced higher rates of CSA compared to white lesbians (26.9%) (Descamps et al., 2000). And another study comparing two-spirit (see adult LGBTQ Health Care Delivery Chapter, p. x) Native Americans with heterosexual Native Americans found that "two-spirit" women and men experienced more childhood physical abuse and CSA than heterosexual women and men (Balsam, Huang, Fieland, Simoni, & Walters, 2004). A study on Puerto Rican drug users revealed that sexual minority orientation was associated with childhood physical abuse and CSA among men, and CSA among women (Finlinson et al., 2003).

A study in NYC found that transfeminine people of color had experienced more gender-related abuse during adolescence than White transfeminine people (58.6% of African Americans and 63% of Latinas versus 33.5% of Whites) (Hwahng & Nuttbrock, 2010). Findings also revealed that perpetrators of abuse during adolescence were often parents or other family members (Nuttbrock et al., 2010). Findings from a small qualitative study of transfeminine people of color in NYC also found that 40% had experienced parental hostility and aggression, and 40% had experienced parental indifference and neglect because of their gender identity (Koken, Bimbi, & Parsons, 2009). In interpreting these findings, it is especially important to contextualize these findings within socio-structural frameworks such as historical trauma, poverty, and racism so as not to pathologize families or communities of color as inherently homo- or transphobic (see discussions on historical trauma in the chapter on Adult LGBTQ, and also Hwahng & Lin, 2009). Researchers who do not make linkages between sociostructural and interpersonal phenomena may end up stereotyping or repathologizing people and families of color.

Targeted Victimization and Sexual Orientation

Balsam and colleagues (2005) also discuss possible factors for greater victimization of LGB people during childhood and adolescence. These include sexual minority boys being unable to access other same-sex peers to explore their sexuality, thus turning to older men to explore their same-sex attractions, and rendering these boys vulnerable to potential sexual abuse by older men. Sexual minority girls, on the other hand, may respond to same-sex feelings or rejection by family and peers by acting out behaviors such as truancy, substance use, or running away from home that may also render them vulnerable to sexual abuse by predatory men, and a general increase in physical and sexual victimization (Balsam, 2003; Balsam et al., 2005).

It is also unclear whether childhood and adolescent abuse is a direct consequence of SMY disclosing their orientation, gender atypicality, or a response to a youth's subtle behavioral cues without any overt disclosure, since most research does not determine causality for abuse. For both sexual minority boys and girls, gender-atypical appearance and behavior may make them more visible and vulnerable to aggression by adults (Balsam, 2003; Hall, 1998; Waldo, Hesson-McInnis, & D'Augelli, 1998). Sometimes SMY experienced decreased family protection and support even before these youth recognize their own same-sex attractions and self-identities, and there may be an as-yet unmeasured trait of emerging gay or bisexual orientation to account for this family maltreatment (Corliss, Cochran, & Mays, 2002; Saewyc et al., 2006). High prevalence of youth maltreatment appears to occur during adolescence (Snyder & Sickmund, 2000), which is concurrent with the years of developing sexual orientation; therefore, it is often impossible to determine if coming out preceded being abused or vice versa (Saewyc et al., 2006).

Researchers have also discussed the developmental impact of childhood and adolescent abuse on sexual identity formation, in which the trauma from abuse may delay the coming out process for sexual minority adolescents and women (Balsam, 2003). One hypothesis alludes that

CSA may "cause" homosexuality in women (Butke, 1995). Balsam (2003) refers to this as hypothesis as a "cultural myth," which may further impede the coming out process for sexual minority girls and women, who may then believe that their same-sex attractions are merely "symptoms" of abuse perpetrated by men. Sexual minority female survivors of childhood abuse may also internalize beliefs that they are "bad" and do not deserve to be happy, therefore denying themselves the opportunity to pursue same-sex relationships or functional same-sex relationships; they may also be less psychologically resilient to confront interpersonal and social rejection if they come out in public. Saewyc and colleagues (2006) assert that childhood and adolescent sexual and physical abuse are not the causes of same-sex orientation. Childhood and adolescent sexual and physical abuse are among the most predominant predictors of youth risk behaviors such as substance use and abuse, suicide attempts, running away from home, and teen pregnancy, and studies have reported a higher prevalence of these risk behaviors among SMY (Anderson, Teicher, Polcari, & Renshaw, 2002; Borowsky, Ireland, & Resnick, 2001; De Bellis, 2002; DuRant, Krowchuk, & Sinal, 1998; Hershberger & D'Augelli, 1995; Robin et al., 2002; Rotheram-Borus, Marelich, & Srinivasan, 1999; Russell & Joyner, 2001; Saewyc, Magee, & Pettingel, 2004). Some studies indicate that bisexual adolescents, or those with attractions to both genders, are at higher risk for victimization compared to gay and lesbian peers (Robin et al., 2002; Russell, Franz, & Driscoll, 2001).

With regard to policy implications, professionals who work with families of SMY in crisis should help these families to respond in caring ways (Saewyc et al., 2006). Therapy that attempts to change the sexual orientation of children and adolescents is considered unethical since the methods may cause great harm, and little credible evidence for their effectiveness exists (American Psychiatric Association, 2000). Families should be encouraged to support their sexual minority child or children, rather than further stigmatizing them, and individual and community interventions should also incorporate messages that emotional pressure or corporal punishment will not change a child's gender expression or sexual orientation. Organizations and case workers must raise awareness about the extremely high levels of violence directed at SMY, both in families and in communities. Educational institutions can play an important role in supporting SMY, for positive youth development, and linking SMY to supportive community resources. For religious families and SMY, it is useful to provide information about safe, open, and affirming religious institutions in their local area. And finally, legal efforts to reduce the stigma of sexual minority orientation and protect the rights of sexual minorities will also have a positive effect on SMY. Legal efforts can be truly effective if augmented with advocacy and interventions to increase community acceptance, reduce violence, and increase respect for SMY and diversity.

HOMELESS YOUTH

Saewyc and colleagues (2006) state that because SMY experience higher prevalence of abuse, they represent a greater proportion among runaway, homeless, juvenile justice, and foster care populations. It is not uncommon for LGBTQ youth to run away from home after being rejected by their families. Higher rates of sexual abuse, physical abuse, and/or neglect are also reported among homeless LGB youth compared to homeless hetero-sexual youth (Cochran, Stewart, Ginzler, & Cauce, 2002; Kruks, 1991; Whitbeck, Chen, Hoyt, Tyler, & Johnson, 2004) resulting in a disproportion-ate number of them becoming homeless and street involved, and therefore, less likely to be in school (Saewyc, 2005). There are very few shelters or "safe spaces" specifically for youth with same-sex attractions (von Wormer & McKinney, 2003). (An exception, discussed below, is the HOTT program at Callen–Lorde Community Health Center in NYC.) In order to survive, homeless, street-involved youth may engage in sex work, drug dealing, and other delinquent behaviors potentially deleterious to their health (Cohen et al., 1981; Kruks, 1991; Silbert & Pines, 1982; Simons & Whitbeck, 1991; Tyler, Hoyt, Whitbeck, & Cauce, 2001a; Winters, Rema-fedi, & Chan, 1996) and SMY are more likely to experience physical and sexual victimization on the street compared to their heterosexual peers (Cochran et al., 2002; Tyler, 2008; Whitbeck et al., 2004). SMY are vulnerable through multiple factors; earlier experiences of abuse and victimization in the home have been linked to later revictimization among homeless youth (Ryan, Kilmer, Cauce, Watanabe, & Hoyt, 2000; Simons & Whitbeck, 1991; Tyler, Hoyt, & Whitbec, 2000; Tyler, Hoyt, Whitbeck, & Cauce, 2001b; Whit-beck, Hoyt, & Yoder, 1999; Whitbeck & Simons, 1993), while an indirect effect occurs through high-risk behaviors such as trading sex, prostitution, and associating with deviant peers.

Heterosexual parents may be ill-equipped to respond to their chil-dren's nonheterosexual emerging sexual identities. A primary intervention includes providing therapeutic assistance to families to help them cope with their child's sexual/gender identities, improve the home environment, and help prevent initial and recurrent homelessness (Cochran et al., 2002).

Other policy implications (Tyler, 2008) include interventions that take into account specific stressors that SMY are experiencing, such as sexual orientation victimization, negative mental health outcomes, and trading sex. Shelters and other agencies should also advertise that SMY are welcome. They should encourage SMY to seek out their services, and hire visibly open LGBT staff members. Case workers and service providers also need to work with SMY to change negative self-images that have developed from years of abuse, victimization, and neglect. Ideally, services such as counseling, job training, and employment opportunities would help to prepare SMY in establishing functional work patterns and intimate relationships.

TEEN PREGNANCY

In population-based surveys in the United States and Canada, researchers have found a higher rate of teen pregnancy among sexual minority female adolescents than among their heterosexual counterparts, from 2 to as much as 7 times higher (Blake et al., 2001; Saewyc et al., 1999; Saewyc, Pettingell, & Skay, 2004). Population-based surveys on SMY in the United States suggest similar disparities (Blake et al., 2001; Saewyc et al., 1999; Saewyc, Pettingell, & Skay, 2004). Researchers attribute this disparity in pregnancies in large part to greater risk factors for teen pregnancy which includes "higher rates of ever having sexual intercourse, higher odds of early sexual initiation (often in the context of sexual abuse), multiple lifetime partners, substance use before sex, and lack of condom use or other effective contraception" (Saewyc, Poon, Homma, & Skay, 2008). This research further indicated that teen pregnancy involvement for lesbian and bisexual youth was significantly associated with sexual orientation discrimination as well as experiences of exclusion, harassment, and violence. Lesbian and bisexual adolescent girls and young women were also five times more likely to report recent involvement in commercial sex work compared to heterosexual adolescent girls and young women (Saewyc et al., 1999).

SEXUAL ORIENTATION AND MENTAL HEALTH

The experience of "minority stress" (Meyer, 2003) resulting from sexual minority marginalization, abuse, and victimization has been demonstrated to cause negative health outcomes, and is especially associated with negative mental health. For example, one study on lesbian and bisexual female youth (D'Augelli, 2003) found that related to their sexual orientation, 46% experienced fears of losing friends, 42% experienced fears of verbal abuse at school, 28% experienced fears of physical abuse at school, and 15% experienced fears of physical abuse at home. Having fears related to sexual orientation violence (SOV) was significantly associated with negative mental health and suicidal ideation. Higher self-esteem was associated with more same-sex sexual partners and fewer fears regarding violence relative to sexual orientation.

Negative reactions from mothers regarding sexual orientation was also associated with negative mental health outcomes. In addition, female youth who had not lost friends due to their sexual orientation had significantly higher self-esteem than youths who had lost friends. Loss of friends was also strongly associated with past suicide attempts. Youth who had supportive parents and friends had less negative mental health outcomes and were less likely to report past suicide attempts compared to youths who had two unsupportive parents and had lost friends due to their sexual orientation (D'Augelli, 2003).

In a sample of both female and male SMY, gender atypicality was associated with significantly more negative symptoms on both the Brief Symptom Inventory and Trauma Symptom Checklist scales; 9% met the criteria for PTSD in the last year and was associated with past physical SOV, marginally associated with sexual SOV. Three times the number of sexual minority girls had PTSD compared to sexual minority boys (D'Augelli et al., 2006).

SMY of color may be particularly vulnerable to negative mental health outcomes. One study indicated that 41% of female SMY of color and 35% of male SMY of color had attempted suicide (Advocates for Youth, 1999a). Native American youth have been measured to live stressful lives in which many are suffering from depression, substance use, and suicidality; suicide is particularly high among young Native American men, especially those who are HIV infected (Dinges & Quang, D.-T., 1993; Sullivan, 1991).

In addition, a study of transfeminine people in NYC found statistically significant very strong "dose response" associations between gender-related psychological and physical abuse and major depression/suicidality during early and late adolescence (Nuttbrock et al., 2010). Since a majority of African-American and Latina transfeminine people experienced gender-related abuse during their adolescence, an alarming number of African-American and Latina transfeminine people also experienced major depression and suicidality during their adolescence, which is also a critical time of identity development (Hwahng & Nuttbrock, 2010).

SEXUAL ORIENTATION AND PHYSICAL HEALTH

HIV Risk

The Centers for Disease Control and Prevention (CDC) released a report that emphasizes the disproportionate impact of HIV and syphilis among gay and bisexual men in the United States (CDC, 2010). Among US racial/ethnic groups, Blacks are at the highest risk of acquiring HIV/ AIDS. Although Blacks made up 13% of the US population in 2006, they accounted for 46% of new HIV infections that year (CDC, 2008). At CDC's 2010 National STD Prevention Conference, the data indicated that the rate of new HIV diagnoses among MSM is more than 44 times that of other men and more than 40 times that of women (CDC, 2010). Among the complex factors contributing to the high rates of HIV and syphilis among gay and bisexual men are the high prevalence of HIV and other STDs among MSM, which increases the risk of disease exposure, limited access to prevention services, complacency about HIV risk, and difficulty of consistently maintaining safe behaviors with every sexual encounter over the course of a lifetime, particularly among young gay and bisexual men. In comparison with other sexual practices, receptive anal intercourse is highly risky especially if protective strategies do not consistently include condom use. These risk factors are compounded by a lack of awareness of syphilis symptoms and how it can be transmitted (e.g., oral sex) as well as how homophobia and stigma can prevent MSM from seeking prevention, testing, and treatment services.

In order to explain and understand HIV risk, what is crucially needed are holistic models that can synthesize various data to examine various levels of "health ecology" within "health ecosystems" (Honari, 1999) in order to create innovative solutions for issues such as HIV risk. A health ecological perspective includes a global view that takes into account the microenvironment (such as family, home, and communication with others), macroenvironment (such as neighborhoods, community, cultures, educational systems, and political and economic systems), the history of microlevel and macrolevel relations, the present and future directions of cultural diversity, and would also include both qualitative and quantitative conceptions of populations and resources.

Nuttbrock and colleagues (epub ahead of print) found that one of the major differences of HIV rates among ethnicities in the transfeminine population was due to sexual orientation, in which androphilia (sexual attraction to males) was highly correlated to increased risk of HIV. Interestingly, African-American and Latina transfeminine people were 90–91%

androphilic, whereas White transfeminine people were only 19.9% androphilic. Previous discussions in this chapter have noted the high rates of adolescent gender-related abuse, and adolescent depression and suicidality, generally, and in this study among African-American and Latina transfeminine people. There may be a correlation between experiences of adolescent gender-related abuse, adolescent depression/suicidality, and androphilia during this critical identity development period that may impact the formation of a gender identity that is prone to revictimization (Hwahng & Nuttbrock, 2010). It thus appears that gender-related adolescent abuse may affect the development of gender identity for transfeminine people of color and that this type of abuse within families of color may be a vehicle for the intergenerational transmission of historical trauma (Hwahng & Nuttbrock, 2010).

Given this evidence, SMY of color may thus be disproportionately vulnerable to risk of HIV compared to Euro-American SMY. For example, young Native American MSM often feel socially isolated from their communities and home and often attend Euro-American or non-Native gay bars to explore their sexuality, which may leave them vulnerable to victimization and engaging in sex while under the influence of substances (Advocates for Youth, 1999b; "Darrell Joe," 1995; Gilley, 2006). In addition, 64% of young Native Americans, MSM reported unprotected anal intercourse, which was higher than any other racial group (Advocates for Youth, 1999b).

Research that has focused mostly on female youth of color often indicates high levels of risky behavior. In Herrick, Matthews, and Garofalo (2010) study of racially diverse sexual minority female youth, 16–24 years, 94% were sexually active, 50% had unprotected vaginal sex in the past year, 25% had receptive anal sex with a male partner in their lifetime, and 19% had receptive anal sex with a male partner in the past year, 88% had sex while intoxicated, 42% had participated in public sex, 20% had engaged in intercourse resulting in pregnancy, 20% had shared sex toys, 30% had experienced forced sex, 7% had exchanged sex for resources, and 3.6% tested positive for HIV. Another study on a low-income majority women of color sample, 18–29 years, revealed that WSWM compared to WSMO were significantly more likely to report past and recent high-risk sexual behavior, including sex with an HIV-positive man, multiple male sexual partners, sex with MSM, sex with an Intravenous Drug User (IDU), trading sex for drugs or money, and anal receptive intercourse (Scheer et al., 2002). WSWM also had much greater number of lifetime male partners and male partners within the past 6 months compared to WSMO (307 versus 16 in lifetime, 9 versus 2 in the past 6 months) and

WSWM were also more likely to have serological markers for both hepatitis B and hepatitis C viruses.

Young WSW who are illicit drug users are at particular risk for HIV and young women of color are disproportionately represented among young WSW illicit drug users. In one study on young Latino IDUs in Harlem, 18–30 years, young Latina WSW had 42% HIV seroprevalence, which was significantly higher than young MSM (18%), young WSMO (16%), and young men who have sex with women only (5%) (Diaz, Vlahov, Greenberg, Cuevas, & Garfein, 2001). Both young Latina WSW and young Latino MSM were more likely to engage in receptive syringe sharing and trading sex for money or drugs than heterosexual women or men. Another study of racially diverse young women IDUs, 18–30 years, compared WSW IDUs to non-WSW IDUs among five US cities and found that WSW IDUs compared to non-WSW were at higher risk and more likely to participate in sex work and to test positive for HIV and Hepatitis B. The researchers concluded that HIV seroprevalence among young WSW IDUs cannot be explained by their greater involvement in sex work (Friedman et al., 2003).

INNOVATION IN HEALTH-CARE PARADIGMS

Optimal Structure and Content of Health-Care Delivery Services for SMY

Dr. Robert Garofalo (n.d.), the former President of the Gay and Lesbian Medical Association, considers what structure and content of health-care delivery to LGBTQ youth will produce the optimal outcomes. More important than disclosing sexual orientations or gender identities is the general lack of discussion about sexual health topics with teens. Structurally, health-care delivery systems need to be multifaceted since LGBTQ youth exist in all communities. Culturally competent services are needed beyond specialized clinics or drop-in centers as well as in private practice, schools, emergency departments, and public health clinics (Garofalo, n.d.). The content of health-care delivery needs to be grounded in the unique aspects of being LGBTQ, for example, homosexual stigma.

With the exception of HIV prevention data among YMSM there is little data on extant health-care delivery services and needs for SMY, yet an abundance of research exists regarding risk behaviors and clinical outcomes for these highly heterogeneous youth (Garofalo, 2010; Savin-Williams &

Cohen, 2009). Some researchers and providers advocate a shift in focus from adolescent high-risk behaviors and outcomes to their pride, self-determination, and resilience (Savin-Williams & Cohen, 2009; 1990; Garofalo, n.d.). Nonetheless, LGBTQ adolescents do have a disproportionate risk of health problems related to medical and nonmedical risk-taking behaviors including suicide attempts, drug use, and high-risk sexual behaviors in addition to school truancy and dropout that can lead to high-risk choices (Garofalo Wolf, Kessel, Palfrey, & DuRant, 1998). Further, SMY also are more likely to engage in multiple risk-taking behaviors in comparison with their heterosexual peers. Their health care is complicated by a lack of training for providers in addition to the discomfort they may feel talking about their sexuality in front of their parents. With the exception of the Gay and Lesbian Medical Association and the Society for Adolescents Medicine, for examples, few groups of clinicians take special interest in LGBTQ adolescents, possibly due to stigma and funding issues (National Research Council and Institute of Medicine, 2007).

Chicago's Broadway Youth Center (BYC) offers a multitude of barrier-free services 6 days a week from 1 p.m.–8 p.m. and is located in heavily trafficked geographic areas targeting high-risk LGBTQ and homeless youth and offer services such as housing assistance, case management, HIV/STD testing and medical management, counseling, food/shower/laundry, General Education Development (GED)/job training, and a mentorship program. BYC offers community space, which is youth owned and operated. During its first two years of operation (2004–2006) between nearly 4000–5000 youth were served annually with over 500 medical cases. More than 90% of the youth reported having difficulty accessing health care elsewhere and over 70% returned for services.

Promising future directions in health care include decreasing stigma around SMY and increasing cultural competency of staff. Training issues for staff include debunking misconceptions about SMY and learning how to approach and include sexual orientation in their medical histories. However, Garofalo (n.d.) wonders whether training will be enough in the face of moral and religious mores. Future research needs to move on from small non-population-based samples from one geographic area to multisite studies that include women and racial/ethnic minorities, and to consider alternate data collection methods such as using the Internet. The funding needs to be specific to health-care delivery and models of care that go beyond the "spectrum of dysfunction" (HIV, drugs, suicide). Large national studies need to include sexual orientations and gender identities measures as a demographic, not risk variable (Garofalo, n.d.).

CALLEN–LORDE COMMUNITY HEALTH CENTER: HOTT

Callen–Lorde's adolescent health-care program, "HOTT," is a progressive, innovative health-care program for LGBTQ youth (and young adults) and presented here in detail as a model of an effective strategy in the provision of health services for this vulnerable population. HOTT includes a mobile medical van and provides low- or no-cost medical and mental health services for LGBTQ youth and runaway/homeless youth, including comprehensive primary care, HIV care, trans/gender-variant care, counseling, HIV/STI prevention services, and health education. The HOTT mobile medical van goes to meet the adolescents at multiple locations in NYC where the youth are known to spend time. The medical van is free, ensures confidentiality, and provides clean, safe space to engage a difficult-to-reach population that Callen–Lorde would otherwise not be able to engage.

Callen–Lorde's HOTT Program serves predominantly LGBTQ youth, many of whom are homeless from 13 to 24 years of age. A significant proportion of the homeless youth may identify with the identities and behaviors of LGBTQ persons but do not necessarily think of, or refer to themselves as gay, lesbian, bisexual, or transgender. Although some youth do not refer to themselves as gay, they may have same-sex relations, while others who identify as gay may not be exclusively engaging in same-sex relations. Because adolescents' sense of self, gender identities, and sexual orientations are ever-evolving as is developmentally appropriate for their age, the staff must maintain a delicate balance in their ways of communicating with their clients. One of the major challenges in serving LGBTQ youth is to understand what it means to care for those who are vulnerable on so many different levels at once, immersed in a heterosexist world at home, in school, and the community. The staff must understand how to talk about the rejection, stigma, and pejorative comments they experience as well as know the language and behaviors relevant to these youth. While conveying a sense of openness and safety when interacting with LGBTQ youth, staff must simultaneously maintain a clear understanding of the politics and history of the labeling of LGBTQ persons. Most importantly, the staff never needs to impose those identities on the youth. Adolescents are young and can change—multiple times—in their developing sense of sexuality and selves. Staff must be prepared to tolerate what may appear to be contradictions as the youth evolves. It is also recommended that all staff be comfortable articulating all parts of sexual anatomy and every sexual act while maintaining a poker face. Part of health care is being able to talk about sex comfortably.

Harm Reduction

Harm reduction is most commonly known in the field of addictions, where the underlying philosophy is "to meet clients where they are" and help protect themselves from harm (Denning, 2000; von Wormer & McKinney, 2003). The harm reduction approach originally was developed to help people with addictive behavior problems to develop the skills to maintain their treatment goals, even in high-risk situations, and to deal effectively with setbacks (Marlatt, 1985). Youth with same-sex attractions and gender-variant behaviors are just like other youth when it comes to potentially high-risk behaviors involved with, for example, early initiation of sexual activity that is often accompanied by alcohol and other drug use (von Wormer & McKinney, 2003). For many LGBTQ youth, these problems are compounded by the lack of social support, relevant sex education in high school, adult role models, and mistreatment by other youth. Even with family support, many LGBTQ youth still feel shame about their sexual orientation and lack the necessary tools to negotiate high-risk situations, especially where a power differential is involved as is the case in their interactions with adults.

At the HOTT program, instead of implementing a medical model approach to patient care, medical providers implement a nonjudgmental harm reduction philosophy in their approach to serving LGBTQ youth. Although there is a role for using the "medical model" in the interpretation of medical data, the medical model is otherwise an authoritarian and prescriptive approach to treating pathology by diagnosing symptoms and syndromes, and deemed not optimum for working with youth. Developmentally, youth are supposed to be questioning authority, to individuate, and separate from parents and authority. Medical care providers are specifically trained to be authorities, which in the context of treating youth, is not a functional approach. Callen–Lorde staff feel that the approach must be shifted from a hierarchical (vertical), authoritarian staff model to a more horizontal, team-centered approach in which the patient is a member of the team. Some core values, from a harm reduction approach to youth health care include providing a nonjudgmental environment; shifting the locus of control inward so that the patient has agency of control; establishing an environment where consequences of behavior and choices are clear, including negative outcomes; modifying the medical model approach to the patient, and considering the role of the patient, how the patient perceives the problem, and what feels right. Finally, the staff engages in a dialogue around the patient's goals: Are the goals reasonable? What are the consequences? And, what are optimal outcomes?

For those youth who live at home, the medical provider engages in a dialogue with their patients where the adolescents become part of the conversation, but are not being told what to do. Rather, the provider finds out what the patient wants to do and helps him/her get there. One of the goals is to help the youth learn how to problem solve, to think their problems through, and turn a solution into actionable behavior. In uncontrolled epidemics, such as HIV/AIDS, the prescriptive model does not work for adults either. This clash is only amplified among LGBTQ youth if their experiences of authority have been rejection and ostracism. When they come into contact with another authority, such as a physician, they will expect the same authoritarian scripts to be played out and will never talk about what they are really doing.

Healthy Boundaries

Boundaries are a monumental issue in youth work. Adolescents and young adults who come to Callen–Lorde for services are frequently survivors. That is, these youth have had to make choices that a typical young person (in an industrialized country) does not have to make in order to stay alive. As an example, a young man comes out to his mother at age 16 as being gay, she tells him he has to move out immediately. With no notion of where to go or what to eat, he goes to the village and quickly learns that he can get money or shelter in exchange for sex (an example of survival sex versus "sex work," "prostitution," or "escorting"). As such, it is a healthy and adaptive response to an untenable situation. Another example involves a teenage woman who is found making out with another teenage girl by her older brother and cousin. In an attempt to "make her straight," they sexually assault her. This pattern continues undiscovered or unacknowledged by her parents. As a means of making her situation more bearable, she begins to use alcohol and marijuana daily to feel better. (While she will eventually be labeled an "alcoholic," at this moment, she is engaging in, what could be referred to as "survival drinking.")

What may appear to be "youth problems" can sometimes be unresolved problems or contradictions within health-care staffs' own lives. At Callen–Lorde, the staff are encouraged to do their best to become aware of and filter out their own internal issues that may affect their perceptions of or interactions with the adolescent clients. As Anderson (1998) points out, in order to work effectively with youth with same-sex attractions, care providers need "to examine their own beliefs and values about gay people, to be comfortable with their own sexuality, to educate themselves as to what it means to be gay, and to understand what it means to a parent to have a gay child."

Providers may experience a strong pull to want to rescue the patients, especially those who are homeless and struggling. Instead it is the role of health-care providers to help patients develop agency around their own decisions. To do otherwise is to disempower the youth, communicating in essence, that "you cannot take care of yourself so I will take care of you." This approach is counterproductive because it does not encourage the development of control and self-determination.

Trauma is another enormous issue in youth work. Youth who have experienced any type of abuse while growing up have already experienced poor boundaries in adult relationships, especially in the case of sexual abuse. Depending on the population, as many as one in three teens may experience sexual violence before reaching adulthood (Saewyc, Pettingell, & Magee, 2003; Saewyc et al., 2006; Tonkin, Murphy, Lee, Saewyc, & the McCreary Centre Society, 2005). If a staff member tries to rescue these youth, they are often seen as just another person who does not establish a healthy boundary.

In the HOTT Mobile Medical Van as well as in the clinic, the staffs' primary goal with their adolescent patients is to treat the illness, not to be their friend. The staff do not date, have sex, or share their personal life with their patients. It is important for the youth to know that staff will always be professional, and the focus of the dialogue will be on the patient, not the health-care provider. Youth might want to know, for example, if a particular medical provider is gay or married. The physician will assert that the primary focus is the patient, especially if the client has only been a patient with HOTT for less than a year. However, if the patient and the provider developed a relationship over 3 or 4 years and have established a healthy boundary in their relationship, the provider might consider revealing their marital status, for example, once s/he understands why the patient wants to know. This evolution in the provider–patient relationship may be instructive for youth in demonstrating how healthy boundaries evolve over time. This is especially important for young people who engage in sex work (as do many clients in the HOTT Program) and are approached by older people, to see and hear how healthy boundary dynamics are developed.

Rethinking Roles: Not Authority, Not Friend

HOTT staff strives to maintain the delicate balance in their roles as "not authority, not friend." As staff, they must be clear with adolescent clients that they will not be friends, who would, for example, call them on the phone at night. But what they will do is provide safe space for reflection, something the teens likely have never done before. How staff try to work with youth who come for their services is to provide a safe space for reflection, to help them think about their problems, shed light on them, but not tell them what to do.

VERTICAL AND HORIZONTAL KNOWLEDGE

The team model can benefit patients of all ages as people have affinities for some individuals over others. It generates vertical, in-depth knowledge about the patient, and horizontal knowledge about the patient shared by all staff. Furthermore, a lone staff person could hear complete falsehoods from a patient which are then challenged by the experiences of another team member with that same patient. The same patient might show respect for one provider and complete disrespect for another. Certain dynamics may play out in the waiting room differently than in the patient care room. HOTT staff meetings are horizontally inclusive: all staff who come in contact with the adolescents attend staff meetings. As an example, the social worker will know a patient's diagnosis; the physician will know the case management needs. The receptionist has a unique opportunity to observe behaviors, hear patient interactions that may not come up in the patient care room while they are waiting, and share these at the next staff meeting. The HOTT staff team functions essentially as one person; a patient may have different stories for each of them but the team pools the information for a more complete and comprehensive sense of the individual. Most importantly, the staff needs to learn how to talk about patients' identities and behaviors and the relationship between the two. Taking a bio-psycho-social approach, the goal is neither to over-medicalize nor overpsychosocialize the adolescents' health problems. Medical providers must know their patients at all levels in order to really understand them.

Low-Threshold Approach

Services for adolescent patients should be "low threshold," meaning that the staff needs to encourage and acknowledge patients' small, incremental steps toward accomplishing an agreed-upon goal created by the patient. Many youth who find their way to the HOTT Program have extraordinarily stressful, complex lives. Some do not even know what day it is, not to mention being able to keep their appointment time. The staff need be able to read patients, know their comfort zone, and find the balance between those who genuinely cannot organize themselves versus those who try to "work the system." The Clinical Director of HOTT commented that, "society has no place for these youth; you create one safe space but their lives are so much more complex than that. A low threshold approach means that sometimes the marker of success is that the youth stay connected to the HOTT Program and don't die."

CONCLUSION

LGBTQ youth are not a homogenous group. The literature paints a portrait of youth who are more distressed, substance misusing, homeless, and suicidal than their heterosexual counterparts (Almeida et al., 2009; Cochran et al., 2002; Fergusson et al., 1999; Lock & Steiner, 1999; Rosario et al., 1997; Savin-Williams & Cohen, 1996). Issues for trans/gender-variant youth are more complicated (Mallon, 2009). Sexual minority and trans/gender-variant youth of color may be at particularly high risk for a number of adverse outcomes and may need special attention and interventions that also take into account multiple jeopardy stress arising from factors such as historical trauma, racism, and poverty (Balsam et al., 2004; Bowleg et al., 2003; Duran & Walter, 2004). Garofalo and colleagues (1998) and Savin-Williams (2009) among others (Owens, 1998) emphasize the importance of broadening our view of LGBTQ youth from one that focuses on dysfunction—for instance, suicide, depression, mental health, homelessness, and HIV—to a strengths-based perspective that emphasizes pride, self-determination, agency, creativity, and resilience. Perhaps the best approach is one that recognizes and integrates vulnerability, risk, resiliency, and the full spectrum of LGBTQ youth experiences.

REFERENCES

"Darrell Joe" (1995). *Seasons*, 4–8, Autumn.

Advocates for Youth. (1999a). *Issues at a glance: Adolescent sexual health and the dynamics of oppression: A call for cultural competency.* Washington, DC: Advocates for Youth.

Advocates for Youth. (1999b). *Issues at a glance: HIV/STD prevention and young men who have sex with men.* Washington, DC: Advocates for Youth.

Almeida, J., Johnson, R. M., Corliss, H. L., Molnar, B. E., & Azrael, D. (2009). Emotional distress among LGBT youth: The influence of perceived discrimination based on sexual orientation. *Journal of Youth and Adolescence, 38*(7), 1001–1014.

American Boyz. (2002, February 16–19). *Race and racism: Town hall meeting.* Paper presented at the Sixth Annual True Spirit Conference: Letting Our True Spirits Soar ... Washington, DC.

Anderson, A. (1998). Strengths of gay male youths: An untold story. *Child and Adolescent Social Work Journal, 15*(1), 55–71.

Anderson, C. M., Teicher, M. H., Polcari, A., & Renshaw, P. F. (2002). Abnormal T2 relaxation time in the cerbellar vermis of adults sexually abused in childhood: Potential role of the vermis in stress-enhanced risk for drug abuse. *Psychoneuro-endocrinology, 27,* 231–244.

Appleby, G. A., & Anastas, J. W. (1995). Social work practice with lesbians and gays. In A. T. Morales & B. W. Sheafor (Eds), *Scoial work: A profession of many faces* (7th edn, pp. 333–366). Boston, MA: Allyn and Bacon.

Association, A. P. (2000). *Therapies focused on attempts to change sexual orientation (reparative or conversion therapies).* Position statement. APA Document Reference No. 200001, May 2000. Retrieved April 21, 2006, from http://www.psych. org/Departments/EDU/Library/APAOfficialDocumentsandRelated/Position Statements/200001.aspx

Austin, S. B., Jun, H.-J., Jackson, B., Spiegelman, D., Rich-Edwards, J., Corliss, H. L., et al. (2008). Disparities in child abuse victimization in lesbian, bisexual, and heterosexual women in the Nurses' Health Study II. *Journal of Women's Health, 17*(4), 597–606.

Baker, J. A., Derrer, R. D., Davis, S. M., Dinklage-Travis, H. E., Linder, D. S., & Nicholson, M. D. (2001). The flip side of the coin: Understanding the school's contribution to dropout and completion. *School Psychology Quarterly, 16*(4), 406–426.

Balsam, K. F. (2003). Traumatic victimization in the lives of lesbian and bisexual women: A contextual approach. *Journal of Lesbian Studies, 7*(1), 1–14.

Balsam, K. F., Huang, B., Fieland, K. C., Simoni, J. M., & Walters, K. L. (2004). Culture, trauma, and wellness: A comparison of heterosexual and lesbian, gay, bisexual, and two-spirit Native Americans. *Cultural Diversity and Ethnic Minority Psychology, 10*(3), 287–301.

Balsam, K. F., Rothblum, E. D., & Beauchaine, T. P. (2005). Victimization over the life span: A comparison of lesbian, gay, bisexual, and heterosexual siblings. *Journal of Consulting and Clinical Psychology, 73*(3), 477–487.

Barlow, J. Z. (2002, February 16–19). *Occupying the middle: The no/low-hormone, non-operative transsexual.* Paper presented at the Sixth Annual True Spirit Conference: Letting Our True Spirits Soar ... Washington, DC.

Birkett, M., Espelage, D. L., & Koenig, B. (2009). LGB and questioning students in schools: The moderating effects of homophobic bullying and school climate on negative outcomes. *Journal of Youth and Adolescence, 38,* 989–1000.

Blake, S. M., Ledsky, R., Lehman, T., Goodenow, C., Sawyer, R., & Hack, T. (2001). Preventing sexual risk behaviors among gay, lesbian, and bisexual adolescents: The benefits of gay-sensitive HIV instruction in schools. *American Journal of Public Health, 91,* 940–946.

Blumenstein, R., & Hansbury, G. (2002, February 16–19). *The construction, de-construction, and re-construction of gender identity mergers and the power of language*. Paper presented at the Sixth Annual True Spirit Conference: Letting Our True Spirits Soar . . . Washington, DC.

Bontempo, D. E., & D'Augelli, A. R. (2002). Effects of at-school victimization and sexual orientation on lesbian, gay, or bisexual youths' health risk behavior. *The Journal of Adolescent Health, 30*, 364–374.

Borowsky, I. W., Ireland, M., & Resnick, M. D. (2001). Adolescent suicide attempts: Risks and protectors. *Pediatrics, 107*, 485–493.

Boswell, H. (2002, February 16–19). *Transcending gender*. Paper presented at the Sixth Annual True Spirit Conference: Letting Our True Spirits Soar . . . Washington, DC.

Bowleg, L., Huang, J., Brooks, K., Black, A., & Burkholder, G. (2003). Triple jeopardy and beyond: Multiple minority stress and resilience among black lesbians. *Journal of Lesbian Studies, 7*(4), 87 –108.

Broadus, K. (2003, February 16–19). *People of color only (POC): Community-driven meeting*. Paper presented at the Seventh Annual True Spirit Conference: Masculinity: The Magical Mystery Tour, Washington, DC.

Brown, M., & Colbourne, M. (2005). Bent but not broken: Exploring queer youth resilience. In M. Ungar (Ed.), *Handbook for working with children and youth: Pathways to resilience across cultures and contexts*. Thousand Oaks, CA: Sage Publications.

Butke, M. (1995). Lesbians and sexual child abuse. In L. A. Fuentes (Ed.), *Sexual abuse in nine North American cultures* (pp. 236–258). Thousand Oaks, CA: Sage Publications.

Cabaj, R. P. (2000). Substance abuse, internalized homophobia, and gay men and lesbians: Psychodynamic issues and clinical implications, pp. 5–24. *Journal of Gay and Lesbian Psychotherapy, 3* (3–4).

Carlson, E. B., & Dalenberg, C. J. (2000). A conceptual framework for the impact of traumatic experiences. *Trauma, Violence, & Abuse, 1*(1), 4–28.

Clatts, M. C. (1999). Case six: Does "nonjudgmental" care include prescribing sex hormones? In J. Blustein, C. Levine, & N. N. Dubler (Eds), *The adolescent alone: Decision making in health care in the United States*. New York, NY: Cambridge University Press.

Cochran, B. N., Stewart, A. J., Ginzler, J. A., & Cauce, A. M. (2002). Challenges faced by homeless sexual minorities: Comparison of gay, lesbian, bisexual, and transgender homeless adolescents with their heterosexual counterparts. *American Journal of Public Health, 92*, 773–777.

Cohen, L. E., Kluegel, J. R., & Land, K. C. (1981). Social inequality and predatory criminal victimization: An exposition and test of a formal theory. *American Sociology Review, 46*, 505–524.

Corliss, H. L., Cochran, S. D., & Mays, V. M. (2002). Reports of parental maltreatment during childhood in a United States population-based survey of homosexual, bisexual, and heterosexual adults. *Child Abuse & Neglect, 26*(11), 1165–1178.

Costain, E. (2002, February 16–19). *Beyond binaries: Youth and gender identity*. Paper presented at the Sixth Annual True Spirit Conference: Letting Our True Spirits Soar . . . Washington, DC.

D'Augelli, A. R. (2003). Lesbian and bisexual female youths aged 14 to 21: Developmental challenges and victimization experiences. *Journal of Lesbian Studies, 7*(4), 9–29.

D'Augelli, A. R., Grossman, A. H., & Starks, M. T. (2006). Childhood gender atypicality, victimization, and PTSD among lesbian, gay, and bisexual youth. *Journal of Interpersonal Violence, 21*(11), 1462–1482.

D'Augelli, A. R., Hershberger, S. L., & Pilkington, M. W. (1998). Lesbian, gay, and bisexual youth and their families: Disclosure of sexual orientation and its consequences. *American Journal of Orthopsychiatry, 68*, 361–371.

D'Augelli, A. R., Pilkington, N. W., & Hershberger, S. L. (2002). Incidence and mental health impact of sexual orientation victimization of lesbian, gay, and bisexual youths in high school. *School Psychology Quarterly, 17*(2), 148–167.

Davis, T. S., Saltzburg, S., & Locke, C. R. (2009). Supporting the emotional and psychological well being of sexual minority youth: Youth ideas for action. *Children and Youth Services Review, 31*, 1030–1041.

De Bellis, M. D. (2002). Developmental traumatology: A contributory mechanism for alcohol and substance use disorders. *Psychoneuroendocrinology, 27*, 155–170.

Descamps, M. J., Rothblum, E., Bradford, J., & Ryan, C. (2000). Mental health impact of child sexual abuse, rape, intimate partner violence, and hate crimes in the National Lesbian Health Care Survey. *Journal of Gay and Lesbian Social Services, 11*(1), 27–55.

Denning, P. (2000). *Practicing harm reduction psychotherapy: An alternative approach to addictions.* New York, NY: Guilford Press.

Diaz, T., Vlahov, D., Greenberg, B., Cuevas, Y., & Garfein, R. (2001). Sexual orientation and HIV infection prevalence among young Latino injection drug users in Harlem. *Journal of Women's Health & Gender-Based Medicine, 10*(4), 371–380.

Dinges, N. G., & Quang, D.-T. (1992/1993). Stressful life events and co-occurring depression, substance abuse and suicidality among American Indian and Alaska native adolescents. *Culture, Medicine, and Psychiatry, 16*, 487–502.

Duran, B., & Walters, K. L. (2004). HIV/AIDS prevention in "Indian Country." Current practice, indigenist etiology models, and postcolonial approaches to change. *AIDS Education and Prevention, 16*(3), 187–201.

DuRant, R. H., Krowchuk, D. P., & Sinal, S. H. (1998). Victimization, use of violence, and drug use at school among male adolescents who engage in same-sex sexual behavior. *Journal of Pediatrics, 133*(1), 113–118.

Eccles, J. S., Midgley, C., Wigfield, A., Buchanan, C. M., Reuman, D., Flanagan, C., et al. (1993). Development during adolescence: The impact of stage-environment fit on young adolescents' experiences in schools and in families. *The American Psychologist, 48*, 90–101.

Eliason, M. J., & Schope, R. (2001). Does "don't ask don't tell" apply to health care? Lesbian, gay, and bisexual people's disclosure to health care providers, pp. 125–134. *Journal of the Gay and Lesbian Medical Association, 5*(4), December.

Fassinger, R. E. (1991). The hidden minority: Issues and challenges working with lesbian women and gay men. *The Counseling Psychologist, 19*(2), 157–176.

Fergusson, D. M., Horwood, L. J., & Beautrais, A. L. (1999). Is sexual orientation related to mental health problems and suicidality in young people? *Archives of General Psychiatry, 56,* 876–880.

Fish, J. (2006). Heterosexism in health and social care. New York, NY: Palgrave Macmillan, xi, 236 p.

Finlinson, H. A., Robles, R. R., Colon, H. M., Lopez, M. S., Negron, M. C., Oliver-Velez, D., et al. (2003). Puerto-Rican drug users' experiences of physical and sexual abuse: Comparisons based on sexual identities. *Journal of Sex Research, 40,* 277–285.

Friedman, S. R., Ompad, D. C., Maslow, C., Young, R., Case, P., Hudson, S. M., et al. (2003). HIV prevalence, risk behaviors, and high-risk sexual and injection networks among young women injectors who have sex with women. *American Journal of Public Health, 93*(6), 902–906.

Garofalo, R. (n.d.). Adolescent health care service and systems: Issues of LGBT youth. Children's memorial hospital, Howard Brown Health Center, Northwestern University (*Powerpoint presentation*). Accessed June 28, 2010, from http://www.bocyf.org/garofalo_presentation.pdf

Garofalo, R., Wolf, C., Kessel, S., Palfrey, J., & DuRant, R. H. (1998). The association between health risk behaviors and sexual orientation among a school-based sample of adolescents. *Pediatrics, 101*(5), 895–898.

Gilley, B. J. (2006). *Becoming two-spirit: Gay identity and social acceptance in Indian country.* Lincoln, NE: University of Nebraska Press.

Gino, A. (2001, February 16–19). *Living liminally.* Paper presented at the Fifth Annual True Spirit Conference: Celebrating Human Diversity, Washington, DC.

Goffman, E. (1963). *Stigma: Notes on the management of spoiled identity.* Englewood Cliffs, NJ: Prentice-Hall.

Goodenow, C., Szalacha, L., & Westheimer, K. (2006). School support groups, other school factors, and the safety of sexual minority adolescents. *Psychology in the Schools, 43,* 573–589.

Griffey, C., Giordano, M., & Terry, J. (2002, February 16–19). *The invisibility of FTM youth.* Paper presented at the Sixth Annual True Spirit Conference: Letting Our True Spirits Soar . . . Washington, DC.

Gwadz, M. V., Clatts, M. C., Leonard, N. R., & Goldsamt, L. (2004). Attachment style, childhood adversity, and behavioral risk among young men who have sex with men. *Journal of Adolescent Health, 34*(5), 402–413.

Hahm, H. C., Wong, F. Y., Huang, Z. J., Ozonoff, A., & Lee, J. (2008). Substance use among Asian Americans and Pacific Islanders sexual minority adolescents: Findings from the National Longitudinal Study of Adolescent Health. *Journal of Adolescent Health, 42*(3), 275–283.

Hall, J. (1998). Lesbians surviving childhood sexual abuse: Pivotal experiences related to sexual orientation, gender, and race. *Journal of Lesbian Studies, 2*(1), 7–28.

Herdt, G., & Koff, B. (2000). *Something to tell you.* New York, NY: Columbia University Press.

Herek, G. (1988). Heterosexual's attitudes toward lesbians and gay men: Correlates and differences. *Journal of Sex Research, 25,* 451–477.

Herrick, A. L., Matthews, A. K., & Garofalo, R. (2010). Health risk behaviors in an urban sample of young women who have sex with women. *Journal of Lesbian Studies, 14,* 80–92.

Hershberger, S. L., & D'Augelli, A. R. (1995). The impact of victimization on the mental health and suicidality of lesbian, gay, and bisexual youths. *Developmental Psychology, 31,* 65–74.

Honari, M. (1999). Health ecology: An introduction. In M. Honari & T. Boleyn (Eds.), *Health ecology: Health, culture and human–environment interaction.* New York, NY: Routledge.

Howard Brown Health Center. (2010). Broadway youth center. Accessed June 28, 2010, from http://www.howardbrown.org/hb_services.asp

Hunter, J., & Schaecher, R. (1987). Stresses on lesbian and gay adolescents in school. *Social Work in Education, 9*(3), 180–190.

Hwahng, S. (2002, February 16–19). *LoHo FTMs and other hormonal alternatives.* Paper presented at the Sixth Annual True Spirit Conference: Letting Our True Spirits Soar . . . Washington, DC.

Hwahng, S. (2003, February 16–19). *Race, ethnicity and transmasculinity.* Paper presented at the Seventh Annual True Spirit Conference: Masculinity: The Magical Mystery Tour, Washington, DC.

Hwahng, S. J., & Lin, A. J. (2009). The health of lesbian, gay, bisexual, transgender, queer, and questioning people. In C. Trinh-Shevrin, N. Islam, & M. Rey (Eds.), *Asian American communities and health: Context, research, policy, and action* (pp. 226–282). San Francisco, CA: Jossey-Bass Publishers.

Hwahng, S. J., & Nuttbrock, L. (2007). Sex workers, fem queens, and cross-dressers: Differential marginalizations and HIV vulnerabilities among three ethno-cultural male-to-female transgender communities in New York City. *Sexuality Research & Social Policy, 4*(4), 36–59.

Hwahng, S. J., & Nuttbrock, L. (2010). *Adolescent gender-related abuse, androphilia, and HIV risk among transfeminine people of color.* Paper presented at the Working Group on Gender, New York State Psychiatric Institute and Columbia University.

Jessup/Beautiful Thunder, G. (2001, February 16–19). *Winkte in a Wasicu world.* Paper presented at the Fifth Annual True Spirit Conference: Celebrating Human Diversity, Washington, DC.

Koken, J. A., Bimbi, D. S., & Parsons, J. T. (2009). Experiences of familial acceptance–rejection among transwomen of color. *Journal of Family Psychology, 23*(6), 853–860.

Kosciw, J. G., & Diaz, E. M. (2006). *The 2005 National School Climate Survey: The experiences of lesbian, gay, bisexual, and transgender youth in our nation's schools.* New York, NY: Gay, Lesbian and Straight Education Network. Retrieved on April, 24, 2010 from http://www.glsen.org

Kosciw, J. G., Diaz, E. M., & Greytak, E. A. (2008). *The 2007 National School Climate Survey: The experiences of lesbian, gay, bisexual, and transgender youth in our nation's school.* New York, NY: Gay, Lesbian and Straight Education Network.

Kosciw, J. G., Greytak, E. A., & Diaz, E. M. (2009). Who, what, where, when, and why: Demographic and ecological factors contributing to hostile school climate for lesbian, gay, bisexual, and transgender youth. *Journal of Youth Adolescence, 38,* 976–988.

Krieglstein, M. (2003). Heterosexism and social work: An ethical issue. In S. Michael (Ed.), *Sexual minorities: Discrimination, challenges, and development in America* (pp. 75–91). New York, NY: The Haworth Press, Inc.

Kruks, G. (1991). Gay and lesbian homeless/street youth: Special issues and concerns. *Journal of Adolescent Health, 12,* 515–518.

La Gaipa, D., Percival, T., Bell, A., & Rosen, L. (2001, February 16–19). *Transqueer evolution—Living as a gay man.* Paper presented at the Fifth Annual True Spirit Conference: Celebrating Human Diversity, Washington, DC.

Lewis, Y. (2002, February 16–19). *People of color meeting.* Paper presented at the Sixth Annual True Spirit Conference: Letting Our True Spirits Soar ... Washington, DC.

Lock, J., & Steiner, H. (1999). Relationships between sexual orientation and coping styles of gay, lesbian, and bisexual adolescents from a community high school. *Journal of the Gay and Lesbian Medical Association, 3*(3), 77–82.

Mallon, G. (2009). *Social work practice with transgender and gender variant youth.* New York, NY: Routledge.

Mallon, G. P. (1992). Gay and no place to go: Assessing the needs of gay and lesbian adolescents in out-of-home care settings. *Child Welfare, 71*(6), 547–556.

Marlatt, A. (1985). Relapse prevention: Maintenance strategies in the treatment of addictive behaviors, Paris: Lavoisier.

Marshall, K. (2001, February 16–19). *Blurring the lines: Creating our own identities.* Paper presented at the Fifth Annual True Spirit Conference: Celebrating Human Diversity, Washington, DC.

Marshall, K. (2002, February 16–19). *Blurring the lines: Creating our own identities.* Paper presented at the Sixth Annual True Spirit Conference: Letting Our True Spirits Soar ... Washington, DC.

Martin, A. D., & Hetrick, E. S. (1988). The stigmatization of the gay and lesbian adolescent. *Journal of Homosexuality, 15,* 163–183.

McCabe, S. E., Hughes, T. L., Bostwick, W. B., West, B. T., & Boyd, C. J. (2009). Sexual orientation, substance use behaviors and substance dependence in the United States, pp. 1333–1345. *Addiction. 104*(8), August.

Meyer, I. J. (2003). Prejudice, social stress, and mental health in lesbian, gay, and bisexual populations: Conceptual issues and research evidence, 674–697, *Psychological Bulletin, 129*(5), September.

Mitchell, L. J. (2003, February 16–19). *Filling the void(s)—POC only: Community-driven meetings.* Paper presented at the Seventh Annual True Spirit Conference: Masculinity: The Magical Mystery Tour, Washington, DC.

National Gay & Lesbian Task Force Policy Institute. (1991). *Anti-gay/lesbian violence, victimization, and defamation.* Washington, DC: Author.

Nuccitelli, A., & McAdams, R. (2002, February 16–19). *Femme boy caucus.* Paper presented at the Sixth Annual True Spirit Conference: Letting Our True Spirits Soar ... Washington, DC.

Nuccitelli, A., & Todd, M. (2002, February 16–19). *MultiGenderPlicity.* Paper presented at the Sixth Annual True Spirit Conference: Letting Our True Spirits Soar . . . Washington, DC.

Nuttbrock, L., Bockting, W., Mason, M., Hwahng, S., Rosenblum, A., Macri, M., et al. ([Epub ahead of print]). A further assessment of Blanchard's typology of homosexual versus non-homosexual or autogynephilic gender dysphoria. *Archives of Sexual behavior.*

Nuttbrock, L., Hwahng, S., Bockting, W., Rosenblum, A., Mason, M., Macri, M., et al. (2010). Psychiatric impact of gender-related abuse across the life course of male-to-female transgender persons. *Journal of Sex Research, 47*(1), 12–23.

Owens, R. E. (1998). *Queer kids: The challenge and promise for lesbian, gay, and bisexual youth.* New York, NY: The Hawthorn Press.

Otis, M. D., & Skinner, W. F. (1996). The prevalence of victimization and its effect on mental well-being among lesbian and gay people. *Journal of Homosexuality, 30,* 93–117.

Patton, J., & Libman, A. (2003, February 16–19). *Bookends: FTM youth and elders bridging the years.* Paper presented at the Seventh Annual True Spirit Conference: Masculinity: The Magical Mystery Tour, Washington, DC.

Pazos, S. (2009). Social work practice with female-to-male transgender and gender variant youth. In Ge. P. Mallon (Ed.), *Social work practice with transgender and gender variant youth* (2nd edn, pp. 87–103). New York: NY: Routledge/Taylor & Francis Group.

Peddle, D. (2005). *The aggressives.* USA: Seventh Art Releasing.

Pilkington, N. W., & D'Augelli, A. R. (1995). Victimization of lesbian, gay, and bisexual youth in community settings. *Journal of Community Psychology, 23*(1), 34–56.

Poteat, V. P., Espelage, D. L., & Koenig, B. W. (2009). Willingness to remain friends and attend school with lesbian and gay peers: Relational expressions of prejudice among heterosexual youth. *Journal of Youth and Adolescence, 38*(7), 952–962.

Ringeisen, H., Henderson, K., & Hoagwood, K. (2003). Context matters: Schools and the "research to practice gap" in children's mental health. *School Psychology Review, 32*(2), 153–168.

Robin, L., Brener, N. D., Donahue, S. F., Hack, T., Hale, K., & Goodenow, C. (2002). Associations between health risk behaviors and opposite-, same-, and both-sex sexual partners in representative samples of Vermont and Massachusetts high school students. *Archives of Pediatric and Adolescent Medicine, 156,* 349–355.

Rosario, M., Hunter, J., & Gwadz, M. (1997). The coming-out process and its adaptational and health-related associations among gay, lesbian, and bisexual youths: Stipulation and exploration of a model. *Journal of Adolescent Research, 12*(4), 454–476.

Rothblum, E. D., & Factor, R. (2001). Lesbians and their sisters as a control group: Demographic and mental health factors. *Psychological Science, 12*(1), 63–69.

Rotheram-Borus, M. J., Marelich, W. D., & Srinivasan, S. (1999). HIV risk among homosexual, bisexual, and heterosexual male and female youths. *Archives of Sexual Behavior, 28,* 159–177.

Russell, S. T., Franz, B. T., & Driscoll, A. K. (2001). Same-sex romantic attraction and experiences of violence in adolescence. *American Journal of Public Health, 91,* 903–906.

Russell, S. T., & Joyner, K. (2001). Adolescent sexual orientation and suicide risk: Evidence from a national study. *American Journal of Public Health, 91,* 1276–1281.

Ryan, C., & Futterman, D. (1998). *Lesbian and gay youth: Care and counseling.* Philadelphia, PA: Hanley & Belfus.

Ryan, K. D., Kilmer, R. P., Cauce, A. M., Watanabe, H., & Hoyt, D. R. (2000). Psychological consequences of child maltreatment in homeless adolescents: Untangling the unique effects of maltreatment and family environment. *Child Abuse & Neglect, 24,* 333–352.

Saewyc, E. M. (2005). Teen pregnancy among gay, lesbian, and bisexual youths: Influences of stigma, sexual abuse, and sexual orientation. In A. Omoto & H. Kurtzman (Eds.), *Sexual orientation and mental health: Examining identity and development in lesbian, gay, and bisexual people* (pp. 95–116, Chapter 5). Washington, DC: APA Press.

Saewyc, E. M., Bearinger, L. H., Blum, R. W., & Resnick, M. D. (1999). Sexual intercourse, abuse and pregnancy among adolescent women: Does sexual orientation make a difference? *Family Planning Perspectives, 31*(3), 127–131.

Saewyc, E. M., Magee, L. L., & Pettingell, S. (2004). Teenage pregnancy and associated risk behaviors among sexually abused adolescents. *Perspective on Sexual and Reproductive Health, 36*(3), 98–105.

Saewyc, E. M., Pettingell, S. L., & Magee, L. L. (2003). The prevalence of sexual abuse among adolescents in school. *Journal of School Nursing, 19,* 266–272.

Saewyc, E. M., Pettingell, S. L., & Skay, C. L. (2004). Teen pregnancy among sexual minority youth in population based surveys of the 1990s: Countertrends in a population at risk. *Journal of Adolescent Health, 34,* 125–126.

Saewyc, E. M., Poon, C. S., Homma, Y., & Skay, C. L. (2008). Stigma management? The links between enacted stigma and teen pregnancy trends among gay, lesbian, and bisexual students in British Columbia. *The Canadian Journal of Human Sexuality, 17*(3), 123–139.

Saewyc, E. M., Skay, C. L., Pettingell, S. L., Reis, E. A., Bearinger, L., Resnick, M., et al. (2006). Hazards of stigma: The sexual and physical abuse of gay, lesbian, and bisexual adolescents in the United States and Canada. *Child Welfare, 85*(2), 195–213.

Savin-Williams, R. C. (1994). Verbal and physical abuse as stressors in the lives of lesbian, gaymale and bisexual youths: Associations with school problems, running away, substance abuse, prostitution, suicide. *Journal of Consulting and Clinical Practice, 62,* 261–269.

Savin-Williams, R. C. (2001). A critique of research on sexual-minority youths. *Journal of Adolescence, 24*(1), 5–13, February.

Savin-Williams, R. C., & Cohen, K. M. (1996). Psychosocial outcomes of verbal and physical abuse among lesbian, gay, and bisexual youths. In R. C. Savin-Williams & K. M. Cohen (Eds.), *The lives of lesbians, gays, and bisexuals: Children to adults* (pp. 181–200). Fort Worth, TX: Harcourt Brace College Publishers.

Savin-Williams, R. C., & Cohen, K. M. (2009). Development of same sex attracted youth. In I. H. Meyer, & M. E. Northridge (Eds.), *The health of sexual minorities: Public health perspectives on lesbian, gay, bisexual and transgender populations* (pp. 27–47). New York, NY: Springer Publishing.

Savin-Williams, R. C., & Cohen, K. M. (1996). The lives of lesbians, gays, and bisexuals: Children to adults (pp. 181–200). Orlando, FL, US: Harcourt Brace College Publishers.

Saltzburg, S. (2004). Learning that an adolescent child is gay or lesbian: The parent experience. *Social Work, 49*(1), 109–118.

Sanchez, D. (2003, February 16–19). *Trans health—POC only.* Paper presented at the Seventh Annual True Spirit Conference: Masculinity: The Magical Mystery Tour, Washington, DC.

Scheer, S., Parks, C. A., McFarland, W., Page-Shafer, K., Delgado, V., Ruiz, J. D., et al. (2003). Self-reported sexual identity, sexual behaviors and health risks: Examples from a population-based survey of young women. *Journal of Lesbian Studies, 7*(1), 69–83.

Scheer, S., Peterson, I., Page-Shafer, K., Delgado, V., Gleghorn, A., Ruiz, J. D., et al. (2002). Sexual and drug use behavior among women who have sex with both women and men: Results of a population-based survey. *American Journal of Public Health, 92*(7), 1110–1112.

Sears, J. T. (1997). *Overcoming heterosexism and homophobia.* New York, NY: Columbia.

Silbert, M. H., & Pines, A. M. (1982). Entrance into prostitution. *Youth & Society, 13*, 471–500.

Simons, R. L., & Whitbeck, L. B. (1991). Sexual abuse as a precursor to prostitution and victimization among adolescent and adult homeless women. *Journal of Family Issues, 12*, 361–379.

Smith, M. R., & Gordon, R. A. (1998). Personal need for structure and attitudes towards homosexuality. *The Journal of Social Psychology, 138*(1), 83–87.

Snyder, H., & Sickmund, M. (2000). Sexual assault of young children as reported to law enforcement: Victim, incident, and offender characteristics. July 2000. Retrieved April 4, 2006, from www.unh.edu/ccrc/factsheet.html#3

Solik, S., & O'Malley, H. (2002, February 16–19). *Transqueer evolution—Living as a gay man.* Paper presented at the Sixth Annual True Spirit Conference: Letting Our True Spirits Soar . . . Washington, DC.

Stone, L., & Harvey, R. G. (2005). *Nurturing queer youth: Family therapy transformed.* New York, NY: W.W. Norton and Co.

Sullivan, C. (1991). Pathways to infection: AIDS vulnerability among the Navajo. *AIDS Education and Prevention, 3*, 241–257.

Sullivan, M. (2003). Homophobia, history and homosexuality: Trends for sexual minorities. In S. Michael (Ed.), *Sexual Minorities: Discrimination, Challenges, and Development in America* (pp. 75–91). New York, NY: The Haworth Press, Inc.

Swann, S. K., & Herbert, S. E. (2009). Ethical issues in the mental health treatment of trans adolescents. In G. P. Mallon (Ed.), *Social work practice with transgender and gender variant youth* (2nd edn). New York, NY: Routledge.

Tonkin, R., Murphy, A., Lee, Z., Saewyc, E., & McCreary Centre Society. (2005). *British Columbia youth health trends: A retrospective, 1992–2003.* Vancouver, BC: McCreary Centre Society. ISBN #: 1-895438-71-3. Available at http://www.mcs.bc.ca

Tyler, K. A. (2008). A comparison of risk factors for sexual victimization among gay, lesbian, bisexual, and heterosexual homeless young adults. *Violence and Victims, 23*(5), 586–602.

Tyler, K. A., Hoyt, D. R., & Whitbeck, L. B. (2000). The effects of early sexual abuse on later sexual victimization among female homeless and runaway youth. *Journal of Interpersonal Violence, 15,* 235–250.

Tyler, K. A., Hoyt, D. R., Whitbeck, L. B., & Cauce, A. M. (2001a). The effects of a high-risk environment on the sexual victimization of homeless and runaway youth. *Violence and Victims, 16,* 441–455.

Tyler, K. A., Hoyt, D. R., Whitbeck, L. B., & Cauce, A. M. (2001b). The impact of childhood sexual abuse on later sexual victimization among runaway youth. *Journal of Research on Adolescence, 11,* 151–176.

Uribe, V., & Harbeck, K. M. (1992). Project 10 addresses needs of gay and lesbian youth. *Educational Digest, 58*(2), 50–54.

von Wormer, K., & McKinney, R. (2003). What schools can do to help gay/lesbian/bisexual youth: A harm reduction approach. *Adolescence, 30*(151), 132.

Waldo, C. R., Hesson-McInnis, M. S., & D'Augelli, A. R. (1998). Antecedents and consequences of victimization of lesbian, gay, and bisexual young people: A structural model comparing rural university and urban samples. *American Journal of Community Psychology, 26,* 307–334.

Walters, K. L. (1999). Urban American Indian identity attitudes and acculturative styles. *Journal of Human Behavior and the Social Environment, 2*(1–2), 163–178.

Welle, D. L., Fuller, S. S., Mauk, D., & Clatts, M. C. (2006). The invisible body of queer youth: Identity and health in the margins of lesbian and trans communities. *Journal of Lesbian studies, 10*(1–2), 43–71.

Whitbeck, L. B., Chen, X., Hoyt, D. R., Tyler, K. A., & Johnson, K. D. (2004). Mental disorder, subsistence strategies, and victimization among gay, lesbian, and bisexual homeless and runaway adolescents. *The Journal of Sex Research, 41,* 329–342.

Whitbeck, L. B., Hoyt, D. R., & Yoder, K. A. (1999). A risk-amplification model of victimization and depressive symptoms among runaway and homeless adolescents. *American Journal of Community Psychology, 27,* 274–296.

Whitbeck, L. B., & Simons, R. L. (1993). A comparison of adaptive strategies and patterns of victimization among homeless adolescents and adults. *Violence and Victims, 8,* 135–152.

Whitlock, K., & Kamel, R. (Ed.). (1989). *Bridges of respect: Creating support for gay and lesbian youth.* Philadelphia, PA: American Friends Service Committee.

Winters, K. C., Remafedi, G., & Chan, B. Y. (1996). Assessing drug abuse among gay/bisexual young men. *Psychology of Addictive Behaviors, 10,* 228–236.

Yarbrough, D. G. (2003). Gay adolescents in rural areas: Experiences and coping strategies. *Journal of Human Behavior in the Social Environment, 8*(2–3), 129–144.

Zimmerman, M. A., Washienko, K. M., Walters, B., & Dyer, S. (1996). The development of a measure of enculturation for Native American youth. *American Journal of Community Psychology, 24,* 295–310.

CHAPTER SIX

Sexual Minority and Gender-Variant Adults

Resiliencies and Vulnerabilities in Health Care

Maria Messina and Sel L. Hwahng

INTRODUCTION

Although there may be no obvious physical, social, or linguistic markers that distinguish lesbian, gay, bisexual, trans/gender-variant[1] and queer or questioning (LGBTQ) persons from their heterosexual counterparts, outside major cities such as New York, Chicago, or San Francisco, and other metropolitan areas in the United States, social exposure to and interpersonal contact with LGBTQ persons are likely to occur with much less frequency. For those unfamiliar with LGBTQ people, this chapter begins with a section titled "Definition of Terms: Sexual Minority Nomenclature," which provides a general introduction to issues related to sexual self-perceptions, sexual orientations, and gender identities. This section outlines particular vulnerabilities related to physical and mental health morbidity and resiliency within various subpopulations. It is, therefore, not exhaustive of any one topic.

Based on epidemiological and social scientific data, the next section ("Challenges") identifies health-care needs for LGBTQ populations, with particular emphasis on LGBTQ people of color. It pinpoints potential stressors and barriers to seeking health care for LGBTQ populations as well as

---

[1]"Gender-variant" is to "transgender" what "MSM" is to "gay men." Both "gender-variant" and "MSM" are descriptive (versus identity) terms, and "gender-variant" connotes a much broader spectrum beyond the assumption of a binary sex/gender system where an individual crosses over from one gender to the other, often through hormone therapy and/or sexual reassignment surgery.

recognizes unique concerns for each subpopulation (e.g., Hwahng & Lin, 2009). A stressor is a stimulus or circumstance that causes a mentally or emotionally disruptive or upsetting condition that is capable of affecting physical or mental health, usually characterized by increased heart rate, a rise in blood pressure, muscular tension, irritability, and depression (Meyer, 1995, 2003). Within the context of health-care needs, the general diversity within LGBTQ communities, or the specific diversity within each subpopulation, whether by geographic locale, socioeconomic status, ethnicity, education, or individual proclivities, is emphasized.

Over the past few decades, researchers, public health practitioners and clinicians have come to realize that LGBTQ persons have unique health concerns (Dean et al., 2000; GLMA, 2001; Harcourt, 2006; Mayer et al., 2008). The *Journal of the American Medical Association* (1996) states that same-sex partners have the same concerns as opposite-sex partners across the lifespan, but some diseases are particularly relevant to men and women who have same-sex partners. Areas of unique exposure to risk are related to sexual behaviors, sexual orientation, and gender identity (Meyer, 2001).

There is a compendium of terms or labels to identify individuals attracted to the same gender or same sex. Inherent to this discussion is the understanding that these labels, LGBTQ, reflect highly diverse individuals who have been classified by "expert others," that is, doctors and scientists, who historically pathologized same-sex relations (Epstein, 2003). This inclination to classify (Needham, 1978), in particular, the continuum of sexual behaviors, orientations, and desires is a modern western proclivity where sexuality has become an important part of identity (Caplan, 1987).

The acronyms Lesbian, Gay, Bisexual, Transgender, Questioning (LGBTQ), women who have sex with women (WSW), men who have sex with men (MSM), as well as sexual minorities (SM) are used here. In referring to ethnic minorities, Black with a capital "B" is used instead of African American, because it subsumes African and Afro-Caribbean Americans, White, "W," refers to European or Caucasian Americans, Latino refers to those from Latin America, "API" refers to Asian Americans and Pacific Islander Americans, and Native Americans refer to the indigenous people in North America. However, the ethnic and gender identity terminologies used by individual researchers are retained.

Diversity

Despite the remarkable diversity within LGBTQ populations, experiences of stigma, discrimination, rejection, hostility, and violence unite them across cultures and geographic locales (Northridge, 2001) and are discussed below. Although the body of literature is growing, knowledge about LGBTQ health-care needs and experiences is relatively new, demographically uneven, and at times conflicting (Sullivan & Losberg, 2003). Data often cannot be generalized because the research methodologies vary (Cochran, Keenan, Schober, & Mays, 2000; Solarz, 1999) and key issues are imprecisely conceptualized or measured (Swann & Anastas, 2003). Because of the AIDS epidemic in the 1980s, more research has been conducted on HIV among gay men and to a lesser extent lesbians, than research on other public health issues. Where there is research addressing LGBTQ health (LaSala, 2003) it generally excludes bisexual and trans/gender-variant persons and underrepresents ethnic/racial minorities, the poor, and uneducated.

Trans/gender-variant health in general has not been a focus of specialized clinical care because of an even greater lack of data and resources than with gay and lesbian health as well as resistance to identification due to potential for discrimination or social isolation (Elze, 2006; Sullivan & Losberg, 2003; Swann & Anastas, 2003). There is also a dearth of research on aspects of trans/gender-variant people of color populations including API trans/gender-variant people (Hwahng & Lin, 2009; Nemoto, Operario, Keatley, Han, & Soma, 2004).

Moreover, identities are complex, multifaceted, and should not be reduced to a single dimension (Caplan, 1987; Herek, 2004). Sexuality is but one facet of human identity, the importance of which may vary from context to context as well as from person to person (JAMA, 1996). In certain contexts, for example, ethnic identity may take precedence over sexual orientation. A lesbian Asian American might emphasize her ethnicity rather than her sexual orientation when with family, because she cannot risk losing their social support or being ostracized within a racially biased world.

Great variation also exists within the more marginalized Latino, Black/African- and Asian-American subpopulations who do not necessarily experience or define sexual orientation or relate to the world in the same way (Hwahng & Nuttbrock, 2007). Research indicates that men of color are less likely to identify as gay even though they have sex with other men (Hunter, Shannon, Knox, & Martin's, 1998).

Barriers to Care

Fearing real or perceived discrimination from medical providers prevents many LGBTQ persons from revealing their sexual orientations and gender identities (Mayer et al., 2008; Weisz, 2009). One of the most significant health risks among LGBTQ is avoidance of seeking routine medical care and dissatisfaction with services (Bovicini & Perlin, 2003). Although great progress has been made in health care for LGBTQ persons, research shows that there are still doctors who are reluctant or refuse to treat them, or who think it better for patients to withhold their sexual orientation (Finlon, 2002). Including disclosure of sexual behavior and activity in a medical exam is crucial for the provider in determining risk for particular diseases and prevention strategies.

Trans/gender-variant persons may have an even greater struggle to receive adequate medical care than do WSW and MSM. Some doctors refuse treatment, insist on using wrong pronouns, or do not provide necessary services (Lombardi, 2001). Physicians who willingly provide services may fail to distinguish sexual orientation from gender identity and think trans/gender-variant persons' health-care needs are the same as gay and lesbian patients (Finlon, 2002).

Similar to trans/gender-variant populations, bisexual person's health-care needs are inadequately addressed; they are frequently viewed as incomplete lesbians or gay men (Finlon, 2002). Substandard health care is inevitable when providers focus on the labels instead of the person, behaviors, or symptoms (Dean et al., 2000). Health-care providers may not be aware of or trained for understanding specific health experiences for lesbian, gay, bisexual, transgender, queer, or questioning persons (Garnets & D'Augelli, 1994; Johnson, Mimiaga, & Bradford, 2008; Rothblum, 1994; Wolfe, 1998). To address these gaps and educate the new generation of physicians on sexual minorities and health, the American College of Physicians has issued the Fenway Guide to Lesbian, Gay, Bisexual, and Transgender patients (Mayer et al., 2008).

Systemic barriers to adequate health care for LGBTQ persons are often informed by homophobia and transphobia in mainstream U.S. culture. These barriers include lack of benefits for same-sex partners or children of nonheterosexual couples. Unlike other industrialized countries, sex reassignment surgery is not covered by insurance in the United States (Dean et al., 2000). Unless advance directives such as health-care proxies or power of attorney are arranged, same-sex partners have no say in the disposition of an incapacitated partner in most states, and are restricted or denied access in emergency rooms, inpatient units, or foster care agencies (Dean et al., 2000). Although much progress has been made in providing specialized health care for LGBTQ populations in urban areas, the same is not true for LGBTQ clients in the more sparsely populated rural areas (Finlon, 2002).

LGBTQ and Family

In addition to clinical care issues, LGBTQ's relationship with their families can affect their engagement with health care (Mayer et al., 2008). Regulatory, programmatic, and legislative/policy definitions need LGBTQ-inclusive definitions of family since they lack access to rights and benefits of legal marriage. Increasingly, LGBTQ persons are raising families or adopting children and seek LGBTQ-friendly adoption agencies and legal services. LGBTQ persons are coming out at an earlier age and seeking support from clinicians (D'Augelli & Hershberger, 1993) further emphasizing the need for clinicians to be educated about and sensitized to the needs of sexual and gender minorities. Because LGBTQ elders are not legally sanctioned partners, they have less support than non-LGBTQ elders and less security regarding care of partners when they are catastrophically ill (Cahill, South, & Spade, 2000).

DEFINITION OF TERMS: SEXUAL MINORITY NOMENCLATURE

Defining sexuality is problematic. The terms sex, gender, and gender identity are used in different ways and can be confusing. The way in which cultures define the nature of human sexuality and of masculinity and femininity are notions that do not entirely reflect biology, but are largely the result of socio-cultural processes (Ortner & Whitehead, 1981). Even the emphasis placed on biological factors and the perception of the biological body and its "natural" divisions is not the same in all cultures (Ardener, 1977). Most societies tend to use a limited set of physical features (particularly sex organs) as the primary way of determining the sex of a person as well as their assumed gender (Butler, 1993). However, many societies also have alternative systems in which the "materiality" of the body is based on social attributes such as spirituality and role specialization as primary sources for selecting sex and gender (Gilley, 2006; Johnson, 1997; Kulick, 1998; Morris, 1994; Nanda, 1999; Prieur, 1998; Reddy, 2005; Roscoe, 1998; Sinnott, 2004).

The most familiar binary sex and gender model uses "sex" to describe the body—the biological (chromosomal) and anatomical (internal and external genitalia) that society recognizes as male or female (Makadon, Mayer, Potter, & Goldhammer, 2007). According to this dichotomous model, every person is defined as either male or female; gender is fixed and rooted in biological sex and the accepted gender identity and role reflect the apparent physical sex. Due to advocacy by trans/gender-variant and intersex people and social movements, new models that could be described as "polysexual" or "polygender" are developing that venture away from the fixed, dichotomous depiction of men and women that excludes intersex people, those who perceive themselves as being a gender different from the one assigned at birth, or feel "other" than male or female (Beemyn, 2005).

In addition, a cross-cultural perspective indicates that some cultures include more than two sexes/genders. For example, alternative, third-sex/gender and fourth-sex/gender roles that are neither man nor woman and/or may combine the roles of man and woman, have been described among the *hijras* in India (Nanda, 1999; Reddy, 2005), berdaches/two-spirits[2] among Native American societies (Jacobs, Thomas, & Lang, 1997; Roscoe, 1998; Williams, 1992) and the Sambia in New Guinea (Herdt, 1994).

Moreover, because U.S. culture has been mostly influenced by Euro-American values and systems, there is a long tradition of pathologizing same-sex orientation and behavior (Cochran, 2001). Interestingly enough, the binary sex and gender system embedded in our society does not fully encompass the complete spectrum of what is found in nature. For every 1000 children born, about 17 have ambiguous genitalia that neither fits neatly into the category of male nor female and are referred to as "intersexuals" (Fausto-Sterling, 2000). Intersex individuals are born with sex chromosomes, external genitalia, and/or internal reproductive organs that are not exclusively male or female. Previously, genital variations were surgically altered to conform to male or female in infancy, but current guidelines now advocate waiting until adulthood for intersex individuals to choose their identity since forming a gender identity is a complex biological and social process that may take years (Lee et al., 2006).

---

[2]*Two-spirit* is a contemporary term adopted in 1990 from the Northern Algonquin word *niizh manitoag*, which means "two-spirits." This term signified the embodiment of both feminine and masculine spirits within one person (Anguksuar, 1997). It is implied, then, that heterosexual women and men primarily embody one spirit, a feminine or masculine spirit, respectively. Traditionally, indigenous values had respected sexual and gender diversity and many two-spirits had sacred, ceremonial, and/or leadership roles in their communities (Gilley, 2006; Lang, 1997; Roscoe, 1998). European colonization imposed compulsory Christianity and the suppression of two-spirit roles in many Native American communities (Balsam, Huang, Fieland, Simoni, & Walters, 2004; Gilley, 2006).

Sexual Orientation and Gender Variance

Here, sexual orientation refers to whom one is attracted: androphilic (attracted to males), gynephilic (attracted to females) as well as gay, lesbian, bisexual, and heterosexual. According to Sell (2007) sexual orientation has three dimensions: desire/attraction, behavior and identity. Sexual behavior might not correspond to sexual orientation, identity or attraction (Marrazzo, 2004; Sell, 1997/2007). Moreover, individual sexual behavior and orientation might vary over time (JAMA, 1996). Gender identity refers to the self-perception of being a man, woman, or another sex or gender.

Generally speaking, homosexual refers to persons engaging in "same-sex" relations and tends to refer more specifically to males. Originally, "homosexual" was a medical term used to classify "deviant" sexual behavior as a "disease" in the 19th century where the primary purpose was to cure homosexual "perversions" through hormonal injection, genital manipulation, brain surgery, hypnosis, and shock therapy (Katz, 1992; Stein, 2007). Homosexuality was considered as mental illness until the American Psychiatric Association took it out of the Diagnostic and Statistical Manual of Mental Illnesses (DSM) in 1973 and The American Psychological Association Council of Representatives, in 1975. It was not until the late 20th century that same-sex behaviors were decriminalized in the United States. In Lawrence v. Texas, in 2003, Justice Kennedy of the U.S. Supreme Court removed legislation criminalizing same-gender sexual relations throughout the country. Moreover, in its revised policy statement of 2008, the American Psychological Association (2008) recognized the benefit and medical necessity of gender transition treatments, resolved to support the provision of these treatments, and called upon public and private insurers to cover them (APA, 2008).

"Gay" antedates "homosexual" by several centuries and has a rich history of meanings (Boswell, 1980). In contemporary usage, gay is different from homosexual in that it is a "self-assigned" characterization of persons who have a conscious erotic preference for their own gender (Boswell, 1980). "Lesbian" is a 20th-century construct used to differentiate women with romantic and sexual desire for women. However, not all women who engage in sexual relations with other women identify as lesbian (Laumann, Gagnon, Michael, & Michael, 1994; Marrazzo, Coffey, & Bingham, 2005). Earlier on the AIDS epidemic, scientific and medical experts identified being gay as a risk factor for HIV (Epstein, 1996; Padilla, Vasquez, & Parker, 2007; Patton, 1990; Treichler, 1988; Watney, 1988). However, health researchers soon discovered that there were many individuals participating in same-sex behavior who did not identify as "gay." The acronym "MSM," for "men who have sex with men," is currently used to characterize sexual behavior, not identity. Likewise, the acronym, "WSW" for "women who have sex with women" characterizes and emphasizes sexual practice and not identify self-perception. "MSMW" ("men who have sex with men and women") and WSWM ("women who have sex with women and men") apply to individuals who have sexual relations with both the same and opposite sex.

Trans/gender-variant persons are those who live part time or full time in the gender role of the opposite biologic sex (Lawrence, Shaffer, Snow, Chase, & Headlam, 1996; Lawrence, 2007). Some trans/gender-variant persons (both MTF and FTM) are only attracted to males (androphilic), some only to females (gynephilic), some are attracted to both males and females (androphilic/gynephilic), and there are even some attracted neither to males nor females (asexual) (American Boyz, 2001; Nuttbrock et al., 2009b). There also appears to be racial differences in relation to sexual attraction. A recent New York City study found that 90% of Black and Latina transfeminine people were androphilic while only 20% of White transfeminine people were androphilic (Nuttbrock et al., Epub ahead of print). Self-identifying trans/gender-variant nomenclature is vast and ever evolving.[3] Male-to-female trans/gender-variant persons, "MTFs," or transfeminine people are biological males who, with or without sex reassignment surgery, often identify and live as women part time or full time. Female-to-male trans/gender-variant persons, "FTMs," or transmasculine people are biological females who, with or without sex reassignment surgery, often live and identify as men part or full time. Research among gender-variant immigrant Southeast Asian and Latina/o MTF participants revealed a mixing of genders where some participants identified either as a "gay man" and a "queen," or as "male" and a "woman," and at the same time strongly identified with their male genitalia (Hwahng &

---

[3]Mason (2006) cites over 60 terms, including: Androgyne, Autogynephillic, Bi-Gendered, Bio Man, Bio Woman, Butch Queen, Butch Queen Up in Drags, Conceptually Gendered, Crossdresser, Differently Gendered, Femme, Femme Male, Femme Queen, Full Time, Gender Bender, Gender Curious, Gender Dualist, Gender Dysphoric, Gender Emerging, Gender Euphoric, Gender Evolving, Gender Fluid, Gender Fuck, Gender inverted, Gender Migrator, Gender Queer, Gender Questioning, Gender Variant, Homosexual Transsexual, Hormonally Challenged, Intergendered, Liminal Gendered, Non Op Transsexual, Non Passing, Omni-Gendered, Out, Closeted, Over Dresser, Pan Gendered, Part Time, Passing, Poly Gendered, Post Op Transsexual, Pre Op Transsexual, Queen, T-Girl, Trannie, Trans Lesbian, Transbian, Transdyke, Transgenderist, Transman, Transsexual, Transvestite, and Transwoman.

Nuttbrock, 2007). The term "trans/gender-variant" itself can be confusing as it is a colloquial yet widely accepted umbrella term applied to a wide variety of individuals who see themselves as partly or completely the opposite sex or gender than that of their natal sex. Many trans/gender-variant persons can become emotionally and/or physically ill when unable to live their desired gender. Placed under this trans/gender-variant umbrella, are cross dressers, preoperative transsexuals, postoperative transsexuals, and those who identify as nonoperative transsexuals. Trans/gender-variant people may or may not live full time in their preferred social presentation of gender. Some individuals attracted to the same-sex reject any of the LGBTQ labels and self-identify as "queer," emphasizing that they are atypical, "unusual," or "odd." "Questioning," particularly refers to youth who are not yet certain of their sexual orientation or gender identity.

Labeling Practices

Having said this, there are still some epistemological and epidemiological concerns with labeling practices. Although some people choose lesbian, gay, bisexual, and trans/gender-variant, others choose queer, or other labels, and some gender-variant individuals may not relate to these labels at all (Eliason & Schope, 2007). Gender identity formation is a highly individualized process. Some may develop a gender or sexual identity but may not affiliate, or do not have the opportunity to participate within a larger LGBTQ community, especially in rural areas (Finlon, 2002). To further emphasize the problematic nature of labeling, Herek (2004) challenges the utility of even using the acronym "LGBTQ." On the other hand, some intersex persons would like to see "intersex" added, thus "LGBTQI" (Pattatuchi-Aragon, 2006). Those classified as deviant or other seek to establish the terms of their own identities (Herek, 2004).

CHALLENGES

Although existing research on sexual and gender minorities is limited, data indicate clinical issues that disproportionately affect LGBTQ persons include substance abuse, tobacco use, and body mass index issues, such as being overweight and obese (Dean et al., 2000; Makadon et al., 2007; Wolitski, Stall, Valdiserri, Denning, & Levine, 2007; Cochran et al., 2001) as well as depression and anxiety disorders (Cochran, 2001; Mayer et al., 2008). For example, LGBTQ persons collectively are 40–70% more likely to smoke than non-LGBT persons (Makadon et al., 2007). These disorders are not inherently pathological to LGBTQ persons but are more likely to result from living marginalized lives, concealing sexual identity, or enduring stress from rejection, hostility or violence expressed verbally, emotionally or physically by intolerant family or community members (Cochran, 2001; Meyer, 2003; Mills et al., 2004; Safren & Heimberg, 1999). Among the leading indicators by Healthy People 2010 (GLMA, 2001, p. 1), the "prevention agenda" and "roadmap for improving the health of all people in the United States during the first decade of the twenty-first century," states that as a group, MSM are at increased risk for sexually transmitted infections (STIs), anal cancer, and mental health disorders (Royal, 2006).

STIGMA

LGBTQ individuals still suffer disproportionately from social stigma, violence, and exclusion from health care based on sexual orientations and gender identities and expression, which have adversely impacted their overall health (Cochran, 2001; Herek, Chopp, & Strohl, 2007; National Coalition LGBT Health, 2009; Padilla et al., 2007). LGBTQ may also be members of other communities with health disparities which introduce more vulnerability: racial/ethnic, linguistic, geographic, and in some cases, must also cope with poverty or immigration status (Hwahng & Nuttbrock, 2007; National Coalition for LBGT Health, 2009). LGBTQ people of color are often described as experiencing "multiple-minority status" or "multiple jeopardy," which are compounded stressors resulting from socioeconomic status, racism, discrimination, homophobia, immigration and migration experiences, and other stressors that may work in tandem with each other (Balsam et al., 2004; Bowleg, Huang, Brooks, Black, & Burkholder, 2003; King, 1998). For example, specific stressors for the API LGBTQ population include trauma from war and violence, racism, and factors related to acculturation (Hwahng & Lin, 2009).

Stigma and MSM Ethnic/Racial Minorities

Some African Americans, API, and other ethnic minorities experience the gay and lesbian community as racist and their ethnic communities as homophobic (Battle & Crum, 2007; Chan, 1989; Dang & Vianney, 2007; Diaz, Ayala, Bein, Henne, & Marin, 2001a; Mays & Cochran, 1988).

Social epidemiologists have studied how social marginalization compromises mental and physical health of already marginalized people (Krieger, 2001; Link & Phelan, 2001). Compared to White Americans,

Black Americans have suffered from greater morbidity and mortality from diabetes, hypertension, cardiovascular diseases, HIV/AIDS, renal disease, many types of cancer, and other maladies (Battle & Crum, 2007; Krieger, Rowley, Herman, Avery, & Philip, 1993). Scholars hypothesize three pathways through which stigma and marginalization lead to poorer health and well-being: perceived discrimination, disadvantageous social structures, and internalized stigma (Battle & Crum, 2007). Structural determinants or institutionalized racism, for example, affect the material environment which "then becomes the pathway—through differential exposure to pollution, crime, neighborhood services, food availability, good schools, information, and the like—to the health disparity" (Battle & Crum, 2007, p. 322).

Homosexual and racial stigma may cause negative mental and physical health outcomes (Kessler, Michelson, & Williams, 1999a; Meyer, 1995). As an example, stigma based on homophobia is associated with depression, low self-esteem and sexual risk behaviors among White and Latino gay males (Ramirez-Valles, 2007). Additional cultural barriers for Latino MSM have been identified as machismo, homophobia, family loyalty, sexual silence, poverty, and racism that have led to internalized shame, secrecy, and low self-esteem. It is important to view these barriers not as personal deficits, but as logical outcomes or specific manifestations of socialization processes in the sexual lives of Latino MSM (Diaz, 1998).

Research indicates that there is greater social stigma attached to being gay in African–American communities compared to European–American communities. African Americans are thus, less likely to disclose their gay status (Kennamer, Honnold, Bradford, & Hendricks, 2000). Studies examining how African–American MSM manage their multiple-minority identities, including being both ethnic/racial and sexual minorities, suggest that African–American MSM view ethnicity, gender, and religious beliefs as of primary importance, and sexual orientation and social class as less salient aspects of their identities (Goode-Cross & Good, 2009; Battle & Crum, 2007). In a multiethnic, multisite study of internalized homonegativity (IH) among HIV-positive MSM, higher IH was significantly associated with African–American ethnicity/race (Ross, Rosser, & Neumaier, 2008). IH was also associated with compulsive sexual behavior, openness as MSM, depression, education level, and the importance of religion. Those with higher IH engaged in serodiscordant[4]

---

[4]One partner HIV−, one partner HIV+.

unprotected anal intercourse, disclosed serostatus to secondary partners less frequently, and had lower condom self-efficacy (Ross et al., 2008).

Ethnic Communities, Trauma, and Pathologization

It is important, however, not to pathologize ethnic communities as inherently homophobic. Historically, LGBTQ people of color have been pathologized according to ethnicity. For instance, Asian–American LGBTQ communities and people have been pathologized as inherently asexual and/or sexually passive and docile, and socially submissive (Fung, 1991; Han, 2008; Scott, Gilliam, & Braxton, 2005), whereas low-income African–American and Latino LGBTQ people may be pathologized as inherently sexually irresponsible, and socially dysfunctional and violent (Cohen, 1999; Mercer, 1993). It is thus, imperative to contextualize any measured characteristics, behaviors, and experiences within a multilevel social ecological framework that takes into account the fundamental connections between structural, interpersonal, and intrapsychic forces and dynamics (Duran & Walters, 2004) and utilizes eco-social theory (Krieger, 1994). Previous literature has contextualized contemporary homonegative and sexual-negative norms within historical contexts of trauma (including sexual trauma) that have accumulated over time into current cultural "norms" that are often reinforced within interpersonal and family dynamics that also affect the intrapsychic or "intrapersonal" levels (Simoni, Walters, Balsam, & Meyers, 2006). For instance, among Native Americans the cumulative and intergenerational effects of historical traumas such as genocide, ethnocide, colonization, germ warfare, forced removal from tribal lands, and the forced separation of children from parents are viewed as a "soul wound" and may be related to negative mental health outcomes such as "historical trauma response," posttraumatic stress disorder, alienation, depression, alcohol abuse, and HIV risk, in which Native American two-spirit people experience much more historical trauma compared to heterosexual Native Americans (Duran & Walters, 2004; Simoni, Sehgal, & Walters, 2004).

ETHNIC COMMUNITIES, RESILIENCY, AND CULTURAL BUFFERS

Despite experiences of physical and sexual abuse, discrimination, and substance abuse, cultural factors and personal strengths of LGBTQ people of color may function as buffers and protective mechanisms to negative effects of trauma and other stressors, strengthening mental health and mitigating the effects of stressors (Balsam et al., 2004; Duran & Walters, 2004). Enculturation is the process by which individuals learn about and identify with their ethnic minority culture and express the level of immersion into one's cultural heritage, norms, and traditional values. Zimmerman, Washienko, Walter, and Dyer (1996) suggest that enculturation as a protective mechanism can either mitigate the negative effects of risk factors or stressors or enhance the effects of another variable, such as identity attitudes, to decrease the probability of a negative health outcome.

In one study, Asian–American WSW who identified as Asian, had lower levels of internalized homophobia compared to those identified as Western, indicating greater psychological resiliency among the Asian-identified group (Singh, Chung, & Dean, 2007). Another study encouraged providers to be sensitive to the potential importance of Native American cultural and spiritual practices for two-spirit people (Balsam et al., 2004) that include culturally relevant approaches to healing from substance use, mental health problems, and trauma (Walters, 1997).

ABUSE AND VICTIMIZATION

LGBTQ people may be victims of childhood and/or adult victimization and abuse due to LGBTQ-related discrimination. Abuse and victimization are also often associated with negative health outcomes and behaviors, such as negative mental health, substance use, and high-risk sexual behaviors. Across ethnic groups, Latino/a, Black, two-spirits, and White LGBTQ people experience higher rates of childhood abuse than do their heterosexual counterparts (Corliss, Cochran, & Mays, 2002; Holmes, 1997; Huebner, Rebchook, & Kegeles, 2004; Tjaden, Thoeness, & Allison, 1999). Austin et al. (2008) revealed that in comparison to WSMO (women who have sex with men only), WSW were more likely to report both childhood physical abuse and childhood sexual abuse victimization. In addition, compared to WSMO, WSW who had experienced childhood victimization were also more likely to experience revictimization during adolescence. Other studies also indicate that WSW were more likely to report childhood physical or sexual abuse, childhood and adolescent sexual orientation victimization (verbal, physical, and/or sexual), and lifetime sexual or physical abuse (Cooperman, Simoni, & Lockhart, 2003; D'Augelli, 2003; Descamps, Rothblum, Bradford, & Ryan, 2000; Saewyc, Bearinger, Blum, & Renick, 1999; Scheer et al., 2003). In a study comparing WSW with their WSMO siblings, WSW reported higher levels of psychological, physical, and sexual violence in both childhood and adult-hood (Balsam, Rothblum, & Beauchaine, 2005). Research also indicates that WSW may experience adult abuse and victimization as a continua-tion of the cycle of childhood and adolescent abuse and victimization, and thus adult victimization is actually a "revictimization" arising from prior trauma and abuse (Balsam et al., 2004, 2005). WSW of color often experience higher rates of lifetime victimization compared to White WSW (Descamps et al., 2000; Morris & Balsam, 2003).

Native American two-spirit participants reported experiencing childhood physical abuse from caretakers (40%) nearly twice as high as Native American heterosexual participants (20%) (Balsam et al., 2004). This finding is especially important since the general Native American population already experiences violent victimization more than 2.5 times than that of the overall U.S. population (Greenfield & Smith, 1999). Walters, Simoni, and Howarth (2001) also reported greater lifetime preva-lence of physical assault (36%) and sexual assault (29%) among Native American two-spirit men as compared to non-Native American LGBTQ people. In a national study of 2483 lesbians across the United States, Native American two-spirit females reported the highest rates of physical and sexual abuse and assault, both in childhood and adulthood, compared to Black, Latina, Asian American, and White lesbians (Morris & Balsam, 2003). Transfeminine (MTF trans/gender-variant) people of color reported high levels of gender-related adolescent abuse. In descending order, the highest percentage of adolescent abuse reported by transfeminine people was among Latinas, Blacks and then, Whites (Hwahng & Nuttbrock, 2009).

Domestic Violence

Domestic violence (DV) is also known as "intimate partner violence" or IPV and is a public health concern that greatly impacts women's and men's health (Bornstein, Fawcett, Sullivan, Senturia, & Shiu-Thorton, 2006). Research indicates similar or even higher rates of DV in same-sex couples as in opposite-sex couples (Brown & Groscup, 2009). Research also suggests that severity and types of abuse experienced by same-sex partners follow the same "cycle of violence" as in opposite-sex partners (Renzetti, 1997; Stanley, Bartholomew, Taylor, Oram, & Landolt, 2006). Nonetheless, there is a difference in terms of legal protection and community services available. Delaware, Louisiana, Montana, New York, South Carolina, and Virginia explicitly deny protection to gay and lesbian relationships and 14 states have domestic violence laws that only apply to "household members" (Gay and Lesbian Task Force, 2005). A recent study indicates that male victims of same-sex IPV reported more verbal abuse than male victims of opposite-sex IPV, and higher percentages of women in same-sex relationships experienced more verbal, physical, and sexual IPV than women in opposite-sex relationships. In addition, in urban areas same-sex victims (both male and female) were more than twice as likely to report poor self-perceived health status compared to female opposite-sex victims (Blosnich & Bossarte, 2009).

MENTAL HEALTH

Cochran's 2001 research suggests that the "onset, course, treatment and prevention of mental disorders among gay men and lesbians differ in important ways from those of other individuals" (Bieschke, McClanahan, Tozer, Grzegorek, & Park, 2000; Cabaj & Stein, 1996; Morrow, 2000). Social stigma engendered by homosexuality (or variable gender expression) places gay men, lesbians, (and trans/gender-variant persons) at greater risk for psychiatric morbidity than heterosexuals (Green, 2005; - Haldeman, 1994), especially for depression, and possibly, anxiety (Cochran, 2001). LGBTQ individuals appear to have "heightened risk" for stress-sensitive disorders that are generally related to antihomosexual bias (Cochran & Mays, 2007, 2009).

Yoshikawa, Wilson, Chae, and Cheng (2004) reported that discrimination on racial grounds, immigration status, and homophobia increased depressive symptoms in Asian/Pacific Islander MSM and were associated with high rates of unprotected anal intercourse with secondary partners. Current research indicates that Black MSM are disproportionately burdened by depressive distress and anxiety disorders as compared to their White gay and heterosexual counterparts (Graham, Braithwaite, Spikes, Stephens, & Edu, 2009) due to multiple stigmatized social statuses (Cochran & Mays, 1994).

In a study of African–American gay and bisexual men (GBM), individuals who possess more positive (i.e., integrated) self-identification as African American and gay reported higher levels of self-esteem, HIV prevention self-efficacy, stronger social support networks, greater levels of life satisfaction, and lower levels of psychological distress than their counterparts who reported less positive (i.e., less well integrated) African–American and gay identity development. The more AAGBM are able to integrate and hold positive self-attitudes toward their racial-ethnic and sexual identities, the more likely they are to value themselves, protect their health, and experience greater levels of personal contentment. These findings affirm the importance of successful integration and simultaneous validation of these various identities to the overall psychosocial health of African American GBM (Crawford, Allison, Zamboni, & Soto, 2002). Studies on Asian and Pacific Islander MSM reveal similar findings regarding ethnic and sexual identity integration and health outcomes (Hwahng & Lin, 2009).

Balsam and colleagues (2004) state that Native American two-spirit clients may exhibit PTSD and other psychological symptoms that are also not clearly linked to discrete events but may also experience "secondary trauma," that is, traumas experienced vicariously through their family and community (Amir & Lev-Wiesel, 2004; Hesse, Main, Abrams, & Rifkin, 2003; Rowland-Klein, 2004). Among transfeminine people in New York City, Nuttbrock et al. (2010) found that lifetime major depression was 54% among transfeminine people, which was almost three times higher than the corresponding estimate in the general population (20%) (Kessler, Borges, & Walters, 1999). In addition, among transfeminine people, lifetime suicide ideation was 54%, which was more than 3× higher than in the general population (13.5%), lifetime suicide plan was 35.0%, which was 9× higher than in the general population (3.9%), and lifetime suicide attempts was 27.9%, which was 7× higher than in the general population (4.6%). It thus appears that the transfeminine population in New York City is very depressed and has high rates of negative mental health. A study in San Francisco of transfeminine people of color found that Latinas had the highest levels of depression, followed by Blacks, and then APIs (Nemoto et al., 2004)

Alcohol, Tobacco, and Other Drug Use

Despite the "plethora of methodological problems" with existing research on sexual orientation and alcohol use, Hughes, Wilsnak, Johnson, and Timothy (2006) state that on the whole it appears that lesbians and gay men across ethnicities are more likely to drink alcohol and report related problems than heterosexual counterparts, most likely because of the stigma and marginalization they experience (Burgard, Cochran, & Mays, 2005; Trocki, Drabble, & Midanik, 2005). In general, WSW smoke at approximately twice the rate of heterosexual women (Burgard et al., 2005; Tang et al., 2004). WSWM face a higher risk for excessive alcohol consumption compared to exclusively WSWO (women who have sex with women only) (Burgard et al., 2005). Hahm and colleagues (2008) found that young Asian–American women aged between 18 and 27 years who self-identified as nonheterosexual were more likely to initiate tobacco use, binge drinking, marijuana use, and other drug use than both Asian–American sexual-minority males and heterosexual peers. Two studies in NYC targeting mostly drug-using low-income women of color found that WSW were significantly more likely to have a lifetime history of cocaine use and be cocaine dependent or crack dependent than WSMO (Ompad et al., in press). White LGBTQ people are significantly more likely to engage in lifetime illicit drug use compared to their White heterosexual peers (Cochran, 2001; Hughes & Eliason, 2002).

Male-to-female trans/gender-variant persons may also be at greater risk for substance misuse and risky sexual behaviors (Clements, Wilkinson, Kitano, & Marx, 2001; Nuttbrock et al., 2009a). In contrast to Native American heterosexuals, two-spirit people also showed significantly higher rates of lifetime illicit drug use, had their first alcoholic drink at a younger age, and were significantly more likely to use alcohol to improve sociability, relax, make friends, decrease feelings of inferiority, manage their moods, manage feeling down or depressed, forget, or relieve tension (Balsam et al., 2004). Polydrug use was significantly higher among Vietnamese and Korean MSM compared to Chinese MSM, and also significantly higher among MSM 18–24-years old (Operario et al., 2006).

MSM and Methamphetamine

Recreational drug use, particularly methamphetamine (Speed, Meth, Crystal, Ice, Tina, etc.), is prevalent and a serious public health concern especially among MSM (Colfax et al., 2004, 2005; NIDA, 2009). "Meth" is reported to increase libido and sexual pleasure, the ability to have sex for longer periods of time, and with prolonged use, the inability to ejaculate or achieve an orgasm (Halkitis, Shrem, & Martin, 2005). Meth may also lower inhibitions. Users may exhibit compulsive sexual behavior, be less apt to use condoms, and because of prolonged periods of sex, the delicate linings in the rectum or oral cavities may tear, chafe or become raw greatly increasing the risk for HIV and other STIs (Halkitis et al., 2005). There is a growing body of social and ethnographic research showing that different groups or subpopulations of MSM use crystal methamphetamine and other drugs in different ways that carry different risks (Wainberg, Kolodny, & Drescher, 2006). Clatts, Welle, Goldsamt (2001) caution against making a causal relationship between "speed" (Meth) and risky sexual behaviors and instead emphasize the importance of individual agency of users, who consciously or unconsciously, often have specific expectations about what they want from the experience.

PHYSICAL HEALTH

Sexually Transmitted Infections

STIs are indications of risky sexual practices that facilitate transmission of HIV (Wolitski et al., 2007). The recent increases in STI among men who report sex with men but who do not identify themselves as gay also show that simply asking patients their self-defined sexual orientation is not adequate. JAMA (1996) emphasizes that it is the specific behaviors, not sexual orientation that put people at risk for contracting HIV and other STIs (Mayer et al., 2008). Much research has already indicated how the HIV epidemic has been shaped primarily by the social contextual factors of race, ethnicity, and socio-economic status (Cohen, 1999; Levenson, 2004; Omi & Winant, 1994). More recent research on white, economically privileged transfeminine people, transmasculine people, MSM, and heterosexuals have all indicated low or relatively low HIV seroprevalence (Levenson, 2004; Nuttbrock et al., 2009a, 2009b; Sevelius, 2009). Recent research has indicated that sexual networks and partner concurrency determine HIV risk more than individual sexual behaviors (Bohl, Raymond, Arnold, & McFarland, 2009; Cassels, Pearson, Walters, Simoni, & Morris, 2010; Hart & Elford, 2010).

Based on risk factors, HIV cases were classified in the following hierarchy of transmission categories: (1) male-to-male sexual contact, (2) injection-drug use, (3) both male-to-male sexual contact and injection-drug use, (4) high-risk heterosexual contact (i.e., with a person of the opposite sex known to have HIV or an HIV risk factor) (MMWR, 2008). The highest rate of transmission of HIV to WSW/WSWM is among women who participate in intravenous drug use or have sexual intercourse with MSMW (who may or may not identify as bisexual).

WSW and HIV/STIs

According to the U.S. Department of Health and Human Services (DHHS, 2005) WSW are at risk for the same STIs as heterosexual women and can transmit STIs to each other through skin-to-skin contact, mucosa contact, vaginal fluids, and menstrual blood. Sharing sex toys are another means of STI transmission. The risk for STI transmission among women with same-sex partners depends on the particular STI and the sexual practices involved (Center for Disease Control (CDC), 2006a; Marrazzo, 2004). Although the rate of transmission of STIs between women is probably low relative to WSMO, research indicates that most lesbians have had sexual contact with men, even those who self-identify as lesbians (Diamant, Schuster, McGuigan, & Lever, 1999; van Dam, Koh, & Dibble, 2001). However, there were some significant differences for certain HIV risk factors between the two groups. WSW were significantly younger, more likely to be homeless, have an illegal income source, and have a history of incarceration, less likely to be on public assistance, and less likely to have children than WSMO (Ompad et al., in press).

Transmission of HIV between lesbians is thought to be rare (JAMA, 1996). Some subsets of WSW are at greater risk for HIV than women who only have sex with men due to injection drug use, homelessness, and sexual behaviors with men (Young, Weissman, & Cohen, 1992). In 2008, Hispanic women's rate of HIV infection was nearly four times that the rate of white women (CDC, 2008). The HIV incidence rate for Black women was nearly 23 times as high as that of White women and nearly 4 times as high as that of Hispanic women (CDC, 2008).

WSW who are illicit drug users is one population of WSW who are at high risk for HIV, with seroprevalence ranging from 12.8% to 53% in samples of both noninjection drug users and injection drug users (IDUs) (Diaz, Vlahov, Greenberg, Cuevas, & Garfein, 2001b; Friedman, Curtis, Neaigus, Jose, & Des Jarlais, 1999; Ompad et al., in press). In addition, WSW IDUs constitute 20–30% of women IDUs (Friedman et al., 2003).

WSW's Physical Health

Lesbians face unique challenges that may negatively affect their physical and mental health in ways not shared by opposite-sex partners (Cochran, 2001). Because the risk for HIV infection and other STDs is lower for women who have sex with women (WSW) than for women who also have sex with men (WSWM), some WSW patients and physicians may assume that they are not at risk for gynecologic diseases such as breast, ovarian, or cervical cancer (JAMA, 1996; Marrazzo, 2004; Mayer et al., 2008). However, viruses that cause most cervical cancers can be sexually transmitted between women.

The number one killer among women is heart disease. Lesbian and bisexual women have unique risk factors for smoking (Hughes &

Johnson, 2003), heavy alcohol use and nulliparity. It is hypothesized that lesbians are more likely to be overweight and obese (also known as greater body mass index or BMI) than women of other sexual orientations, putting them at greater risk for cardiovascular disease, lipid abnormalities, glucose intolerance, and other problems due to inactivity (Boehmer, Bowen, & Bauer, 2007; Mayer et al., 2008).

MSM and HIV/STIs

Men who have sex with men (MSM) are at elevated risk for certain sexually transmitted diseases (STDs), including hepatitis A, hepatitis B, HIV/AIDS, syphilis, gonorrhea, and Chlamydia (CDC, 2009). HIV infection and AIDS have had a profound impact on MSM since the beginning of the epidemic. Seventy-one percent of adult male and adolescent new infections are MSM even though only approximately 5–7% identify as MSM (CDC, 2007b).

As mentioned, the literature indicates that MSM experience a disproportionate amount of childhood abuse. Studies suggest a link between childhood sexual abuse and adult HIV risk behaviors among the general MSM population and the Latino MSM population (Arreola, Neilands, & Diaz, 2009; Kalichman et al., 2001; Paul, Catania, Pollock, & Stall, 2001). Among two-spirit men, lifetime victimization significantly predicted lifetime HIV risk behaviors, was associated with sexual partner risk factors, and was associated with the frequency of failure to use a condom because of the influence of alcohol or drugs in the past 12 months (Simoni et al., 2006).

Among MSM overall, there were more new HIV infections in young Black MSM (aged 13–29) than any other age/racial group of MSM, roughly twice that of Whites and Hispanics/Latinos (CDC, 2008). Possible contributing factors include the following: poverty, stigma, high-risk sexual networks, sexual partner concurrency, lack of access to effective HIV prevention services, underestimation of personal risk, not having personally experienced the severity of the early AIDS epidemic, partnering with older men of color (among whom HIV prevalence is high), childhood abuse trauma, and drug use. Studies show that Black MSM have fewer sexual partners than non-Black (White, Latino, and Asian) MSM (Bohl et al., 2009); however, Black MSM test for HIV less frequently, have high rates of undiagnosed infections, higher rates of STDs which can facilitate acquiring or transmitting HIV, and are less likely to be taking antiretroviral medications that make people less infectious.

The CDC (2008) data show that Hispanics/Latinos are disproportionately affected by HIV representing 18% of new HIV infections (in 2006) while representing 15% of the total U.S. population. The CDC (2008) maintains that many of the factors that place African Americans at elevated risk for HIV also contribute to disproportionate rates of infection among Hispanics/Latinos. However, some Hispanics/Latinos face additional unique challenges that place them at increased risk, including language barriers, cultural values that may impede acknowledgment of risk behaviors (e.g., machismo), and migration among those born outside the United States (e.g., long-term separation from the main sexual partner, resulting in new partners).

Native American two-spirit men reported significantly greater exposure to lifetime HIV risk behaviors than Native American heterosexual men in the following categories: anal intercourse without a condom had a sexually transmitted disease, had sex with an HIV+ person, had sex with an injection drug user, and traded sex for money/drugs/favors. Approximately 30% of two-spirit men agreed or strongly agreed with the statement that "AIDS is another form of germ warfare on Indian people." Because of the high level of mistrust of the U.S. government, HIV prevention targeting two-spirit people must be prepared to address high levels of suspicion, and should be developed and delivered in collaboration with community representatives (Simoni et al., 2006). API MSM have the highest proportion of cumulative AIDS cases (72%) among all racial groups of MSM (Chng, Wong, Park, Edberg, & Lai, 2003), and research points to rising levels of risky behaviors among API MSM in certain areas of the United States. There are low rates of HIV testing among APIs, and almost two-thirds of APIs living with HIV are immigrants, and most likely acquired their infection after immigration to the United States (Wong, Campsmith, Nakamura, Crepaz, & Begley, 2004; Zaidi et al., 2005).

API MSM often develop their sense of self in a socio-cultural environment marked by racism, homophobia, and antiimmigrant attitudes, leading to feelings of not fitting in and low self-esteem (Chng et al., 2003; Sanitioso, 1999). Perceptions of Asian–American MSM as submissive, feminine, and sexually available (Han, 2008; Sanitioso, 1999) may result in self-abasing, less assertive, more conforming, less expressive, and less extrovert behavior (Lai, 1998; Wat, 2002). API MSM may choose to engage in unsafe sex in order to appease and protect their partners from uncomfortable feelings rather than protect themselves from HIV risk (Chng et al., 2003). API MSM often practice unprotected anal intercourse (UAI) at very high rates (25–48%) surpassing rates of UAI by white, black, and Latino MSM (Choi, Coates, Catania, Lew, & Chow, 1995; Choi, Operario, Gregorich, & Han, 2003; Chng & Geliga-Vargas, 2000; McFarland, Chen, Weide, Kohn, & Klausner, 2004; Peterson et al., 2001).

Trans/Gender-Variant HIV/STI Risk Factors

Nuttbrock and colleagues (2009a) found exceptionally high levels of HIV, syphilis, hepatitis B and C among Latino and African–American MTFs with significantly lower levels among White Americans: HIV rates were 50%, 48%, and 4%, respectively; syphilis, 22%, 15%, and 1%; hepatitis B, 36%, 36%, and 7%; and hepatitis C: 7%,15%, and 4%. Among the risk factors considered for these STIs was lifetime number of sexual partners, lifetime social expression of trans/gender-variant identity, as well as lifetime casual sex partners. A significant proportion of MTFs report a history of sex work which is highly correlated with higher levels of HIV/STIs (Hwahng & Nuttbrock, 2007; Nuttbrock et al., 2009a). Survival sex work (prostitution) was directly correlated to homelessness and the inability to find employment. Nuttbrock and colleagues (2009b) also found that one of the major differences of HIV rates among ethnicities in the transfeminine population was due to sexual orientation, in which androphilia was highly correlated to increased HIV risk. Black and Latina transfeminine people were 90–91% androphilic, whereas White transfeminine people were less than 20% androphilic. A study in San Francisco found 41%, 23%, and 13% HIV seroprevalence rate among Black, Latina, and API transfeminine people, respectively, and a high prevalence of engagement in survival sex work across all three ethnic populations; the majority of Latinas and APIs were foreign born (82% and 86%, respectively) (Nemoto et al., 2004).

Among API transfeminine people, the majority who engaged in URAS identified as transgender, transsexual, transvestite, androgynous, crossdresser, gender bender, or drag queen (versus female), had not had SRS, were depressed, and/or had attempted suicide (Operario & Nemoto, 2005). Having a consistent female gender identity that fits within the Euro-American gender paradigm may thus have a protective effect; those whose gender identities are based on indigenous Asian gender paradigms may be especially vulnerable to HIV/STIs (Hwahng & Lin, 2009).

Hormones

Hormones are a major health concern for those trans/gender-variant persons seeking alignment between their gendered and physical self (Sanchez, Sanchez, & Danoff, 2009). Access to and the use of feminizing hormones by MTFs, and conversely the use of masculinizing hormones by FTMs, is of extreme importance to many in these groups. While some may seek hormones as part of a complete transition process, there are those who wish only to enhance or maintain their preferred gender presentation (Kirk, 1999; Waddell Clinic Memo, 2006). Regardless of the individual's goal, medical supervision is imperative to properly monitor both external and internal changes.

Intramuscular injection of female hormones was not associated with HIV/STIs, nor was physical and psychological gender abuse. Instead gender-related psychological and physical abuse was associated with major depression especially among adolescents with gender-variant presentation that declined in many instances with age (Nuttbrock et al., 2010). Among Hispanics and African Americans the most "consistent and robust" factor for HIV/STIs was the social expression of trans/gender-variant identity. White, middle-class MTFs who lived their social lives as "heterosexual men" were unlikely to contract HIV/STIs in comparison to those who lived and dressed as "females" from an early age.

Because of exogenous hormone use, trans/gender-variant persons may be at greater risk for cardiovascular disease and complications (Futterweit, 1998). There is also indication that overuse or extended use of hormones may cause or exacerbate depression (Nuttbrock, 2006). Trans/gender-variant patients need careful follow-up of their natal organs and tissue remnants for potential oncological problems after sex reassignment surgery including prostate, breast, cervical, and ovarian cancer (van Haarst, Newling, Gooren, Asscheman, & Prenger, 1998).

Aging

Aging is a significant health concern among LGBTQ people. A brief overview includes the following issues: conflicts between ethnic and sexual minority communities as social support for older LGBTQ people of color; the confluence of heterosexism and ageism that multiply marginalize elderly LGBTQ people; sexuality needs among aging WSW including menopausal changes, sexual satisfaction, and partner availability; transition and health-care complications among older trans/gender-variant people; elevated rates of alcohol and substance use among older LGBTQ people; victimization of elderly LGBTQ people; retirement trajectories for LGBTQ seniors; parenting and grand parenting challenges; and end-of-life issues (Kimmel, Rose, & David, 2006). Clearly, more research and focus are needed on the health-care needs and issues among older and elderly LGBTQ people.

CONCLUSION

Both individual and structural levels of stigma, trauma, and victimization influence risk for morbidity and mortality among LGBTQ persons. Acknowledging these connections, at least as a start, may be the key to developing more effective and innovative interventions for delivery of health-care and other social services. Instead of pathologizing LGBTQ communities as irreparably damaged and traumatized, the resiliency that already exists needs to be augmented as part of such interventions. Health-care delivery for LGBTQ persons needs to be gender affirmative, culturally competent, and embrace compassionate understanding of the needs of vulnerable sexual/gender minorities (National Coalition for LGBT Health, 2009).

REFERENCES

American Boyz. (2001, February 16–19). *Celebrating human diversity,* Paper presented at the Fifth Annual True Spirit Conference. Washington, DC.

American Psychological Association (APA). (2008). *Transgender, gender identity, and gender expression non-discrimination*. APA Policy Statement. Retrieved from http://www.apa.org/about/governance/council/policy/transgender.aspx.

Amir, M., & Lev-Wiesel, R. (2004). The quality of life among survivors' loved ones. In D. R. Catherall (Ed.), *Handbook of stress, trauma, and the family*. New York, NY: Brunner-Routledge.

Ardener, E. (1977). The 'problem' revisited. In Shirley Ardener (Ed.), *Perceiving women* (pp. 19–28). New York, NY: John Wiley & Sons.

Arreola, S. G., Neilands, T. B., & Diaz, R. (2009). Childhood sexual abuse and the sociocultural context of sexual risk among adult Latino gay and bisexual men. *American Journal of Public Health, 99*(S2), S432–S438.

Austin, S. B., Jun, H.-J., Jackson, B., Spiegelman, D., Rich-Edwards, J., Corliss, H. L., et al. (2008). Disparities in child abuse victimization in lesbian, bisexual, and heterosexual women in the Nurses' Health Study II. *Journal of Women's Health, 17*(4), 597–606.

Balsam, K. F., Huang, B., Fieland, K. C., Simoni, J. M., & Walters, K. L. (2004). Culture, trauma, and wellness: A comparison of heterosexual and lesbian, gay, bisexual, and two-spirit native Americans. *Cultural Diversity and Ethnic Minority Psychology, 10*(3), 287–301.

Balsam, K. F., Rothblum, E., & Beauchaine, T. P. (2005). Victimization over the life span: A comparison of lesbian, gay, bisexual, and heterosexual siblings. *Journal of Consulting and Clinical Psychology, 73*(3), 477–487.

Battle, J., & Crum, M. (2007). Black LGB health and well-being. In I. H. Meyer, & M. E. Northridge (Eds.), *The health of sexual minorities: Public health perspectives on lesbian, gay, bisexual and transgender populations* (pp. 320–352). New York, NY: Springer Press.

Beemyn, B. G. (2005). Trans on campus: Measuring, improving the climate for trans/ gender-variant students. *On Campus with Women* [serial online], *34*. http:// www.ocww.org.

Bieschke, K. J., McClanahan, M., Tozer, E., Grzegorek, J. L., & Park, J. (2000). Programmatic research on the treatment of lesbian, gay, and bisexual clients: The past, the present, and the course for the future. In R. M. Perez, K. A. DeBord, & K. J. Bieschke (Eds.), *Handbook of counseling and psychotherapy with lesbian, gay, and bisexual clients* (pp. 309–336). Washington, DC: American Psychological Association.

Blosnich, J. R., & Bossarte, R. M. (2009). Comparisons of intimate partner violence among partners in same-sex and opposite-sex relationships in the United States. *American Journal of Public Health, 99*(12), 2182–2184.

Boehmer, U., Bowen, D. J., & Bauer, G. R. (2007). Overweight and obesity in sexual minority women: Evidence from population-based data. *American Journal of Public Health, 97*, 1134–1140.

Bohl, D. D., Raymond, H. F., Arnold, M., & McFarland, W. (2009). Concurrent sexual partnerships and racial disparities in HIV infection among men who have sex with men. *Sexually Transmitted Infections, 85*(5), 367–369.

Bornstein, D. R., Fawcett, J., Sullivan, M., Senturia, K. D., & Shiu-Thorton, S. (2006). Understanding the experiences of lesbian, bisexual and trans survivors of domestic violence. *Journal of Homosexuality, 51*(1), 159–181.

Boswell, J. (1980). *Christianity, social tolerance, and homosexuality: Gay people in Western Europe from the beginning of the Christian era to the fourteenth century.* Chicago: University of Chicago Press.

Bovicini, K. A., & Perlin, M. J. (2003). The same but different: Clinician–patient communication with gay and lesbians patients. *Patient Education Counseling, 51*(2), 115–122.

Bowleg, L., Huang, J., Brooks, K., Black, A., & Burkholder, G. (2003). Triple jeopardy and beyond: Multiple minority stress and resilience among black lesbians. *Journal of Lesbian Studies, 7*(4), 87–108.

Brown, M. J., & Groscup, J. (2009). Perceptions of same-sex domestic violence among crisis center staff. *Journal of Family Violence, 24*, 87–93.

Burgard, S. A., Cochran, S. D., & Mays, V. M. (2005). Alcohol and tobacco use patterns among heterosexually and homosexually experienced California women. *Drug and Alcohol Dependence, 77*, 61–70.

Butler, J. (1993). *Bodies that Matter: On the discursive limits of "sex".* New York, NY: Routledge.

Cabaj, R. P., & Stein, T. S. (Eds.). (1996). *Textbook of homosexuality and mental health.* Washington, DC: American Psychiatric Press.

Cahill, S., South, K., & Spade, J. (2000). *Outing age: Public policy issues affecting gay, lesbian, bisexual and trans/gender-variant elders.* New York, NY: The Policy Institute of the National Gay and Lesbian Task Force Foundation.

Caplan, P. (Ed.). (1987). *The cultural construction of sexuality.* London: Tavistock.

Cassels, S., Pearson, C. R., Walters, K., Simoni, J. M., & Morris, M. (2010). Sexual partner concurrency and sexual risk among gay, lesbian, bisexual, and transgender American Indian/Alaska natives. *Sexually Transmitted Infections, 37*(4), 272–278.

Center for Disease Control and Prevention (CDC). (2006a). Women who have sex with women (WSW). (*MMWR* August 4, 2006, *55*(RR-11)). Retrieved on July 20, 2009.

Center for Disease Control and Prevention (CDC). (2006b) Proctitus, proctocolitis, enteritis. *Sexually Transmitted Diseases Treatment Guidelines 2006*. Department of Health and Human Services. Retrieved on July 28, 2009 http://www.cdc. gov/std/treatment/2006/proctitis.htm.

Center for Disease Control and Prevention (CDC) and National Center for Health Statistics, HIV Mortality Rates (slides set). (2006c). CDC HIV Update. http:// www.cdc.gov/hiv/topics/surveillance/resources/slides/mortality/slides/ mortality13.pdf

Center for Disease Control and Prevention (CDC). (2007a). *Gynecologic overview*. Division of Cancer Prevention and Control. National Center for Chronic Disease Prevention and Health Promotion.

Center for Disease Control and Prevention (CDC). (2007b). *HIV prevention among men who have sex with men: Risk issues among African American, Latino and young men*. Satellite Broadcast in May 2007 Greg Millet, Rafael Diaz, George Ayala. http://www2c.cdc.gov/podcasts/media/pdf/HIV_03_051707.pdf

Center for Disease Control and Prevention (CDC). (2008). MMWR Analysis Provides New Details on HIV Incidence in U.S. Populations, September, http://www.cdc.gov/hiv/topics/surveillance/resources/factsheets/MMWR-incidence.htm

Center for Disease Control & Prevention (CDC). (2009). Division of viral Hepatitis. National Division for HIV/AIDS, *Viral Hepatitis, STD and TB Prevention*. http:// www.cdc.gov/hepatitis/Populations/msm.htm

Chan, C. (1989). Issues of identity development among Asian American lesbians and gay men. *Journal of Counseling and Development, 68*, 16–20.

Chng, C. L., & Geliga-Vargas, J. (2000). Ethnic identity, gay identity, sexual sensation seeking and HIV risk taking among multiethnic men who have sex with men. *AIDS Education Prevention, 12*(4), 326–339.

Chng, C. L., Wong, F. Y., Park, R. J., Edberg, M. C., & Lai, D. S. (2003). A model for understanding sexual health among Asian American/Pacific islander men who have sex with men (MSM) in the United States. *AIDS Education and Prevention, 15*(1), 21–38.

Choi, K. H., Coates, T. J., Catania, J. A., Lew, S., & Chow, P. (1995). High HIV risk among gay Asian and Pacific Islander men in San Francisco. *AIDS, 9*(3), 306–308.

Choi, K. H., Operario, D., Gregorich, S. E., & Han, L. (2003). Age and race mixing patterns of sexual partnerships among Asian men who have sex with men: Implications for HIV transmission and prevention. *AIDS Education and Prevention, 15*(1), 53–65.

Clatts, M., Welle, D., & Goldsamt, L. A. (2001). Reconceptualizing the interaction of drug and sexual risk among MSM speed users: Notes toward an ethno-epidemiology. *AIDS and Behavior, 5*(2), 115–130.

Clements-Nolle, K., Wilkinson, W., Kitano, K., & Marx, R. (2001). HIV prevention and health service needs of the transgender community in San Francisco.

In W. Bockting & S. Kirk (Eds.), *Transgender and HIV: Risks, prevention, and care* (pp. 69–89). New York, NY: Hawthorne Press.

Cochran, S. D. (2001). Emerging issues in research on lesbians' and gay men's mental health: Does sexual orientation really matter? *American Psychologist, 56,* 931–947.

Cochran, S. D., Keenan, C., Schober, C., & Mays, V. M. (2000). Estimates of alcohol use and clinical treatment needs among homosexually active men and women in the U.S. population. *Journal of Consulting and Clinical Psychology, 68,* 1062–1071.

Cochran, S. D., & Mays, V. M. (1994). Depressive distress among homosexually active African American men and women. *American Journal of Psychiatry, 151*(4), 524–529.

Cochran, S. D., & Mays, V. M. (2007). Physical health complaints among lesbians, gay men, and bisexual and homosexually experienced heterosexuals. *American Journal of Public Health, 97*(11), 2048–2055.

Cochran, S. D., & Mays, V. M. (2009). Burden of psychiatric morbidity among lesbian, gay, and bisexual individuals in the California quality of lifesurvey. *Journal of Abnormal Psychology, 118*(3), 647–658.

Cochran, S. D., Mays, V. M., Bowen, D., Gage, S., Bybee, D., Roberts, S. J., et al. (2001). Cancer-related risk indicators and preventive screening behaviors among lesbians and bisexual women. *American Journal of Public Health, 91*(4), 591–597.

Cohen, C. J. (1999). *The boundaries of blackness: AIDS and the breakdown of Black politics.* Chicago: The University of Chicago Press.

Colfax, G., Coates, T. J., Husnik, M. J., Huang, Y, Buchbinder, S., Koblin, B., et al. (2005). Longitudinal patterns of methamphetamine, popper (amyl nitrite), and cocaine use and high-risk sexual behavior among a cohort of San Francisco men who have sex with men. *Journal of Urban Health, 82,* 162–170.

Colfax, G., Vittinghoff, F., Husnik, M. J., McKirnan, D., Buchbinder, S., Koblin, B., et al. (2004). Substance use and sexual risk: A participant- and episode-level analysis among a cohort of men who have sex with men. *American Journal of Epidemiology, 159,* 1002–1012.

Cooperman, N. A., Simoni, J. M., & Lockhart, D. W. (2003). Abuse, social support, and depression among HIV-positive heterosexual, bisexual, and lesbian women. *Journal of Lesbian Studies, 7*(4), 49–66.

Corliss, H. L., Cochran, S. D., & Mays, V. M. (2002). Reports of parental maltreatment during childhood in a United States population-based survey of homosexual, bisexual, and heterosexual adults. *Child Abuse & Neglect, 26,* 1165–1178.

Crawford, I., Allison, K. W., Zamboni, B. D., & Soto, T. (2002). The influence of dual identity development on psychosocial functioning of African American gay and bisexual men. *Journal of Sex Research, 39*(3), 179–189.

Dang, A., & Vianney, C. (2007). *Living in the margins: A national survey of lesbian, gay, bisexual and transgender Asian and Pacific Islander Americans.* New York, NY: National Gay and Lesbian Task Force Policy Institute.

D'Augelli, A. R. (2003). Lesbian and bisexual female youths aged 14 to 21: Developmental challenges and victimization experiences. *Journal of Lesbian Studies, 7*(4), 9–29.

D'Augelli, A., & Hershberger, S. (1993). Lesbian, gay, and bisexual youth in community settings: Personal challenges and mental health problems. *American Journal of Community Psychology, 21,* 421–448.

Dean, L., Meyer, I. H., Robinson, K., Sell, R. L., Sember, R., Silenzio, V. M., et al. (2000). Lesbian, gay, bisexual, and trans/gender-variant health: Findings and concerns. *Journal of Gay Lesbian Medical Association, 4,* 102–151.

Descamps, M. J., Rothblum, E., Bradford, J., & Ryan, C. (2000). Mental health impact of child sexual abuse, rape, intimate partner violence, and hate crimes in the National Lesbian Health Care Survey. *Journal of Gay & Lesbian Social Services, 11*(1), 27–55.

Diamant, A. L., Schuster, M. A., McGuigan, K., & Lever, J. (1999). Lesbians' sexual history with men: Implications for taking a sexual history. *Archives of Internal Medicine, 159,* 2730–2736.

Diaz, R. (1998). *Latino gay men and HIV: Culture, sexuality, and risk behavior.* New York, NY: Routledge.

Diaz, R., Ayala, G., Bein, E., Henne, J., & Marin, B. (2001a). The impact of homophobia, poverty, and racism on the mental health of gay and bisexual men: Findings from three U.S. cities. *American Journal of Public Health, 91,* 927–933.

Diaz, T., Vlahov, D., Greenberg, B., Cuevas, Y., & Garfein, R. (2001b). Sexual orientation and HIV infection prevalence among young Latino injection drug users in Harlem. *Journal of Women's Health & Gender-Based Medicine, 10*(4), 371–380.

Duran, B., & Walters, K. L. (2004). HIV/AIDS prevention in "Indian Country": Current practice, indigenist etiology models, and postcolonial approaches to change. *AIDS Education and Prevention, 16*(3), 187–201.

Eliason, M. J., & Schope, R. (2007). Shifting sands or solid foundation? Lesbian, gay, bisexual, and transgender identity formation. In H. Meyer & M. E. Northbridge (Eds.), *The health of sexual minorities: Public health perspectives on lesbian, gay bisexual and transgender populations* (pp. 3–26). New York, NY: Springer.

Elze, D. (2006). Oppression, predjudice, and discrimination. In D. F. Morrow & L. Messinger (Eds.), *Sexual orientation and gender expression in social work practice: Working with gay, lesbian, bisexual, & transgender people.* New York, NY: Columbia University Press.

Epstein, S. (1996). *Impure science: AIDS, activism, and the politics of knowledge.* Berkeley: University of California Press.

Epstein, S. (2003). Sexualizing governance and medicalizing identities: The emergence of 'state-centered' LGBT health politics in the United States. *Sexualities 6*(2), 131–171. Thousand Oaks, CA: Sage.

Fausto-Sterling, A. (2000). Five sexes, revisited. *Sciences, 40*(Jul/Aug), 18–23.

Finlon, C. (2002). Health care for all gay, lesbian, bisexual, and trans/gender-variant populations. *Journal of Gay and Lesbian Social Services, 14*(3).

Friedman, S. R., Curtis, R., Neaigus, A., Jose, B., & Des Jarlais, D. C. (1999). *Social networks, drug injectors' lives, and HIV/AIDS.* New York, NY: Kluwer Academic.

Friedman, S. R., Ompad, D. C., Maslow, C., Young, R., Case, P., Hudson, S. M., et al. (2003). HIV prevalence, risk behaviors, and high-risk sexual and injection networks among young women injectors who have sex with women. *American Journal of Public Health, 93*(6), 902–906.

Fung, R. (1991). Looking for my penis: The eroticized Asian in gay video porn. In B. Object-Choices (Ed.), *How Do I Look? Queer Film and Video*. Seattle: Bay Press.

Futterweit, W. (1998). Endocrine therapy of transsexualism and potential complications of long-term treatment. *Archives of Sex Behavior, 27*, 209–226.

Garnets, L. D., & D'Augelli, A. R. (1994). Empowering lesbian and gay communities: A call for collaboration with community psychology. *American Journal of Community Psychology, 22*(4), 447–470.

Gay and Lesbian Medical Association (and LGBT health experts). (2001). *Healthy people 2010: Companion document for Lesbian, Gay, Bisexual, and Transgender (LGBT) Health*. San Francisco, CA: Gay and Lesbian Medical Association.

Gilley, B. J. (2006). *Becoming two-spirit: Gay identity and social acceptance in Indian country*. Lincoln: University of Nebraska Press.

Goode-Cross, D. T., & Good, G. E. (2009). Managing multiple minority identities: African American men who have sex with men at predominantly white colleges. *Journal of Diversity in Higher Education, 2*(2), 103–112.

Graham, L. F., Braithwaite, K., Spikes, P., Stephens, C. F., & Edu, U. F. (2009). Exploring the mental health of black men who have sex with men. *Community Mental Health Journal, 45*(4), 272–284.

Green, B. C. (2005). Homosexual signification: A moral construct in social contexts. *Journal of Homosexuality, 49*(2), 119–134.

Greenfield, L. A., & Smith, S. K. (1999). *American Indians and crime*. Washington, DC: U.S. Department of Justice.

Hahm, H. C., Wong, F. Y., Huang, Z. J., Ozonoff, A., & Lee, J. (2008). Substance use among Asian Americans and Pacific Islanders sexual minority adolescents: Findings from the National Longitudinal Study of Adolescent Health. *Journal of Adolescent Health, 42*(3), 275–283.

Haldeman, D. C. (1994). The practice and ethics of sexual orientation conversion therapy. *Journal of Consulting and Clinical Psychology, 62*, 221–227.

Han, C. S. (2008). A qualitative exploration of the relationship between racism and unsafe sex among Asian Pacific Islander gay men. *Arch Sex Behav, 37*(5), 827–837.

Harcourt, J. (Ed.). (2006). Current issues in lesbian, gay, bisexual and trans/gender-variant (LGBT) health. *Journal of Homosexuality, 51*(1), 1–11.

Hart, G. J., & Elford, J. (2010). Sexual risk behavior of men who have sex with men: Emerging patterns and new challenges. *Current Opinion in Infectious Diseases, 23*(1), 39–44.

Herdt, G. (1994). *Guardians of the flute: Idioms of masculinity*. Chicago: University of Chicago Press.

Herek, G. M. (2004). Beyond "homophobia": Thinking about sexual stigma and prejudice in the twenty-first century. *Sexuality Research and Social Policy, 1*(2), 6–24.

Herek, G. M., Chopp, R., & Strohl, D. (2007). Sexual stigma: Putting sexual minority health issues in context. In I. H. Meyer & M. E. Northbridge (Eds.), *The health of sexual minorities: Public health perspectives on lesbian, gay bisexual and transgender populations* (pp. 171–208). New York, NY: Springer.

Hesse, E., Main, M., Abrams, K. Y., & Rifkin, A. (2003). Unresolved states regarding loss or abuse can have "second-generation" effects: Disorganization, role inversion, and frightening ideation in the offspring of traumatized, non-maltreating parents. In M. F. Solomon & D. J. Siegel (Eds.), *Healing trauma: Attachment, mind, body, and brain.* New York, NY: W.W. Norton.

Holmes, W. C. (1997). Association between a history of childhood sexual abuse and subsequent, adolescent psychoactive substance use disorder in sample of HIV seropositive men. *Journal of Adolescent Health, 20*(6), 414–419.

Huebner, D. M., Rebchook, G. M., & Kegeles, S. M. (2004). Experiences of harassment, discrimination, and physical violence among young gay and bisexual men. *American Journal of Public Health, 94*, 1200–1203.

Hughes, T. L., & Eliason, M. (2002). Substance use and abuse in lesbian, gay, bisexual and transgender populations. *Journal of Primary Prevention, 22*, 263–298.

Hughes, T. L., & Johnson, T. P. (2003). Lesbians and smoking. *Current Women's Health Report, 3*(3), 254–261.

Hughes, T., Wilsnak, S. C., & Johnson, T. P. (2006). Investigating lesbians' mental health and alcohol use: What is an appropriate comparison group? In A. M. Omoto & H. S. Kurtzman (Eds.), *Sexual orientation and mental health: Examining identity and development in lesbian, gay, and bisexual people: Contemporary perspectives on lesbian, gay, and bisexual psychology* (pp. 167–184). Washington, DC: American Psychological Association.

Hunter, S., Shannon, C., Knox, J., & Martin, J. I. (1998). *Lesbian, gay, and bisexual youths and adults: Knowledge for human services practice.* Thousand Oaks, CA: Sage Publications, Inc.

Hwahng, S. J., & Lin, A. J. (2009). The health of lesbian, gay, bisexual, transgender, queer, and questioning people. In C. Trinh-Shevrin, N. Islam & M. Rey (Eds.), *Asian American communities and health: Context, research, policy, and action* (pp. 226–282). San Francisco: Jossey-Bass Publishers.

Hwahng, S. J., & Nuttbrock, L. (2007). Sex workers, fem queens, and cross-dressers: Differential marginalizations and HIV vulnerabilities among three ethnocultural male-to-female transgender communities in New York City. *Sexuality Research & Social Policy, 4*(4), 36–59.

Hwahng, S. J., & Nuttbrock, L. (2009). *Depression and HIV risk among low-income transfeminine people of color in New York City.* Paper presented at the Medical Anthropology at the Intersections: Celebrating 50 Years of Interdisciplinarity conference, Yale University.

Jacobs, S.-E., Thomas, W., & Lang, S. (Eds.). (1997). *Two-spirit people: Native American gender identity, sexuality, and spirituality.* Urbana, IL: University of Illinois Press.

Journal of the American Medical Association (JAMA). (1996). Health care needs of gay men and lesbians in the United States. *Journal of the American Medical Association, 275*(17), 1354–1359.

Johnson, M. (1997). *Beauty and power: Transgendering and cultural transformation in the southern Philippines.* New York, NY: Berg.

Johnson, C. V., Mimiaga, M. J., & Bradford, J. (2008). Health care issues among lesbian, gay, bisexual, transgender and intersex (LGBTI) populations in the United States: Introduction. *Journal of Homosexuality, 54*(3), 213–224.

Kalichman, S. C., Benotsch, E., Rompa, D., Gore-Felton, C., Austin, J., Luke, W., et al. (2001). Unwanted sexual experiences and sexual risks in gay and bisexual men: Associations among revictimization, substance use, and psychiatric symptoms. *Journal of Sex Research, 38*(1), 1–9.

Katz, J. N. (1992). *Gay American history: Lesbians and gay men in the U.S.A.* (rev. Editor). New York, NY: Meridian.

Kennamer, D. J., Honnold, J., Braddford, J., & Hendricks, M. (2000). Differences in disclosure of sexuality among African American and White gay/bisexual men: Implications for HIV/AIDS prevention. *AIDS Education and Prevention, 12*(6), 519–531.

Kessler, R. C., Borges, G., & Walters, E. E. (1999). Prevalence of and risk factors for lifetime suicide attempts in the National Comorbidity Survey. *Archives of General Psychiatry, 56*(7), 617–626.

Kessler, R. C., Michelson, K. D., & Williams, D. R. (1999a). The prevalence, distribution, and mental health correlates of perceived discrimination in the United States. *Journal of Health & Social Behavior, 40,* 208–230.

Kimmel, D., Rose, T., & David, S. (Eds.). (2006). *Lesbian, gay, bisexual, and transgender aging: Research and clinical perspectives.* New York, NY: Columbia University Press.

King, D. (1998). Multiple jeopardy, multiple consciousness: The context of a Black feminist ideology. *Signs, 14*(1), 42–72.

Kirk, S. (1999). *Hormonal feminizing therapy for the transgendered.* Pittsburg: Together Lifeworks.

Krieger, N. (1994). Epidemiology and the web of causation: Has anyone seen the spider? *Social Science and Medicine, 39,* 887–903.

Krieger, N. (2001). Theories for social epidemiology for the 21st century: An ecosocial perspective. *International Journal of Epidemiology, 30,* 668–677.

Krieger, N., Rowley, D. L., Herman, A. A., Avery, B., & Philip, M. T. (1993). Racism, sexism, and social class: Implications for studies of health, disease, and well-being. *American Journal of Preventive Medicine, 9,* 82–122.

Kulick, D. (1998). *Travesti: Sex, gender and culture among Brazilian transgendered prostitutes.* Chicago: The University of Chicago Press.

Lai, D. S. (1998). *Self-esteem and unsafe sex in Chinese-American and Japanese-American gay men.* Unpublished doctoral dissertation, California School of Professional Psychology, Alameda, CA.

LaSala, M. C. (2003). When interviewing "Family": Maximizing the insider advantage in the qualitative study of lesbians and gay men. *Journal of Gay and Lesbian Social Services, 15*(1,2), 15–30.

Laumann, O., Gagnon, J. H., Michael, R. T., & Michael, S. (1994). *The social organization of sexuality: Sexual practices in the United States.* Chicago: University of Chicago Press.

Lawrence, A. A. (2007). Transgender health concerns. In Meyer & Northridge (Eds.), *The health of sexual minorities: Public health perspectives on lesbian, gay, bisexual and transgender populations* (pp. 473–505). New York, NY: Springer.

Lawrence, A. A., Shaffer, J. D., Snow, W. R., Chase, C., & Headlam, B. T. (1996). Health care needs of transgendered patients [letter to the editor]. *JAMA: Journal of American Medical Association, 276,* 874.

Levenson, J. (2004). *The secret epidemic: The story of AIDS and Black America.* New York, NY: Anchor Books.

Lee, P. A., Houk, C. P., Ahtned, S. F., Hughes, I. A., and the International Consensus Conference on Intersex Working Group. (2006). Consensus statement on management of intersex disorders. *Pediatrics, 118,* e488–e500.

Link, B. G., & Phelan, J. C. (2001). Conceptualizing stigma. *Annual Review of Sociology, 27,* 363–385.

Lombardi, E. (2001). Enhancing trans/gender-variant health care [Electronic version]. *American Journal of Public Health, 91,* 869–872.

Makadon, H., Mayer, K., Potter, J., & Goldhammer, H. (Eds.). (2007). *The Fenway guide to lesbian, gay, bisexual, and transgender health.* Philadelphia, PA: American College of Physicians.

Mayer, K. H., Bradford, J. B., Makadon, H. J., Stall, R., Goldhammer, H., et al. (2008). Sexual and gender minority health: What we know and what needs to be done. *American Journal of Public Health, 98*(6), 989–999.

Mays, V. M., & Cochran, S. D. (1988). The Black women's relationship project: A national survey of black lesbians. In M. Shernoff & W. Scott (Eds.), *The Sourcebook on Lesbian/Gay Health Care* (2nd ed., pp. 54–62). Washington, DC: National Lesbian and Gay Health Foundation.

Marrazzo, J. M. (2004). Barriers to infectious disease care among lesbians. *Emerging Infectious Diseases, 10,* 1974–1978.

Marrazzo, J. M., Coffey, P., & Bingham, A. (2005). Sexual practices, risk perception and knowledge of sexually transmitted disease risk among lesbian and bisexual women. *Perspectives on Sexual and Reproductive Health, 37*(1), 6–12.

Mason, M. R. (2006). *Defining our community.* International Foundation for Gender Education, 20th Annual Conference, April, Philadelphia, PA.

McFarland, W., Chen, S., Weide, D., Kohn, R., & Klausner, J. (2004). Gay Asian men in San Francisco follow the international trend: Increases in rates of unprotected anal intercourse and sexually transmitted diseases, 1999–2002. *AIDS Education and Prevention, 16*(1), 13–18.

Mercer, K. (1993). Looking for trouble. In H. Abelove, M. A. Barale, & D. M. Halperin (Eds.), *The lesbian and gay studies reader.* New York, NY: Routledge.

Meyer, I. H. (1995). Minority stress and mental health in gay men. *Journal of Health and Social Behavior, 36*(1), 38–56.

Meyer, I. H. (2001). Why lesbian, gay, bisexual and trans/gender-variant public health? [Electronic version]. *American Journal of Public Health, 91,* 856–859.

Meyer, I. H. (2003). Prejudice, social stress, and mental health in lesbian, gay, and bisexual populations: Conceptual issues and research evidence. *Psychological Bulletin, 129*(5), 674–697.

Mills, T. C., Paul, J., Stall, R., Pollack, L., Canchola, J., Chang, Y. J., et al. (2004). Distress and depression in men who have sex with men: The urban men's health study [published correction appears in *American Journal of Psychiatry*, 2004; *161*(4), 776]. *American Journal of Psychiatry*, *161*, 278–285.

Morris, J. F., & Balsam, K. F. (2003). Lesbian and bisexual women's experiences of victimization: Mental health, revictimization, and sexual identity development. *Journal of Lesbian Studies*, *7*(4), 67–86.

Morris, R. C. (1994). Three sexes and four sexualities: Redressing the discourses on gender and sexuality in contemporary Thailand. *Positions*, *2*(1), 15–43.

Morrow, S. L. (2000). First do no harm: Therapist issues in psychotherapy with lesbian, gay, and bisexual clients. In R. M. Perez, K. A. DeBord, & K. J. Bieschke (Eds.), *Handbook of counseling and psychotherapy with lesbian, gay, and bisexual clients* (pp. 137–156). Washington, DC: American Psychological Association.

Nanda, S. (1999). *Neither man nor woman: The hijras of India*. Belmont, CA: Wadsworth Publishing Company.

National Coalition on LGBT Health. (2009). *Guiding principles on lesbian, gay, bisexual, trans/gender-variant inclusion in health care reform*. http://www.lgbthealth. net/index.shtml, accessed 8/13/2009.

National Institute on Drug Abuse (NIDA). (2009). *Methamphetamine*. Accessed July 19, 2009. http://www.nida.nih.gov/DrugPages/methamphetamine.html

Needham, R. (1978). *Primordial characters*. Virginia: University of Virginia Press.

Nemoto, T., Operario, D., Keatley, J., Han, L., & Soma, T. (2004). HIV risk behaviors among male-to-female transgender persons of color in San Francisco. *American Journal of Public Health*, *94*(7), 1193–1199.

Nemoto, T., Wong, F., Ching, A., Chng, C., Bouey, P., Henrickson, M., et al. (1998). HIV seroprevalence, risk behaviors, and cognitive factors among Asian and Pacific Islander American men who have sex with men: A summary and critique of empirical studies and methodological issues. *AIDS Education and Prevention*, *10*(3 Suppl), 31–47.

Northridge, M. (2001). Editor's note: Advancing gay, lesbian, bisexual and transgender health. *American Journal of Public Health*, *91*, 6.

Nuttbrock, L. (2006). *Report on preliminary findings from the Transgender Project*. New York, NY: Gender Forum/National Development and Research Institutes, Inc.

Nuttbrock, L., Bockting, W., Mason, M., Hwahng, S. J., Rosenblum, A., Macri, M., et al. (Epub ahead of print). A further assessment of Blanchard's typology of homosexual versus non-homosexual or autogrynephilic gender dysphoria. *Archives of Sexual behavior*.

Nuttbrock, L., Hwahng, S., Bockting, W., Rosenblum, A., Mason, M., Macri, M., et al. (2009a). Gender identity affirmation among male-to-female transgender persons: A life course analysis across types of relationships and cultural/lifestyle factors. *Sexual and Relationship Therapy*, *24*(2), 108–125.

Nuttbrock, L., Hwahng, S., Bockting, W., Rosenblum, A., Mason, M., Macri, M., et al. (2009b). Lifetime risk factors for HIV/STI infections among male-to-female transgender persons. *Journal of Acquired Immune Deficiency Syndromes*, *52*(3), 417–421.

Nuttbrock, L., Hwahng, S., Bockting, W., Rosenblum, A., Mason, M., Macri, M., et al. (2010). Psychiatric impact of gender-related abuse across the life course of male-to-female transgender persons. *Journal of Sex Research, 47*(1), 12–23.

Omi, M., & Winant, H. (1994). *Racial formation in the United States: From the 1960s to the 1990s*. New York, NY: Routledge.

Ompad, D., Friedman, S., Hwahng, S. J., Nandi, V., Fuller, C., & Vlahov, D. (in press). Risk behaviors among young drug using women who have sex with women in New York City. *Substance Use and Misuse*.

Operario, D., Choi, K. H., Chu, P. L., McFarland, W., Secura, G. M., Behel, S., et al. (2006). Prevalence and correlates of substance use among young Asian Pacific Islander men who have sex with men. *Prevention Science, 7*(1), 19–29.

Operario, D., & Nemoto, T. (2005). Sexual risk behavior and substance use among a sample of Asian Pacific Islander transgendered women. *AIDS Education and Prevention, 17*(5), 430–443.

Ortner, S. B., & Whitehead, H. (1981). Introduction: Accounting for sexual meanings. In S. B. Ortner & H. Whitehead (Eds.), *Sexual meanings: The cultural construction of gender and sexuality*. Cambridge: Cambridge University Press.

Paul, J. P., Catania, J., Pollock, L., & Stall, R. (2001). Understanding childhood sexual abuse as a predictor of sexual risk-taking among men who have sex with men: The Urban Men's Health Study. *Child Abuse and Neglect, 25*, 557–584.

Padilla, M. B., Vasquez del, A., & Parker, R. G. (2007). Globalization, structural violence and LGBT health: A cross-cultural perspective. In I. H. Meyer, & M. E. Northridge (Eds), *The health of sexual minorities: Public health perspectives on lesbian, gay, bisexual and transgender populations (pp. 209–241)*. New York: Springer.

Pattatuchi-Aragon, A. (Ed.), *Challenging lesbian norms: Intersex, transgender, intersectional, and queer perspectives*. New York, NY: Taylor & Francis, Inc.

Patton, C. (1990). *Inventing AIDS*. New York, NY: Routledge.

Paul, J. P., Catania, J., Pollock, L., & Stall, R. (2001). Understanding childhood sexual abuse as a predictor of sexual risk-taking among men who have sex with men: The Urban Men's Health Study. *Child Abuse and Neglect, 25*, 557–584.

Peterson, J., Bakeman, R., Stokes, J., & the Community Intervention Trial for Youth Study Team. (2001). Racial/ethnic patterns of HIV sexual risk behaviors among young men who have sex with men. *Journal of the Gay and Lesbian Medical Association, 5*, 155–162.

Prieur, A. (1998). *Mema's house, Mexico City: On transvestites, queens, and machos*. Chicago: University of Chicago Press.

Ramirez-Valles, J. (2007). Latino gay and bisexual men's health. In Meyer & Northridge (Eds.), *The health of sexual minorities: Public health perspectives on lesbian, gay, bisexual and transgender populations* (pp. 301–319). New York, NY: Springer Press.

Reddy, G. (2005). *With respect to sex: Negotiating hijra identity in South India*. Chicago: University of Chicago Press.

Renzetti, C. M. (1997). Violence in lesbian and gay relationships. In L. L. O'Toole & J. R. Schiffman (Eds.), *Gender violence: Interdisciplinary perspectives* (pp. 285–293). New York, NY: New York University Press.

Roscoe, W. (1998). *Changing ones: Third and fourth genders in Native North America.* New York, NY: St. Martin's Press.

Ross, M. W., Rosser, B. R. S., & Neumaier, E. R. (2008). The relationship of internalized homonegativity to unsafe sexual behavior in HIV-seropositive men who have sex with men. *AIDS: Education and Prevention, 20*(6), 547–557.

Rothblum, E. D. (1994). Introduction: Lesbianism as a model of a positive lifestyle for women. Special Issue: Lesbianism: Affirming nontraditional roles. *Women and Therapy, 8*(1,2), 1–12.

Rowland-Klein, D. (2004). The transmission of trauma across generations: Identification with parental trauma in children of holocaust survivors. In D. R. Catherall (Ed.), *Handbook of stress, trauma, and the family.* New York, NY: Brunner-Routledge.

Royal, G. (2006). Primary care health issues among men who have sex with men. *Journal of the American Academy of Nurse Practitioners, 18*(4), 144–153.

Saewyc, E. M., Bearinger, L. H., Blum, R. W., & Renick, M. D. (1999). Sexual intercourse, abuse and pregnancy among adolescent women: Does sexual orientation make a difference? *Family Planning Perspectives, 31*(3), 127–131.

Safren, S. A., & Heimberg, K. G. (1999). Depression, hopelessness, *suicidality,* and related factors in sexual minority and heterosexual adolescents. *Journal of Consulting and Clinical Psychology, 67,* 859–866.

Sanchez, N. F., Sanchez, J. P., & Danoff, A. (2009). Health care utilization, barriers to care, and hormone usage among male-to-female transgender persons in New York City. *American Journal of Public Health, 99*(4), 713–719.

Sanitioso, R. (1999). A social psychological perspective on HIV/AIDS and gay or homosexually active Asian men. *Journal of Homosexuality, 36*(3,4), 69–85.

Scheer, S., Parks, C. A., McFarland, W., Page-Shafer, K., Delgado, V., Ruiz, J. D., et al. (2003). Self-reported sexual identity, sexual behaviors and health risks: Examples from a population-based survey of young women. *Journal of Lesbian Studies, 7*(1), 69–83.

Scott, K. D., Gilliam, A., & Braxton, K. (2005). Culturally competent HIV prevention strategies for women of color in the United States. *Health Care Women International, 26*(1), 17–45.

Sell, R. L. (2007). Defining and measuring sexual orientation for research in the health of sexual minorities: Public health perspectives on lesbian, gay, bisexual and transgender populations. In I. H. Meyer & M. E. Northbridge (Eds.), *The health of sexual minorities: Public perspectives on lesbian, gay, bisexual and transgender people* (pp. 355–374). New York, NY: Springer Press.

Sevelius, J. (2009). "There's no pamphlet for the kind of sex I have": HIV-related risk factors and protective behaviors among transgender men who have sex with nontransgender men. *Journal of the Association of Nurses in AIDS Care, 20*(5), 398–410.

Simoni, J. M., Sehgal, S., & Walters, K. L. (2004). Triangle of risk: Urban American Indian women's sexual trauma, injection drug use, and hiv sexual risk behaviors. *AIDS and Behavior, 8*(1), 33–45.

Simoni, J. M., Walters, K. L., Balsam, K. F., & Meyers, S. B. (2006). Victimization, substance use, and HIV risk behaviors among gay/bisexual/two-spirit and heterosexual American Indian men in New York City. *American Journal of Public Health, 96*(12), 2240–2245.

Singh, A., Chung, Y. B., & Dean, J. K. (2007). Acculturation levels and internalized homophobia of Asian American lesbian and bisexual women: An exploratory analysis. *Journal of LGBT Issues in Counseling, 1*(2), 3–19.

Sinnott, M. J. (2004). *Toms and Dees: Transgender identity and female same-sex relationships in Thailand*. Honolulu: University of Hawaii Press.

Solarz, A. L. (Ed.). (1999). *Lesbian health: Current assessment and directions for the future*. Washington, DC: National Academy Press.

Stanley, J. L., Bartholomew, K., Taylor, T., Oram, D., & Landolt, M. (2006). Intimate violence in male same-sex relationships. *Journal of Family Violence, 21*, 31–41.

Stein, E. (2007). Ethical, legal, social, and political implications of scientific research on sexual orientation. In I. H. Meyer & M. E. Northbridge (Eds.), *The health of sexual minorities: Public perspectives on lesbian, gay, bisexual and transgender people*. New York, NY: Springer.

Sullivan, G., & Losberg, W. (2003). A study of sampling in research in the field of lesbian and gay studies. *Journal of Gay & Lesbian Social Services: Issues in Practice, Policy & Research, 15*(1,2), 147–167.

Swann, S. K., & Anastas, J. W. (2003). Dimensions of lesbian identity during adolescence and young adulthood. *Journal of Gay and Lesbian Social Services, 15*(1,2), 109–125.

Tang, H., Greenwood, G. L., Cowling, D. W., Lloyd, J. C., Roeseler, A. G., & Bai, D. G. (2004). Cigarette smoking among lesbians, gays, and bisexuals: How serious a problem? (United States). *Cancer Causes and Control, 15,* 797–803.

Tjaden, P., Thoeness, N., & Allison, C. J. (1999). Comparing violence over the life span in samples of same-sex and opposite-sex cohabitants. *Violence and Victims, 14*, 413–425.

Treichler, P. S. (1988). AIDS, homophobia, and biomedical discourse: An epidemic of signification. In D. Crimp (Ed.), *AIDS: Cultural analysis, cultural activism*. Cambridge, MA: MIT Press.

Trocki, K. F., Drabble, L., & Midanik, L. (2005). Use of heavier drinking contexts among heterosexuals, homosexuals and bisexuals: Results from a national household probability survey. *Journal of Studies on Alcohol, 66*(1), 105–111.

U.S. Department of Health and Human Services (DHHS). (2005). Lesbian health, frequently asked questions. *The National Women's Health Information Center*. The Federal Government Source for Women's Health Information. Womenshealth.gov

U.S. Supreme Court, 2003, Lawrence v. Texas (02-102) 539 U.S. 558. 41 S.W. 3d 349, reversed and remanded. U.S. Department of Health and Human Services (DHHS) (2005). *Lesbian health, frequently asked questions*. The National Women's Health Information Center. The Federal Government source for women's health information. Womenshealth.gov

Van Dam, M. A., Koh, A. S., & Dibble, S. L. (2001). Lesbian disclosure to health care providers and delay of care. *Journal of the Gay and Lesbian Medical Association, 5*(1), 188.

van Haarst, E. P., Newling, D. W., Gooren, L. J., Asscheman, H., & Prenger, D. M. (1998). Metatastic prostatic carcinoma in a male-to-female transsexual. *British Journal of Urology, 81,* 776.

Waddell Clinic Memo. (2006). *Tom Waddell Health Center protocols for hormonal reassignment of gender.* http://www.sfdph.org/dph/comupg/oservices/medSvs/hlthCtrs/TransGendprotocols122006.pdf. Accessed June 24, 2010.

Wainberg, M. L., Kolodny, A. J., & Drescher, J. (2006). Introduction: A look inside the "crystal" ball. *Journal of Gay and Lesbian Psychotherapy, 10*(3,4), 1–7.

Walter, B., Simoni, J. M., & Howarth, P. F. (2001). Sexual orientation bias experiences and service needs of gay, lesbian, bisexual, transgendered, and two-spirited American Indians. *Journal of Gay and Lesbian Social Services, 13,* 133–149.

Walters, K. L. (1997). Urban lesbian and gay American Indian identity: Implications for mental health service delivery. *Journal of Gay and Lesbian Social Services, 6*(2), 43–65.

Wat, E. (2002). *The making of a gay Asian community: An oral history of pre-AIDS Los Angeles.* New York, NY: Rowan & Littlefield.

Watney, S. (1988). AIDS, "moral panic," theory and homophobia. In P. Aggelton & H. Homans (Eds.), *Social aspects of AIDS* (1st ed.). Philadelphia: Falmer Press.

Weisz, V. K. (2009). Social justice considerations for lesbian and bisexual women's health care. *Journal of Obstetrics, Gynecology and Neonatal Nursing, 38*(1), 81–87.

Williams, W. L. 1992. *The spirit and the flesh: Sexual diversity in American-Indian culture.* Boston: Beacon Press.

Wolfe, A. (1998). *One nation, after all: What Americans really think about God, country, family, racism, welfare, immigration, homosexuality, work, the right, the left and each other.* New York, NY: Viking Press.

Wolitski, R. J., Stall, R., Valdiserri, R. O., Denning, P. H., & Levine, W. C. (Eds.). (2007). *Unequal opportunity: Health disparities affecting gay and bisexual men in the United States.* New York, NY: Oxford University Press.

Wong, F. Y., Campsmith, M. L., Nakamura, G. V., Crepaz, N., & Begley, E. (2004). HIV testing and awareness of care-related services among a group of HIV-positive Asian Americans and Pacific Islanders in the United States: Findings from a supplemental HIV/AIDS surveillance project. *AIDS Education and Prevention, 16*(5), 440–447.

Yoshikawa, H., Wilson, P. A. D., Chae, D. H., & Cheng, J. F. (2004). Do family and friendship networks protect against the influence of discrimination on mental health and HIV risk among Asian and Pacific Islander gay men. *AIDS Education and Prevention, 16,* 84–100 10.1521/aeap.16.1.84.27719.

Young, R. M., Weissman, G., & Cohen, J. B. (1992). Assessing risk in the absence of information: HIV risk among women injection drug users who have sex with women. *AIDS Public Policy Journal, 7,* 72–80.

Zaidi, I. F., Crepaz, N., Song, R., Wan, C. K., Lin, L. S., Hu, D. J., et al. (2005). Epidemiology of HIV/AIDS among Asians and Pacific Islanders in the United States. *AIDS Education and Prevention, 17*(5), 405–417.

Zimmerman, M. A., Washienko, K. M., Walter, B., & Dyer, S. (1996). The development of a measure of enculturation for Native American youth. *American Journal of Community Psychology, 24,* 295–310.

CHAPTER SEVEN

Pathways' Housing First

A Consumer-Driven Approach to Ending Homelessness and Promoting Recovery

Sam Tsemberis[1] and Ben Henwood[2]

INTRODUCTION

Homelessness has been a part of the American landscape for the past 30 years. This homelessness "crisis" that started in the early 1980s was a direct result of the federal government's elimination of funding to continue building affordable housing. Homelessness on a large scale continues today, but there has spawned a community of agencies and a lexicon of program interventions aimed at addressing homelessness. In addition to the development of various programs designed to serve those who are homeless, the Unites States Interagency Council on Homelessness (ICH) was founded in the late 1980s to "coordinate the Federal response to homelessness and to create partnerships between the Federal agencies addressing homelessness and every level of government and every element of the private sector" (ICH, 2008). In the 1990s, Homeless Management Information Systems (HMIS) were developed in response to a Congressional mandate requiring states to collect information on homelessness in order to continue receiving federal money from the U.S. Department of Housing and Urban Development (HUD) to serve a homeless population

---

[1]Sam Tsemberis, PhD, Founder and CEO Pathways to Housing, Inc. and Department of Psychiatry, Columbia University Medical Center.

[2]Benjamin Henwood, LCSW, is a mental health services researcher pursuing a PhD in social work at New York University. He most recently served as the Clinical Director of Pathways to Housing in Philadelphia.

(HUD, 2001). These systems were developed to provide a better understanding of homelessness, with better estimates of the number of homeless. This data collection process is now facilitated by the Annual Homeless Assessment Report (AHAR) prepared by HUD.

The 2009 AHAR, which is the fifth and most recent report, concluded that overall homelessness remained largely unchanged from the previous year, with there being roughly 643,000 people nationally who were counted as homeless on a single night in the month of January (HUDs "one night count") and roughly 1.56 million people accessing shelter through homeless services over the course of the year (HUD, 2010). While overall numbers mask wide variation at state and local levels, as well as a growth in the number of homeless families and those living in rural and suburban areas, the 2009 report notes a more than 10% drop in the national number of chronically homeless individuals from the previous year. A working definition of a chronically homeless individual adopted at the federal level is "an unaccompanied homeless individual with a disabling condition who has either been continuously homeless for a year or more, or has had at least four episodes of homelessness in the past three years" (HUD, 2007a, p. 3). In particular, individuals diagnosed with severe mental illnesses disproportionately constitute the chronically homeless population, most of whom have co-occurring addictions (National Coalition for the Homeless, 2008; Susser et al., 1997; U.S. Department of Housing and Urban Development, 2008). It is also the case that people with disabling conditions have significantly reduced incomes and are among the very poorest among the homeless, with little chance of a quick recovery from economic hardship. If a person depends on a monthly SSI disability check for their income, in most places in the United States they would need two or three times the amount of their monthly income to secure housing again. People with disabilities are essentially "priced out" of being housed again (Cooper, Korman, O'Hara, & Zovistoski, 2009). Homelessness can be seen as primarily a problem of poverty, serious mental illness, and substance abuse, but those causes are neither necessary nor sufficient for homelessness to occur. Certainly, however, their combination may hasten the descent into homelessness and impede the recovery from homelessness. Although serious mental illness typically predates homelessness, substance abuse can occur either prior to or post homelessness. Either way, homelessness exacerbates both the symptoms of mental illness and of substance abuse, complicating the relationship between serious mental illness, substance abuse, and homelessness (Drake, Osher, & Wallach, 1991; Mueser, Drake, & Wallach, 1998).

The Pathways' Housing First (PHF) program is an evidence-based practice (NREPP, SAMHSA, 2007) that was developed with this complexity in mind, yet it offers a simple, straightforward solution—provide housing first, and then combine that housing with supportive treatment services. The more than 10% drop in the number of chronically homeless individuals noted in the 2009 AHAR report can be largely attributed to the rapid growth and dissemination of the *Housing First* (HF) approach that originated from the PHF program. In the past 5 years, the number of HF programs has grown from a few dozen to a few hundred. The National Alliance to End Homelessness (NAEH) reports that more than 400 cities and counties have completed 10-year plans to *end* homelessness and 67% of all plans include an HF program (http://www.endhomelessness.org). In California, an estimated 100 HF programs were recently implemented using funds generated by the California Assembly Bill 2034 (the millionaire's tax), which funded the Integrated Services for the Homeless Mentally Ill (Gilmer, Manning, & Ettner, 2009). PHF programs are also growing in Canada and in Europe. The Mental Health Commission of Canada recently funded a $110 million national HF initiative to implement HF programs in five cities and to conduct a cross-site randomized control trial to evaluate its effectiveness (http://www.mentalhealthcommission. ca/english). In Europe, Portugal, France, Finland, Denmark, Ireland, and the Netherlands are planning the implementation of HF programs. This chapter will describe the PHF model, its empirical basis, and its consumer-driven service approach that has been the key to its ongoing success.

PHF Program Model

The design of the PHF program model originated by honoring what most homeless individuals request, which is an apartment of one's own in a normal, community setting. An invitation to be placed in a home of one's own has proven to be an offer of enormous value that many chronically homeless individuals find irresistible. A key feature of PHF is that the program does not require participation in psychiatric treatment or sobriety as a condition for obtaining housing, removing prerequisites to housing that can be insurmountable barriers for the most vulnerable sector of the homeless. Through adopting a harm reduction approach to substance use as opposed to an abstinence-based model, PHF has successfully tested the hypothesis that consumers can move directly from homelessness into independent apartment living though the use of flexible, team-based support services. In addition to paying 30% of their income toward rent, consumers agree to only two conditions: (1) regular staff visits to their apartment and (2) the terms and conditions of a standard lease with full tenant rights.

The PHF program model was born out of frustration with, and stands in stark contrast to, traditional approaches to homeless services in which treatment requirements and expectations of consumer stability have interfered with ending an individual's experience of homelessness. The underlying philosophy of traditional approaches is that change must occur at the individual consumer level before one can transition into permanent housing. Within traditional approaches, consumers must "graduate" through a series of placements typically starting with drop-in centers or shelters, through transitional housing, and finally into permanent housing by demonstrating treatment compliance, psychiatric stability, and abstinence from substance abuse (Kertesz, Crouch, Milby, Cusimano, & Schumacher, 2009; Wong & Stanhope, 2009). If a consumer relapses, becomes unstable, or chooses not to follow rules necessary for congregate living, he/she must leave the program and/or become institutionalized, which by default entails sacrificing their current living situation and the prospect of permanent housing. Success, which is rarely achieved, is attributed to effective treatment and often results in permanent housing in buildings inhabited by other people with psychiatric disabilities (Hopper & Barrow, 2003). The main motivating factor for individual change within this approach is thought to come from a promise of permanent housing. This structurally endorsed incentive presents a high stakes proposition in which an end to homelessness depends on an individual's ability to first learn to manage conditions that by nature are difficult to overcome and often recurring. The nature of this challenge itself may help to explain why the traditional service approach has had limited success at addressing chronic homelessness (U.S. Department of Housing and Urban Development, 2007).

PHF: Empirically Supported

In contrast to the traditional service approach, the PHF program has proven remarkably successful and changed the landscape of what is considered possible for people suffering from chronic homelessness. Research has demonstrated overwhelming evidence that HF is effective for achieving residential stability for people who have remained homeless for years. Initial evaluations of HF in urban areas with primarily street-dwelling samples of chronically homeless persons have yielded convincing results. Using archival data over a five-year period, 88% of HF consumers remained housed as compared to 47% of consumers in traditional residential treatment (Tsemberis & Eisenberg, 2000). In a randomized clinical trial of housing alternatives, individuals assigned to HF spent approximately 80% of their time stably housed compared with only 30% for participants assigned to traditional services after 2 years (Tsemberis, Gulcur, & Nakae, 2004).

In 2004, the U.S. ICH launched its national Initiative to Help End Chronic Homelessness, funded by the Department of HUD, Department of Health and Human Services (HHS), SAMHSA, and the Veterans Administration (VA). Seven of the 11 cities funded used the HF model and achieved 85% housing retention rates after 12 months (Mares, Greenberg, & Rosenheck, 2007). Two years later, HUD published the outcomes of their three-city, 12-month study of HF programs and reported an 84% housing retention rate for 12 months (Pearson, Locke, Montgomery, & Burton, 2007; Pearson, Montgomery, & Locke, 2009). Similar outcomes were replicated for consumers who were long-term shelter dwellers in a suburban county. In that study, approximately 78% of HF participants remained stably housed over a four-year period (Stefancic & Tsemberis, 2007). These studies suggest the model's utility for more than one segment of the homeless population, street dwelling persons, as well as shelter residents, and its effectiveness using housing stock in urban and suburban environments.

While the hallmark of HF's effectiveness has been assessed through success achieved in residential stability, both quantitative and qualitative research has also documented advantages to HF that go beyond residential stability. For instance, consumers rate housing satisfaction significantly higher when living in more independent supported housing settings as compared to congregate or community residences (Siegel et al., 2006). Both choice and scatter-site housing, as part of HF, are significant predictors of consumers' psychological well-being and social integration, respectively (Greenwood, Schaefer-McDaniel, Winkel, & Tsemberis, 2005; Gulcur, Tsemberis, Stefancic, & Greenwood, 2007). HF consumers also describe a greater sense of belonging in the world through having their own home in terms of greater privacy, normalized daily activities, and the presence of a secure base for self-discovery (Padgett, 2007). It is important to note that while some people report feeling lonely in their apartments, they still prefer independent to congregate housing (Yanos, Barrow, & Tsemberis, 2004).

Additionally, although consumers in traditional programs report higher rates of substance use treatment, even those HF consumers with lower rates of treatment utilization yielded no greater rates of alcohol or substance use in a randomized controlled trial (Padgett, Gulcur, & Tsemberis, 2006). Subsequent comparison studies suggest that HF consumers may actually use less drugs and alcohol than those in traditional services (Padgett, Stanhope, Henwood, & Stefancic, 2010), yet there are still those who maintain HF is not appropriate for persons with active addictions (Kertesz et al., 2009). Paradoxically, the traditional service approach that has a program requirement of abstinence is no more effective, or perhaps less effective than HF programs that use a harm reduction approach. These findings reinforce the need to target people's internal motivations for recovery rather than program rules (Prochaska, DiClemente, & Norcross, 1992; Rollnick, Miller, & Butler, 2008). Mandating detoxification or rehabilitation stays for substance use also contributes to higher costs within the traditional service approach (Perez-Pena, 2007).

Indeed, another impetus toward HF has come from cost-effectiveness considerations. Put simply, choosing to leave people on the streets has a price. Culhane (2008) notes that homeless advocates have long argued that providing HF is significantly less costly than having a person remain homeless, and there is now evidence to support this claim. In a HUD-funded review of cost studies dating back to 1998, Culhane (2008) and colleagues found that the average cost for shelter beds nationally is $13,000 or more per year, depending on region and the services available. In New York City, service-enriched shelter beds can range from $23,000 to $33,000 per year and institutional settings such as hospitals or jails can quickly bring those costs well over $100,000 per year. One study found that the combined average annual cost associated with services such as drop-in centers, shelters, emergency services, police interventions, and incarcerations for individuals who are chronically homeless with severe mental illness is $40,500. When this same group is provided HF, the combined rent and service costs range from $17,000 to $24,000, depending on services utilized (Culhane, Gross, Parker, Poppe, & Sykes, 2008). While funding is needed to support rental costs in HF programs, these costs can be offset to some degree through reduction and eventually elimination of outreach, drop-in, shelter, and transitional housing programs since these step by step "housing readiness" programs are unnecessary when using the HF model.

Malcolm Gladwell put a face on this counterintuitive discussion of cost, homeless, mental illness, and service utilization. His memorable

New Yorker profile entitled "Million Dollar Murray" is about a man he met in Reno and his story is briefly summarized below:

Case Vignette: Million Dollar Murray

Murray was a middle-aged homeless man who lived for 10 years in Reno Nevada. He was very well-known figure downtown—a veteran who suffered from schizophrenia. Everyone, it seemed, knew Murray: the Police, the local merchants, homeless outreach teams, the emergency room staff, the detox center staff, and the ambulance drivers all knew Murray well.

Why does Gladwell give him this "Million-Dollar" moniker? Because Gladwell, with the assistance of a local police officer, tallied all of the different services Murray received from the City of Reno over the course of the previous 10 years. He totaled the cost of the emergency medical service transports, police interventions, jail days, detox days, hospital days—all the various services, and calculated that in 10 years, the City of Reno had spent over a million dollars on Murray. And yet Murray remained homeless until the day he passed away.

The service providers in Murray's life repeatedly offered the same services, presumably expecting a different result. Trying to get some people who are homeless into treatment over and over again as an incentive for housing has proven incredibly costly and simply has not, and will not, work for the chronically homeless like Murray.

More than 40 municipalities throughout the United States have conducted cost analysis studies since 2003 to generate strategic planning information as part of their 10-year plans to end chronic homelessness. The findings are striking in their consistency—all demonstrate reduced service use subsequent to housing placement, with cost reductions ranging from $5,266 to $43,045 (Culhane, Parker, Poppe, Gross, & Sykes, 2007). Many find that the reduced costs of services used fully offset the intervention cost. Despite the consistency of these cost studies, Culhane (2008) points out that even when studies of housing solutions clearly indicate that reduced services costs associated with the interventions partially or wholly offset their cost, cost savings do not necessarily transfer between public agencies. Savings accrued from the reduced service utilization of homeless persons are not easily reinvested in housing solutions. Clearly, even when cost savings associated with housing interventions are apparent, there are complicated issues that must be addressed.

Four Essential Program Principles

The HF program is a complex community mental health intervention that includes housing and a clinical component. The program has numerous operational and administrative dimensions and protocols that are well defined (http://www.pathwaystohousing.org). The focus here is to present four of the key program principles upon which this effective intervention is based.

Consumer-Driven Services

PHF's empirical basis and cost effectiveness, which have driven its rapid growth and dissemination, often overshadow the consumer-driven service approach that has been the key to its success. The straightforward, effective solution to the problem of chronic homelessness offered by the PHF program requires creative, flexible staff, since honoring consumer choice does not end with providing people with an apartment; ongoing services must also be "consumer driven." The program's functional separation of housing from support services is intended to make clear that housing is a basic human right and not something that needs to be earned or used as leverage for treatment compliance, yet ongoing support services must continue to match the stated needs of consumers. This requires the consumer to be either the driver of the treatment or at minimum an active collaborator.

The goal of this consumer-driven approach is to *shift the initiative* for setting goals and pursuing solutions from the provider to the consumer. There is a subtle but very important shift in "the battle for initiative" that must take place when attempting to work in a consumer-driven manner. Consumers with a long history of receiving traditional mental health services have been inducted into a system of care where the initiative and drive of the treatment regimen has been prescribed by providers. They have been told (not asked) what ails them (given a diagnosis which may or may not be consistent with their lived experience or beliefs) and what to do about it. Such clinician-driven approaches direct the treatment and interventions and require the client to be either cooperative or complaint. They are instructed on what medications to take, how often to meet with their doctors or case workers, and provided with specific goals and outcomes for their treatments. Rarely have their voices been heard. This renders consumers passive in the decision-making process. In such programs, all they are left with is the option to either comply or not comply. If they fail to comply or *choose* not to comply they are usually labeled as "treatment resistant" or "difficult to serve" as though their failure to agree or respond is a personal failing rather than a difference of opinion. This approach has resulted in an overall system of care that many consumers choose to avoid altogether.

In the HF model, the client is considered to be the expert of their own experience. This is the starting point of consumer-driven services and housing, assuming that consumers (not programs) are the experts of their own needs and wishes. Clients are asked about their priorities and preferences and actively guide the treatment or services from the beginning. They initiate the service approach because services and housing are designed to respond to their needs and priorities.

The consumer-driven clinician is present, actively listening and prepared to take action, but only when the consumer initiates the plan. (This approach is interrupted only in times of crisis when the staff must take an active role intervening to assure the health and safety of the consumer.) Consumers, however, are not used to being active, let alone in charge of clinical interactions. This will take patience and practice for both the consumer and the clinician. For clinicians, there are many instances when it is tempting to point things out to consumers, make suggestions or simply do things for them. This "doing for" approach may seem to be expedient or efficient in the short term but it retains the clinician as the initiator of action and renders the consumers passive. In the long run, it is much more productive to either "do with" or assist the consumer to "do for themselves." In practice, clinicians must be cognizant that while *doing things for* the consumer may be acceptable during the engagement or initial phase of the program, they want to be moving toward *doing things with* consumers, and finally, teaching and supporting consumers *to do things for themselves* (and be ready to provide support when asked).

This fundamental approach is given a significant head start in the PHF program since the program starts by working with consumers to help them achieve their immediate self-stated goal—finding a place of their own to live. Clients actively work with staff to select the neighborhood where they wish to live; they choose their own apartments; they select their own furniture and household items. Providing a person who is homeless with a rent-subsidized furnished apartment with few strings attached also serves as an excellent way to achieve trust—creating a "therapeutic spike"—that then sets the precedent for how all subsequent services are provided. "O.K., you're housed, what can we help you with now?" is how the program should unfold. In order to maintain this approach, clinicians must have the right values including a belief in social justice and compassion, as well as training in a number of different practices known to be effective for this population, including motivational interviewing, integrated dual diagnoses treatment, and supported employment, among others. This well-trained staff member must be prepared to meet the consumers where they are, which may mean to simply be ready to assist, but not necessarily *doing* anything more than that. Ongoing home visits, a part of the program, serve to keep lines of communication between providers and consumers open, so that when consumers are ready they have the support they need.

In fact, the home visit represents the "heart and soul of the program." It is not simply a social call. It is where important communication takes place and where "the change happens"—in the person's own environment. In many ways, the home visit really starts *before* the actual visit. It begins when discussing the need to do a home visit with the client, and it continues while working out a time that is convenient for the client. (Surprise home visits should only be done if there are concerns that a client is in danger or hurt and only after all other ways to contact the client have been exhausted.) Building relationships, after all, takes time—especially when some clients are suspicious of a team's motives and are convinced that the team has the power to take the apartment away (the team does not have that power). During the early phases of the program, clients may deny problems or troubling issues they are facing. To foster trust, team members must convey acceptance and concern—not judgment. Home visits can create an opportunity to connect and work on developing a deeper and more authentic relationship. To do this, team members must be focused but not hurried or rushed. Clients will not open up and ask for help unless they first trust the helper. In fact, unless they trust the helper they may not be home when the helper calls.

Home visits often include the provision of services such as medication delivery, counseling, and nuts-and-bolts things like helping the client fix a leaky faucet. Much of the routine conversation during a home visit centers around specific clinical services, instrumental or housing needs, scheduling new or follow-up appointments, family issues, and other areas discussed at length during the development of the treatment plan. One of the interesting things about a home visit, however, is the way it creates a shift in power dynamics between client and staff. The home visit, after all, occurs on the client's own turf. This, coupled with a PHF program philosophy that does not mandate participation in treatment as a condition for keeping housing, poses an interesting challenge for the team member. Clients will only welcome or tolerate a visit as long as they find it useful or engaging. This is why clinicians must fully embrace and respond to a consumer-driven service approach.

Successful home visits provide staff with an excellent opportunity to assess how someone is doing, as well as examine the condition of the apartment. Team members can learn an enormous amount about clients by carefully observing their living space. What is the meaning of the empty wine bottles on the kitchen counter? Who are the people in that new picture taped to the fridge? The shoes in the doorway are of a different size, who do they belong to? There are still no pictures hanging from these walls ... does the person feel at home? How comfortable is the client in his/her home? Has he/she moved in or are there boxes that are still unpacked since the move? Is that a new crack in the wall near the window? And so on.

Making a home visit provides an opportunity to make innumerable observations about a client's life. In some ways it is a very intimate experience in that it allows the clinician access to the very center of the client's life. The clinician's can not only ask about but actually observe how their client is managing and maintaining their living space; bedrooms, bathrooms, and kitchens that can provide enormous amounts of data to the trained observer. The information obtained during a routine home visit can be stored, noted, asked about, and used as a baseline for the client's *modus operandi* or serve as a reason to intervene. Answers to these questions will inform the way the team approaches the client. This information is also crucial in preventing a possible housing crisis.

There is a lack of formal boundaries when making a home visit and therefore it is essential that the clinician always maintains their clinical and ethical boundaries during such visits. This is a targeted clinical intervention, not a social call. The clinician needs to maintain their professional demeanor at all times and ensure that the visit is consistent with the work the client has agreed to during the treatment plan.

In fact, honoring consumer choice is especially important in times of difficulty or crisis, such as when consumers deplete their financial resources, are under threat of eviction by their landlord, or have relapsed into addiction. Unless there is a danger to the consumer or to others, the staff must support each other to resist desire to control or resolve a chaotic situation. They must make every effort to remain in communication with the consumer, exploring options while allowing the consumer to make the decisions. For example, if a consumer is facing eviction by the landlord because she has invited too many of her homeless friends to stay in her apartment, the staff should work with the consumer to determine the best course of action: What options do we have here? Shall we try to negotiate with landlord? Shall we leave this apartment and start over in another? They discuss the lease violations that led the landlord to file for eviction and how these may be prevented from happening again, and explore what steps should be taken next. By making their own decisions under difficult circumstances, consumers can benefit from their experience and learn to make better decisions in the future. Experiential learning, in which consumers are supported in making their own decisions and observing the consequences of their decisions, is one of the cornerstones of recovery. PHF staff must constantly be offering choices, encouraging self-directed care, and conveying a message of belief that recovery is possible and inevitable.

Separation and Coordination of Housing and Clinical Services

Consumer-driven services are provided by individual clinicians but supported by the appropriate organization structures. As noted, PHF functionally separates treatment options from housing supports, mitigating power differentials between providers and consumers. Consumers have the same rights and responsibilities as all other tenants holding a standard lease. They are required to pay 30% of their income (which typically consists of Supplemental Security Income (SSI)) in rent; the program pays the remainder. Consumer choice also drives the provision of housing (location, type, etc.), but naturally, housing and neighborhood choices are restricted by affordability and suitability of available units. Because the apartments that the program rents consist of rental units available on the open market, there is no need for lengthy project planning and construction. Once the rental stipend is secured, or the housing voucher or other subsidy is obtained, the apartment search begins. HF programs should have the rental stipend or voucher in place before the program begins. To ensure the integration of people with psychiatric disabilities into the community, the program limits leases to no more than 20% of the units in any one building. Apartments are rented at fair market value and meet HUD's Housing Quality standards.

The program may offer to become a consumer's representative payee or offer other budgeting services to help ensure that bills are paid. In PHF programs, however, housing loss occurs only for lease violations, not for treatment noncompliance or hospitalization. Some consumers lose their apartment after they relapse, stop paying bills, and are evicted by the landlord. However, because the housing component is separate from the clinical component, the consumer who is separated from their apartment is not separated from the team's services: eviction from an apartment does not mean being discharged from the program. Rather than an end to the relationship, a consumer's eviction becomes a learning opportunity on how to avoid future mistakes. Program staffs continue to work with the consumer through a housing loss, preventing a return to homelessness and ensuring continuity of care through crises.

Similarly, if a consumer needs in-patient treatment, they go into the hospital, and upon discharge, they return home to their apartment. By separating the criteria for getting and keeping housing from a consumer's treatment status (yet maintaining a close ongoing relationship between these two components), HF programs help prevent the recurrence of homelessness when consumers relapse into substance abuse or a psychiatric crisis. When necessary, team members can provide intensive treatment or facilitate admission to a detox center or hospital to address the clinical crisis. There is no need for eviction; after treatment, the person simply returns home.

Support services are provided through whatever type of model matches consumers needs for which funding can be secured. This is usually provided through a multidisciplinary team approach such as Assertive Community Treatment (ACT) or an intensive case management (ICM) team, in which teams are located off-site, but are available on-call 24 hours a day, 7 days a week and provide most services in a consumer's natural environment (e.g., apartment, workplace, and neighborhood). Teaming is another vital aspect to maintain a consumer-driven approach since colleagues can help keep the "corrective instinct" of providers in check. In addition, team members help when working within a harm reduction approach that considers alternative paths to sobriety as they serve to contain or reduce the many risks associated with behaviors related to addiction such as drug overdose, incarceration, impoverishment, prostitution, malnourishment, unending homelessness, and ill health. Harm reduction is consumer driven and seeks to minimize personal harm and adverse societal effects of substance abuse while the consumer strives toward recovery. Consumer choice is the foundation of the harm reduction approach (Inciardi & Harrison, 2000), in which consumers define their needs and goals as well as the pace and sequence of services.

The choice of ACT or ICM teams is based on current best practices within mental health services and is limited by availability and sustainability of funding. Both of these modalities have excellent outcomes for reducing hospitalization and increasing community tenure while using a recovery-focused approach (Salyers & Tsemberis, 2007). At its core, however, PHF support services need to be flexible and promote consumer choice. This has resulted in the PHF program incorporating such roles as peer providers as well as primary care as part of available services. Peer services are especially important since they help to reduce inherent power differentials between consumers and providers as well as provide consumers a hopeful reminder that recovery is possible. Integrating primary care services through a nurse practitioner or family physician has also become a priority since evidence suggests that chronically homeless individuals represent a stable, aging cohort (Hahn, Kushel, Bangsberg, Riley, & Moss, 2006) with increasing medical needs and a baseline of early mortality (Hibbs et al., 1994; O'Connell, 2005). In addition, as consumers continue to recover they may need fewer services. This can be accomplished by using an ACT step-down team or an enhanced case management team. This flexible adjustment process provides a better match between the consumer and their service needs, increases program capacity, and reduces cost. When the person is fully recovered, there is a complete separation of housing and services because the consumer continues to live in their apartment, and continues paying with no need for program services. The services may be simply discontinued, avoiding the need for a potentially disruptive transition.

Recovery Orientation

PHF consumer-driven approach embodies a recovery orientation that is now the cornerstone of mental health service reform (DHHS, 2003; Stanhope & Solomon, 2008). The rise of the recovery movement itself can be understood as addressing long-held misconceptions that serious mental illness is a lifelong, crippling, degenerative condition (Hopper, 2007). Such misconceptions supported the need for long-term residential care that existed in the United States before deinstitutionalization and contributed to a mental health system that did not support and even discouraged personal growth. In the past 30–40 years, many developments have contributed to a changing view that recovery from serious mental illness is possible. Advances in scientific knowledge, particularly in psychopharmacology and some psychosocial interventions, have provided new ways to address symptoms of mental illness (Dickey et al., 2006; Drake, Mueser, Brunette, & McHugo, 2004). In addition, social movements such as the civil rights and the disability movement have advanced recovery through reframing disadvantage and disability from an individual shortcoming to a lack of fit or problem with the environment (Mitra, 2006; Rioux, 2003). Government policies and judicial court decisions have also supported the idea of recovery through a trend toward community integration and societal accommodation (ADA, 1990; DHHS, 2003; *Olmstead v. L.C.*, 1999).

While many of the aforementioned developments laid the groundwork for the recovery movement, the optimistic shift in thinking that recovery is now a "real possibility" (DHHS, 2003) for persons with serious mental illness came from two distinct sources. The first is longitudinal research that challenged the notion of serious mental illness as a degenerative disease (Harding, 2005). These studies have shown that over time many people achieve either full or partial recovery from schizophrenia. The second and perhaps more influential source of a "recovery-movement" comes from first-person accounts of people who have recovered from serious mental illness (Deegan, 1988; Ridgway, 2001). These accounts have framed recovery in terms of consumer empowerment, hope, and promoting wellness through a rediscovery of the self. Together, these sources have shown that recovery is not only a possibility, but a reasonably attainable goal for persons with serious mental illness.

Although the HF model was not developed explicitly as a recovery-oriented practice, its approach and value base embraces many aspects that are central to the recovery movement. Such recovery principles and their application in practice include: (1) consumer choice and self-direction, (2) person-centered care, (3) empowerment rather than control, (4) strengths-based rather than pathology-based orientation, (5) personal responsibility, and (6) hope for the future (DHHS, 2004; Onken, Craig, Ridgway, Ralph, & Cook, 2007). For people with histories of homelessness, substance abuse, and mental illness, who face complex challenges resulting from years of cumulative disadvantage, such principles within service approaches are equally important. PHF strives to be recovery oriented by placing consumer choice and a shared decision-making process at the forefront (Deegan & Drake, 2006; Drake & Deegan, 2008; Salyers & Tsemberis, 2007).

Community Integration

Essential to the promise of recovery is that individuals with psychiatric disabilities be integrated into society rather than separated into institutional settings or marginalized by limited opportunities that may result in experiencing homelessness. Before deinstitutionalization, state psychiatric hospitals functioned both to house and to treat people with severe mental illness (O'Hara, 2007). Since then, the mental health system has developed several housing models and yet no clear theory of housing and support services has emerged to guide these developments (Newman, 2001). This stands in sharp contrast to housing for people with developmental disabilities where models have been guided by theories of normalization and social valorization (Wolfensberger, 1983; Wong & Stanhope, 2009). Since the

National Institute of Mental Health (NIMH) Community Support System first articulated the goal of providing the necessary skills and support for mental health consumers to live independently in the community in the 1970s (Stroul, 1989), the development of housing approaches has varied from custodial approaches that perpetuate institutional living, to more rehabilitative service intensive models, to recent models that separate housing from services in an effort to provide normalized and permanent housing (Wong & Stanhope, 2009).

PHF promotes community integration by using the scatter-site apartment model and working toward the social inclusion of people with psychiatric disorders (Ridgway & Zipple, 1990; Tsemberis et al., 2004; Yanos, Felton, Tsemberis, & Frye, 2007; Yanos et al., 2004). A scatter-site, normative model, known as supported housing, has been considered the housing approach most conducive to consumer empowerment and community integration (Blanch, Carling, & Ridgway, 1988; Hogan & Carling, 1992; Rog, 2004; Wong et al., 2007). Program staff encourage and foster normative relationships with landlords, neighbors, family, and other natural support networks that promote community living, with services tailored to the individual needs of each consumer. This scatter-site housing design is intended to render consumers virtually indistinguishable from other neighborhood residents with similar socioeconomic and ethnic–racial characteristics (Stefancic & Tsemberis, 2007). The model is also consistent with antidiscriminatory legislation such as the Americans with Disability Act and the Olmstead Supreme Court Decision that mandates that people with disabilities live in the least restrictive settings, both of which are aimed at promoting social inclusion and community integration (ADA, 1990; *Olmstead v. L.C.*, 1999).

CONCLUSION

The PHF program is a systematic attempt to build the programmatic equivalent of unconditional love. The program seeks out among the most vulnerable among the homeless, people who have been homeless for years and who have been diagnosed with psychiatric disabilities, addiction disorders, acute and chronic health problems, and behavioral problems that may interfere with their social functioning or other disabling conditions. The program is committed to providing permanent housing and supports and is designed in a manner that provides each client with multiple chances to succeed. The foundation of the program's success is rooted in its client-driven approach. It is extremely successful in engaging clients that others have failed to engage because it offers housing and services on the client's terms: it provides almost immediate access to one's own apartment without requiring treatment and sobriety as a prerequisite for housing. A well-trained, recovery-focused clinical support staff makes frequent house calls and supports the client in achieving their self-stated goals. While some clients move into their first apartment and manage well right from the onset, others may need to change two or three apartments before they can manage their lives and their housing effectively. The program does not give up; it makes a long-term commitment to do everything possible to help the person leave homelessness and begin their journey of recovery.

REFERENCES

Americans with Disabilities Act of (ADA). (1990). Americans with Disabilities Act of 1990, Pub. L. No. 101–336, Ï 12101(a)(8), 104 Stat. 327, 329 (1990) (amended 2008).

Blanch, A. K., Carling, P. J., & Ridgway, P. (1988). Normal housing with specialized supports: A psychiatric rehabilitation approach to living in the community. *Rehabilitation Psychology, 33*(1), 47–55.

Cooper, E., Korman, H., O'Hara, A., & Zovistoski, A. (2009). Priced out in 2008: The housing crisis for people with disabilities. Retrieved on October 13, 2010 from http://www.tacinc.org/publications_.php

Culhane, D. P., Parker, W. D., Poppe, B., Gross, K. S., & Sykes, E. (2007). Accountability, cost-effectiveness, and program performance: Progress since 1998. Paper presented at the National Symposium on Homelessness Research. Available at http://www.huduser.org/publications/pdf/p12.pdf

Culhane, D. P. (2008). The costs of homelessness: A perspective from the United States. *European Journal of Homelessness, 2,* 97–114.

Deegan, P. (1988). Recovery: The lived experience of rehabilitation. *Psychosocial Rehabilitation Journal, 11*(4), 11–19.

Deegan, P. E., & Drake, R. E. (2006). Shared decision making and medication management in the recovery process. *Psychiatric Services, 57*(11), 1636–1639.

DHHS. (2003). *The President's new freedom commission report: Achieving the promise: Transforming mental health care in America* (No. SMA-03-3832). Rockville, MD: Author.

Dickey, B., Normand, S. L., Eisen, S., Hermann, R., Cleary, P., Cortes, D., et al. (2006). Associations between adherence to guidelines for antipsychotic dose and health status, side effects, and patient care experiences. *Medical Care, 44*(9), 827–834.

Drake, R. E., & Deegan, P. E. (2008). Are assertive community treatment and recovery compatible? Commentary on "ACT and recovery: Integrating evidence-based practice and recovery orientation on assertive community treatment teams." *Community Mental Health Journal, 44*(1), 75–77.

Drake, R. E., Mueser, K. T., Brunette, M. F., & McHugo, G. J. (2004). A review of treatments for people with severe mental illnesses and co-occurring substance use disorders. *Psychiatric Rehabilitation Journal, 27*(4), 360–374.

Drake, R. E., Osher, F. C., & Wallach, M. A. (1991). Homelessness and dual diagnosis. *American Psychologist, 36*, 1149–1158.

Gilmer, T., Manning, W., & Ettner, S. (2009). A cost analysis of San Diego County's REACH Program for homeless persons. *Psychiatric Services, 60*, 445–450.

Hahn, J. A., Kushel, M. B., Bangsberg, D. R., Riley, E., & Moss, A. R. (2006). Brief report: The aging of the homeless population: Fourteen-year trends in San Francisco. *Journal of General Internal Medicine, 21*(7), 775–778.

Harding, C. (2005). Changes in schizophrenia across time: Paradoxes, patterns, and predictors. In L. Davidson, C. Harding, & L. Spaniol (Eds.), *Recovery from severe mental illness: Research evidence and implications for practice* (Vol. 1). Boston, MA: Center for Psychiatric Rehabilitation.

Hibbs, J. R., Benner, L., Klugman, L., Spencer, R., Macchia, I., Mellinger, A., et al. (1994). Mortality in a cohort of homeless adults in Philadelphia. *The New England Journal of Medicine, 331*(5), 304–309.

Hogan, M. F., & Carling, P. J. (1992). Normal housing: A key element of a supported housing approach for people with psychiatric disabilities. *Community Mental Health Journal, 28*(3), 215–226.

Hopper, K. (2007). Rethinking social recovery in schizophrenia: What a capabilities approach might offer. *Social Science & Medicine, 65*, 868–879.

Hopper, K., & Barrow, S. M. (2003). Two genealogies of supported housing and their implications for outcome assessment *Psychiatric Services, 54*(1), 50–54.

Greenwood, R. M., Schaefer-McDaniel, N. J., Winkel, G., & Tsemberis, S. J. (2005). Decreasing psychiatric symptoms by increasing choice in services for adults with histories of homelessness. *American Journal of Community Psychology, 36*(3–4), 223–238.

Gulcur, L., Tsemberis, S., Stefancic, A., & Greenwood, R. M. (2007). Community integration of adults with psychiatric disabilities and histories of homelessness. *Community Mental Health Journal, 43*(3), 211–228.

Inciardi, J. A., & Harrison, L. D. (Eds) 2000). *Harm reduction: National and international perspectives.* Thousand Oaks, CA: Sage.

Kertesz, S. G., Crouch, K., Milby, J., Cusimano, R. A., & Schumacher, J. (2009). Housing first for homeless persons with active addiction: Are we overreaching? *The Milbank Quarterly, 87*(2), 1–52.

Mares, A. S., Greenberg, G., & Rosenheck, R. A. (2007). HUD/HHS/VA Collaborative initiative to help end chronic homelessness National performance outcomes assessment: Is system integration associated with client outcomes? West Haven, CT: Northeast Program Evaluation Center. Accessed November 30, 2008, from http://aspe.hhs.gov/hsp/homelessness/CICH07/index.htm

Mitra, S. (2006). The capability approach and disability. *Journal of Disability Policy Studies, 16*(4), 236–247.

Mueser, K. T., Drake, R. E., & Wallach, M. A. (1998). Dual diagnosis: A review of etiological theories. *Addictive Behaviors, 23*(6), 717–734.

National Coalition for the Homeless. (2008). *Mental illness and homelessness.* Washington, DC: National Resource Center on Homelessness and Mental Illness.

Newman, S. J. (2001). Housing attributes and serious mental illness: Implications for research and practice. *Psychiatric Services, 52*(10), 1309–1317.

O'Connell, J. J. (2005). Premature mortality in homeless populations: A review of the literature. Nashville, TN: National Health Care for the Homeless Council, Inc. Accessed March 7, 2010, from http://www.nhchc.org/PrematureMortalityFinal.pdf

O'Hara, A. (2007). Housing for people with mental illness: Update of a report to the President's New Freedom Commission. *Psychiatric Services, 58,* 907–913.

Olmstead, v. L.C. (98-536) 527 U.S. 581 (1999).

Onken, S. J., Craig, C. M., Ridgway, P., Ralph, R. O., & Cook, J. A. (2007). An analysis of the definitions and elements of recovery: A review of the literature. *Psychiatric Rehabilitation Journal, 31*(1), 9–22.

Padgett, D. K. (2007). There's no place like (a) home: Ontological security among persons with serious mental illness in the United States. *Social Science Medicine, 64*(9), 1925–1936.

Padgett, D., Gulcur, L., & Tsemberis, S. (2006). Housing first services for people who are homeless with co-occurring serious mental illness and substance abuse. *Research on Social Work Practice, 16*(1), 74–83.

Padgett, D., Stanhope, V., Henwood, B., & Stefancic, A. (2010). Substance use outcomes among homeless clients with serious mental illness: Comparing housing first with treatment first programs. *Community Mental Health Journal,* Online First™ Published online 9 January 2010. Accessed on October 13, 2010 from http://www.springerlink.com/

Pearson, C. L., Locke, G., Montgomery, A. E., & Burton, L. (2007). The applicability of Housing First models to homeless persons with serious mental illness, United States Department of Housing and Urban Development Office of Policy Development and Research, Rockville. Available at and accessed May 15, 2008, from http://www.huduser.org/publications/homeless/hsgfirst.html

Pearson, C., Montgomery, A. E., & Locke, G. (2009). Housing stability among homeless individuals with serious mental illness participating in housing first programs. *Journal of Community Psychology, 37*(3), 404–417.

Perez-Pena, R. (2007, April 17). Revolving door for addicts adds to Medicaid cost. *The New York Times,* Front page.

Prochaska, J. O., & DiClemente, C. C. (1992). Stages of change in the modification of problem behaviors. *Progress in Behavior Modification, 28,* 183–218.

Ridgway, P. (2001). Re-storying psychiatric disability: Learning from first person recovery narratives. *Psychiatric Rehabilitation Journal, 24*(4), 335–343.

Ridgway, P., & Zipple, A. M. (1990). The paradigm shift in residential services: From the linear continuum to supported housing approaches. *Rehabilitation Journal, 13*(4), 11–31.

Rioux, M. (2003). On second thought: Constructing knowledge, law, disability, and inequality. In S. Herr, L. Gostin, & H. Koh (Eds.), *The human rights of persons with intellectual disabilities.* New York, NY: Oxford University Press.

Rog, D. J. (2004). The evidence on supported housing. *Psychiatric Rehabilitation Journal, 27*(4), 334–344.

Rollnick, S., Miller, W. R., & Butler, C. (2008). *Motivational interviewing in health care: Helping patients change behavior.* New York, NY: Guilford Press.

SAMHSA's National Registry of Evidence-based Program and Practices: Pathways' Housing First Program. (2007). Available at http://www.nrepp.samhsa.gov/programfulldetails.asp?PROGRAM_ID=195

Salyers, M. P., & Tsemberis, S. (2007). ACT and recovery: Integrating evidence-based practice and recovery orientation on assertive community treatment teams. *Community Mental Health Journal, 43*(6), 619–641.

Siegel, C. E., Samuels, J., Tang, D. I., Berg, I., Jones, K., & Hopper, K. (2006). Tenant outcomes in supported housing and community residences in New York City. *Psychiatric Services, 57*(7), 982–991.

Stanhope, V., & Solomon, P. (2008). Getting to the heart of recovery: Research methods for recovery oriented practice and their implications for evidence based practice. *British Journal of Social Work, 38,* 885–899.

Stefancic, A., & Tsemberis, S. (2007). Housing first for long-term shelter dwellers with psychiatric disabilities in a suburban county: A four-year study of housing access and retention. *Journal of Primary Prevention, 28*(3–4), 265–279.

Stroul, B. A. (1989). Community support systems for persons with long-term mental illness: A conceptual framework. *Psychosocial Rehabilitation Journal, 12*(3), 9–26.

Susser, E., Valencia, E., Conover, S., Felix, A., Tsai, W., & Wyatt, R. (1997). Preventing recurrent homelessness among mentally ill men: A "critical time" intervention after discharge from a shelter. *American Journal of Public Health, 87*(2), 256–262.

Tsemberis, S., & Eisenberg, R. F. (2000). Pathways to housing: Supported housing for street-dwelling homeless individuals with psychiatric disabilities. *Psychiatric Services, 51*(4), 487–493.

Tsemberis, S., Gulcur, L., & Nakae, M. (2004). Housing first, consumer choice, and harm reduction for homeless individuals with a dual diagnosis. *American Journal of Public Health, 94*(4), 651–656.

U.S. Department of Health and Human Services. (2004). *Strategic prevention framework overview.* Rockville, MD: U.S. Department of Health and Human Services, Substance Abuse Mental Health Services Administration. Retrieved April 12, 2006, from http://alt.samhsa.gov/Hottopics/spf_overview.htm

U.S. Department of Housing and Urban Development, Office of Special Needs Assistance Programs. (2007a). Defining chronic homelessness: a technical guide for HUD programs, Washington, DC.

U.S. Department of Housing and Urban Development. (2007b). The Annual Homeless Assessment Report to Congress, Washington, DC. Available at and accessed January 11, 2008, from http://www.huduser.org/intercept.asp?loc=/Publications/pdf/ahar.pdf

U.S. Department of Housing and Urban Development. (2010). *The Fifth Annual Homeless Assessment: Report to Congress.* Washington, DC.

U.S. Interagency Council on Homelessness. (2008). *Innovations in 10-year plans to end chronic homelessness in your community.* Washington, DC. Downloaded October 28, 2008, from http://www.ich.gov/slocal/Innovations-in-10-Year-Plans.pdf

U.S. White House, Office of Management and Budget (2006). U.S. Interagency Council on Homelessness Assessment. Washington D.C. Downloaded October 13, 2010 http://www.whitehouse.gov/omb/expectmore/detail/10006246.2006.html

Wolfensberger, W. (1983). Social role valorization: A proposed new term for the principle of normalization. *Mental Retardation, 21,* 234–239.

Wong, Y.-L. I., Filoromo, M., & Tennille, J. (2007). From principles to practice: A study of implementation of supported housing for psychiatric consumers. *Administration and Policy in Mental Health and Mental Health Services Research, 34*(1), 13–28.

Wong, Y. L. I., & Stanhope, V. (2009). Conceptualizing community: A comparison of neighborhood characteristics of supportive housing for persons with psychiatric and developmental disabilities. *Social Science & Medicine, 68,* 1376–1387.

Yanos, P. T., Barrow, S. M., & Tsemberis, S. (2004). Community integration in the early phase of housing among homeless persons diagnosed with severe mental illness: Successes and challenges. *Community Mental Health Journal, 40*(2), 133–150.

Yanos, P., Felton, B., Tsemberis, S., & Frye, V. (2007). Exploring the role of housing type, neighborhood characteristics, and lifestyle factors in the community integration of formerly homeless persons diagnosed with mental illness. *Journal of Mental Health 16.6:* 703–717.

CHAPTER EIGHT

Homeless Veterans

The Big Picture and the New York Experience

Henrietta Fishman

INTRODUCTION

With many public and private institutions struggling with cost containment and budget constriction, new methods for cross-system coordination are needed to eliminate barriers and ensure access to homeless services. Although homeless veterans are overrepresented in the United States population, there is a misperception that their veteran status entitles them to the resources they need to escape homelessness, and has often mitigated against their receiving access to programs and services available for nonveterans. This is the story of the VA-New York City experience in developing an integrated system of care for homeless veterans.

While much attention to homeless veterans has been generated recently, the common denominator among them is that they are veterans. Their needs, issues, and responses are diverse, but the tie that binds them together is military service—a powerful and unique connection. Homeless veterans are not a new phenomenon. The combination of transient living arrangements, poverty, illness, and lack of support systems are major risk factors in the etiology of homelessness. The high visibility of homeless veterans in the 1970s and 1980s along with the current military conflicts in Iraq and Afghanistan, have focused growing attention on this subpopulation. Following war and economic upheaval, veterans have not always had a home they could return to.

HISTORY

"For tens of thousands of Union veterans the Civil War never ended. Prominent among this group were Federal soldiers who returned to civilian life suffering the long-term physical consequences of battlefield wounds or wartime disease" according to historian Patrick Kelly, author of *Creating a National Home: Building the Veterans' Welfare State 1860–1900*. Near the end of the Civil War, Congress established the National Home for Disabled Volunteer Soldiers to develop a network of federal institutions where Union soldiers could recover from the perils of war. Ultimately, the eligible included elderly veterans and veterans unable to function in civilian life. By 1900, over 100,000 Union soldiers had received care in federal institutions and many remained for the rest of their lives. These soldiers were not markedly different from today's homeless veterans. Residents were either single, widowed, or divorced, lacked family support, and had some type of disability rendering them unable to reenter civilian life either on a temporary or permanent basis. Although about half were unskilled, half were from skilled professions. But there were few opportunities for employment immediately after the war and many of these veterans were too ill or war-weary to seek employment. Indeed, many of these veterans were homeless and federal institutions diverted them from alms or poor houses. Ultimately, many of these facilities evolved into VA residential treatment centers.

Why Are They Homeless?

In exploring the causes of homelessness among veterans, it is necessary to include the impact and meaning of the war itself, the socioeconomic environment and veterans' personal vulnerabilities. We might ask: When Johnny or Jane comes marching home, what is the public perception of the war, and how does this affect veterans' sense of worth and self esteem? What effect does this perception have on the availability of resources and social supports? And how does this interact with the political and economic climates of the time? This is particularly relevant in 2009, when a lack of affordable housing and unemployment reaching over 10% nationally have a profound effect on homelessness.

A number of studies have indicated that the risk factors for homelessness are the same among veteran and nonveteran populations: poverty, housing instability, joblessness or underemployment, substance abuse, mental illness, and medical problems. While combat experience has been identified by many as a major factor in the etiology of homelessness,

Rosenheck, Gallup & Leda (1991) noted that "Post military social isolation, psychiatric disorder, and substance abuse had the strongest direct effects on homelessness..." among male Vietnam veterans. This researcher was unable to identify a causal relationship, except for postmilitary isolation, in comparing combat and noncombat veterans. This finding continues to be controversial, particularly with the attention being given to the mental health of the OIF/OEF veterans and the small, but growing, incidence of homelessness.

With the high rate of PTSD among veterans returning from Iraq and Afghanistan and the incidence of this diagnosis among this newly homeless population, implications exist for the prevention of homelessness. The incidence of PTSD among returning veterans is reflected in data collected from VA Residential Treatment Programs. In 2008, over 20% of the veterans in residential PTSD programs were from the Operation Enduring and Iraqi Freedom (OEF/OIF) eras. For veterans returning from Iraq and Afghanistan in this All Volunteer Army, National Guard and Reserves may be scattered throughout a wide geographic area, so that these veterans may lack access to the support and structure they had in the regular Army. Within the VA, active intervention to prevent homelessness among this new population of veterans has been recognized and implemented with a number of programs.

A major population-based study identified socioeconomic disadvantage, mental illness and addiction as major risk factors for homelessness (Shelton et al., 2009). Of interest are his findings on childhood experiences associated with dysfunctional families, poverty, abuse, and separation from parents or caregivers as major risk factors for homelessness among nonveterans. These findings are consistent with VA data. Rosenheck and Fontana (1994) also noted that premilitary exposure to traumatic experiences, physical or sexual abuse prior to age 18, and foster care placement before age 16 had a substantial impact on homelessness.

Who Are They?

Earlier studies identified the typical homeless veteran as white, older, high-school educated, and likely to have been hospitalized for substance abuse or psychiatric disorders, as compared to the nonveteran population. Since 2000, some of these characteristics have begun to shift among VA programs, with over half of the homeless veterans treated in Fiscal Year 2008 (October 2007–September 2008) representing minorities, predominately Afro-Americans. While no change has been noted among veterans homeless for less than a month, the percentage of veterans homeless for more than two years continues to increase. The majority of veterans seen in specialized homeless programs still are from the Vietnam and Post Vietnam eras, averaging about 50 years of age. These veterans increasingly suffer from comorbid substance abuse and mental illness, physical disabilities, poverty, and unemployment. An extremely diverse population of homeless veterans is evolving: a growing number of women and OIF/OEF veterans, a growing number of chronically homeless from streets and encampments and an aging population with extensive medical problems. Given gender, age and life-cycle needs and attributes, as well as disabilities, a one-size-fits-all approach is tantamount to failure. Programs are challenged to engage these veterans. This often requires developing a new set of knowledge and skills to provide the services they need.

What Do They Want?

Like their nonveteran counterparts, veterans tend to want the same things: a job and a place to live. Legal assistance, emergency financial help, transportation, childcare, credit counseling, and access to treatment and rehabilitation are cited as needs. Often veterans express a sense of shame, despair, hopelessness, anger, and failure. A study of focus interviews with homeless veterans from the Vietnam era noted that they often felt powerless and victimized because of a distorted public perception, thus feeling abandoned and maligned as a result of their military service and homelessness (Applewhite, 1997). They expressed a need for respect for their military service. With increasing age and medical and mental health disabilities, veterans also want and need a source of income, access to treatment, and community supports. When housed, these veterans are at risk for spiraling back into homelessness without a support network.

Addressing the Needs of Homeless Veterans

Although homeless veterans are not new to the VA, a range of specialized programs was implemented by the Veterans Health Administration, beginning in 1987. Programs providing outreach, contract community residential care and rehabilitation were implemented. The initial initiative, the Homeless Chronically Mentally Ill Program (later to be identified under the umbrella of Health Care for Homeless Veterans) consisted of street outreach with linkage to contract residential care. The goal was to engage these veterans in treatment to help them through successful transition from the streets to the community. This core grew to include residential treatment (Domiciliary Care for Homeless Veterans), transitional and supported housing (the Grant and Per Diem and Supported Housing Programs) the HUD-VA-Supported Housing Program (subsidized section 8 housing with VA case management) and Compensated Work Therapy (prevocational therapeutic employment). The Department of Labor established the Homeless Veterans Reintegration Program to help homeless veterans obtain employment.

How Many Are Homeless?

As the largest network of direct services to homeless veterans in the country, the VA provided services to approximately 80,000 homeless veterans in Fiscal Year 2008. In its 2008 CHALENG Report, the VA estimated that the number of homeless veterans in America dropped from almost 196,000 in 2006 to 131,000 in 2008. It should be noted that this dramatic change was affected by a change in the methodology. The VA, through its Northeast Program Evaluation Center (NEPEC), has been collecting extensive data since 1987, when the first programs specifically designated for homeless veterans were implemented.

Because a means of accurately identifying the number of homeless veterans is not available, estimates vary widely. Several authors have noted that homeless veterans represent a disproportionate share of homeless persons over the age of 18. While approximately 11% of the United States' population is homeless nonveterans, almost 23% of the population are homeless veterans. In August 2007, Levitt and Associates conducted in Manhattan a one-month study comparing of the health and social characteristics of chronically unsheltered with sheltered homeless adults. Among the chronically unsheltered, a significant number were old, sick and veterans (with an average age of 53). This group had been chronically homeless for a cumulative average of ten years. Their characteristics mirrored those identified among nonstreet sheltered homeless veterans: histories of psychiatric and substance abuse problems as well as serious medical problems. Through self-reports 20% were identified as veterans. Among the sheltered homeless, 13% were veterans. The Point in Time Study conducted annually by the HUD Continuum of Cares nationally does not identify veterans at this point. However, HUD does offer a count of sheltered veterans. The 2008 Annual Homeless Assessment Report indicated Veterans represented 15% nationally. The Report noted that these numbers essentially were consistent from 2006 through 2008.

For a one-year period (2006–2007) the VA, in collaboration with Veterans Benefits Administration (VBA) and the New York City

Department of Homeless Services (DHS), conducted a data match between the DHS SCIMS and the VBA's Compensation and Pension Master Record to identify veterans who might be eligible for VA benefits. The target group was the population at a New York City (NYC) shelter for 410 homeless male veterans. Although homeless veterans were scattered throughout the shelter system, this site provided a more stable population who could be linked to services. In a sample of 960, approximately 21% were identified as possibly entitled to a VA pension, indicating the extent of disability as well as age.

Although NYC estimated that 9% in the adult shelter system were veterans, a match between DHS and VBA data for 2006 indicated that somewhat more than 11% of adult males were veterans. Veterans tended to stay in shelters for longer periods of time. Nonveterans in 2006 stayed an average of 353 nights and veterans stayed 587 nights. It is not clear as to what this means.

THE NEW YORK EXPERIENCE

All of these reports suggested the need for a more comprehensive and aggressive outreach and linkage to services for homeless Veterans in New York City. Although VA was providing extensive specialized services to homeless veterans in the metropolitan NYC area in 2006, it became increasingly clear that more intensive, targeted efforts were needed to address the needs of homeless veterans. A number of partnerships with community agencies had been developed, but the urgency of the numbers of homeless in NYC had eclipsed the needs of these veterans. There was a widespread and incorrect belief that the VA could provide all the services these veterans needed, including housing.

For over 20 years, the VA has worked closely with New York City (NYC) programs and agencies in a number of venues. Throughout this time, and through several mayoral administrations, VA has established a credible reputation, forging relationships with career as well as appointed officials. Although they consistently advocated for the needs of homeless veterans, VA staff were unable to obtain support at the highest levels of NYC government for a system specifically targeting the needs of veterans. Despite large numbers of veterans within the total homeless population—both individuals and families—homeless veterans were viewed as a minority. Ultimately, intense pressure from veterans' organizations, elected officials, and the New York City Council led to the development of a NYC shelter specifically for homeless veterans in 1987. Since its inception, VA has been the major service provider in this shelter, providing outreach and comprehensive services to eligible veterans.

In New York City, aware of the difficulty in engaging homeless veterans in shelters or on the streets, Project TORCH (The Outreach and Rehabilitation Center for Homeless Veterans) was designed to offer a "Welcome Home" invitation to these veterans, providing the portal of entry to VA and community services.

Project TORCH

Project TORCH was the first drop-in, multiservice center for homeless veterans in the national VA system. Located in a VA community-based outpatient center in downtown Brooklyn, New York, it serves homeless veterans from throughout the metropolitan New York City area. It is the gateway to VA and community services. While drop-in centers are not a new phenomenon, Project TORCH has a number of unique components. The milieu is warm and welcoming. Veterans had a major role in selecting the pictures and décor. At the reception desk, homeless veterans are greeted by other homeless veterans who provide an orientation to the program. Overall, the program is veteran centered, with an emphasis on creating a supportive environment to engage veterans. A veterans' advisory group meets regularly to provide input and their recommendations have helped shape the program. Applewhite describes three types of problems identified by homeless veterans in focus group meetings: health and mental health problems, resource-related problems, and public perception problems. Essentially, veterans' advisory group members cited barriers in all of these areas that affected their access and utilization of services. They were discouraged by their symptoms and vulnerability, by dehumanizing bureaucratic systems and by insensitive service providers. The structure processes and activities of Project TORCH are designed to enhance and sustain veterans' affiliation with the TORCH community of veterans: to help them develop self-esteem and a sense of hope.

Access to primary medical care is of major importance. Homeless veterans tend to under report medical or physical problems that, left untreated, can lead to emergency room visits and serious complications. Chronic illnesses such as hypertension, diabetes, and asthma are endemic. Studies have demonstrated that homeless veterans have excessive rates of mortality and morbidity and high rates of acute hospitalization. Because homeless veterans tend to seek emergency room treatment and often are hospitalized for longer periods than other veterans, their health-care costs are excessive. At Project TORCH, early medical intervention and follow-up are provided, along with considerable education about health, wellness, and medication.

Case managers link veterans to primary medical and mental health care as well as substance abuse treatment services. Access to resources is provided by an on-site VA benefits counselor, an expedited process to apply for Social Security benefits, and linkage with other benefits and entitlements. Breakfast and lunch, clothing and facilities to shower and wash clothes are on site. Psycho-educational groups, life skills training, AA and NA, art therapy, and an exercise room also are available. This wraparound package of services is available to all homeless veterans eligible for VA services

Aware that the environment in which these services are offered has an impact on veterans' willingness to accept services, a veteran-centric milieu has been created. Homeless veterans have a major role in the program, including meal preparation and group leadership. In a sense, Project TORCH becomes a "home" for homeless veterans. This is particularly apparent when veterans fail to complete residential programs, generally because of relapse or lose their jobs, or face other adversities. They come back to Project TORCH to stabilize their lives. In this nonjudgmental and supportive venue, veterans can cope with their sense of failure and shame and move on with getting their lives together.

Because of its commitment to providing peer support, a pilot initiative was developed to train veterans to provide peer-assisted case management to homeless mentally ill veterans transitioning to housing in the community. For homeless veterans, the movement into independent housing can present a multitude of environmental stressors, such as paying rent, shopping and maintaining their apartment. This has the potential of discontinuing their connection with the support offered by professional staff and peers, leading to isolation and relapse into homelessness.

A cohort of formerly homeless veterans, who had benefitted from the treatment of their mental illness and substance abuse, and were leading stable lives in the community, was selected to participate. These peer advisors received training and supervision from clinical staff. Beginning one month before the veteran moved into housing and continuing for 12 months, peer counselors' roles were to help the veterans develop social networks and integrate into the community. This pilot program, one of the earliest recovery-oriented initiatives in the VA, was successful for advisors as well as peers, improving self-esteem and quality of life. Outreach at NYC shelters, including Borden Avenue, the all veterans' shelter created an opportunity for collaboration with NYC agencies, including DHS. Among other accomplishments, NYC arranged to shuttle veterans from Borden Avenue to Project TORCH, and VA provided shuttle service from NYC shelters to TORCH. Step by step, VA began to enter the radar screen of leadership in NYC and the community. This improved homeless veterans' access to VA services. However, VA had minimal access to services available to nonveterans in the shelter system, such as housing. Over time, with advocacy and support, VA began to have a place at the table with NYC leadership.

The Process

In 1994, a plan for reforming New York City's homeless services system was developed. This included a continuum of care providing outreach and drop-in centers, assessment centers for the shelter system, service programs both within the shelter system and by community agencies, and access to housing. However, this plan focused on a restructuring of the emergency shelter system which, at that point, was housing over 6000 adults nightly.

With the national emphasis on developing 10-year action plans to end homelessness, New York City convened a Coordinating Council representing the public, business, and nonprofit sectors. The VA was invited to participate on one of the task forces. Intensive collaboration among NYC, VA, and community agencies led to the development of *"Uniting for Solutions Beyond Shelter"* (2004) — a 5-year plan for ending homelessness in NYC. This far-reaching plan presented a 10-point strategy: overcome street homelessness, prevent homelessness, coordinate discharge planning, coordinate city services and benefits, minimize disruptions to families whose homelessness cannot be prevented, minimize the duration of homelessness, shift resources into preferred solutions, provide resources for vulnerable populations to access and afford housing and measure progress, evaluate success, and invest in continuous improvement. During the planning process, NYC officials appeared to be more sensitized to the needs of veterans, their sensitivity intensified by the war and publicity about the returning OIF/OEF veterans. However, veteran-specific services were not supported.

Two years later, the Mayor selected a veteran to head up the NYC DHS. The Commissioner had an extensive background of involvement with homeless initiatives and was eager to develop a national model to end homelessness among veterans. To this end, his deputies linked the Commissioner to the VA Network Director in order to explore the possibility of partnering to develop a model of integrated services for homeless veterans. Initially, there was the hope from NYC that VA was able to provide housing and the initial work was to inform NYC of the resources that VA actually could provide. This began a process that culminated in December 2006 with an announcement by VA Secretary Nicholson and NYC Mayor Bloomberg about a new partnership between VA and New York City to end homelessness among veterans. The Mayor issued a 100-day challenge to create a strategic plan to achieve this goal. In addition, DHS committed to housing 100 homeless veterans within the 100 days, exceeding this challenge by housing 135 veterans.

A task force cochaired by the VA Network Director and the Commissioner was appointed, along with a steering committee co-chaired by VA and DHS leadership; were charged with creating a new system to meet the goals identified by the Secretary and the Mayor. Homeless veterans in NYC shelters were also involved in this phase of the process, meeting in focus groups to give input into the planning. The Steering Committee developed workgroups cochaired by VA and DHS and provided oversight and guidance. With clearly defined "deliverables," each workgroup provided a written report. These were reviewed and revised and were coordinated into a report "Operation Home," approved by the Task Force and the Mayor.

While some workgroup members knew each other, the majority did not. In addition to creating an action plan, a major outcome of this process was VA and DHS developing trust in one another. Working as a team developed relationships that carried over into the implementation phase. Trust had to occur in tandem with risk taking if innovative solutions were to be developed. Finding a common "language" was imperative, given that agency-specific acronyms, program names, and verbal "shorthand" often hindered communication. Many staff had spent most of their careers in direct contact with homeless people and the systems that serve them. They understood the advantages and limitations of available resources on a different level than staff in administrative positions. The challenge was to identify a new system that could effectively integrate VA, NYC, NYS, and community providers in order to overcome impediments that had previously fragmented service delivery for veterans.

For example, VA had a definition of "veteran" that differed from NYC's. Eligibility requirements for NYC, NYS, and VA programs and services often were different. Community agencies generally required periods of sobriety and stability that created waits of several months for housing, a major barrier to veterans' community integration. Coordinating and integrating the different systems was a formidable task.

Operation Home

This new model would provide immediate assessment for homeless veterans at a multiservice center colocated with a VA drop-in center, Project TORCH. VA and DHS staff would work as a team at this site, which would be a single point of entry into the DHS and VA systems. Veterans eligible for VA services would receive health care and assistance with benefits. Veterans who were not eligible would be linked with DHS resources. All homeless veterans would be assigned to temporary housing, if appropriate. NYC would provide much needed prevention and diversion resources for those at risk for homelessness. In addition, VA and NYC would provide street outreach together. Safe havens would be developed for veterans needing a low-demand facility. Homeless veterans in VA hospitals would be eligible for these services as well as homeless veterans completing VA residential treatment programs. For this model to work, housing and treatment resources had to be expanded. During the planning process, several steps were taken to expand resources. DHS closed the 410-bed Borden Avenue shelter and completely renovated it, creating 243 modular units of transitional housing for homeless male and female veterans. The runway to this housing would be the multiservice center. VA added additional clinical staff at the multiservice center site. Hours of operation were extended to accommodate the program.

The available housing stock—a critical element—was sparse. A total of 138 transitional beds were available through the VA Grant per Diem Program. At the point when the multiservice center became operational, the HUD/VASH program had been funded and 1100 subsidized housing vouchers became available for homeless veterans and their families. This program involved a partnership between VA and the New York City Housing Authority (NYCHA). With the success of its partnership with VA and its experience in working with NYCHA, DHS made its staff available to expedite the HUD-required housing site inspections, which shortened the length of time for veterans to move into housing.

CONCLUSION: WHERE ARE WE NOW?

In a statement before the U.S. House of Representatives Committee on Veterans Affairs, DHS Commissioner Hess stated "... we believe that this system will serve as a national model for permanently ending veterans' homelessness." Access to NYC and VA services has been a positive outcome. In the three years that VA has worked with NYC to develop a new service system for homeless veterans, the number of veterans in shelters has been reduced by 60%. From August 2008 until May 2009, 3622 homeless veterans were seen in the multiservice center and linked to services. Project TORCH has seen the number of veterans in their program double during this time.

While many challenges remain, the infrastructure has been established and the partnerships between NYC and VA community agencies have strengthened, adding to the resources available for homeless veterans. While no one in America should be homeless, that any veteran in this country would not have a home is unacceptable.

REFERENCES

The Operation Home Ending Veteran Homelessness Task Force. (2007). *A new way home for veterans experiencing homelessness in New York City.* A Report. New York City Department of Homeless Services.

A Progress Report on A New Way Home for Veterans Experiencing Homelessness in New York City by the Joint NYC-VA Task Force. (2008). New York City Department of Homeless Services.

Applewhite, S. L. (1997). Homeless veterans: Perspectives on social services use. *Social Work, 42,* 19–30.

Characteristics of the Manhattan Street Homeless Population. (2008). Center for Urban Community Services.

Kelly, P. J. (1997). *Creating a national home: Building the Veterans' Welfare State 1860–1900.* Cambridge: Harvard University Press.

Health Care for Homeless Veterans Programs: The Twenty-Second Annual Report. (2009). Department of Veterans Affairs Northeast Program Evaluation Center. http://vaww.nepec.mentalhealth.med.va.gov

FURTHER READING

Cunningham, M., Henry, M., & Lyons, W. (2007). *Vital mission: Ending homelessness among veterans.* Washington, DC: National Alliance to End Homelessness.

Fairweather, A. (2006). *Risk and protective factors for homelessness among OIF/OEF veterans.* Swords to Plowshares Iraq Veteran Project.

Henderson, C., Bainbridge, J., Keaton, K., Kenton, M., Guz, M., & Kanis, B. (2008). The use of data to assist in the design of a new service system for homeless veterans in New York City. *Psychiatric Quarterly, 79,* 3–17.

Hess, R. J. (2009). *A national commitment to end veterans' homelessness.* Testimony before the U.S. House of Representatives June 3, 2009.

Kuhn, J., & Nakashima, J. (2009). *Community Homelessness Assessment, Local Education and Networking Group (CHALENG) for Veterans.* Washington, DC: U.S. Department of Veterans Affairs.

Levitt, A. J., Culhane, D. P., DeGenova, J., O'Quinn, P., & Bainbridge, J. (2009). Health and social characteristics of homeless adults in Manhattan who were chronically or not chronically sheltered. *Psychiatric Services, 60,* 978–981.

McGuire, J., Rosenheck, R., & Burnette, C. (2002). Expanding service delivery: Does it improve relationships among agencies serving homeless people with mental illness? *Administration and Policy in Mental Health, 29,* 243–256.

Morrissey, J. P., Calloway, M. O., Thakur, N., Cocozza, J., Steadman, H. J., Dennis, D., et al. (2002). Integration of service systems for homeless persons with serious mental illness through the ACCESS program. *Psychiatric Services, 53,* 949–957.

O'Connell, M. J., Kasprow, W., & Rosenheck, R. (2008). Rates and risk factors for homelessness after successful housing in a sample of formerly homeless veterans. *Psychiatric Services, 59,* 268–275.

Perl, L. (2007). *Congressional Research Service Report for Congress.* Veterans and Homelessness.

Rosenheck, R., Bassuk, E., & Salomon, A. (2002). *Special populations of homeless Americans: The 2002 National Symposium on Homelessness Research.* U.S. Department of Health and Human Services. Available at http://aspe.hhs.gov/progsys/homeless/symposium/2-Spclpop.htm

Rosenheck, R., Gallup, P., & Leda, C. A. (1991). Vietnam era and Vietnam combat veterans among the homeless. *American Journal of Public Health, 81,* 643–646.

Rosenheck, R., & Kizer, K. (1998). Hospitalizations and the homeless. *New England Journal of Medicine, 339,* 1166.

Rosenheck, R., & Koegel, P. (1993). Characteristics of veterans and nonveterans in three samples of homeless men. *Hospital and Community Psychiatry, 44,* 858–863.

Seibyl, C. (2009). *Evaluating MHRRTPs: How to use data to improve program outcomes.* Presentation of Northeast Program Evaluation Center (NEPEC) data at a national VA conference July 2009.

Sadowski, L. S., Kee, R. A., Vander Weele, T. J., & Buchanan, D. (2009). Effect of a housing and case management program on emergency department visits and hospitalizations among chronically ill homeless adults: A randomized trial. *Journal of the American Medical Society, 17,* 1771–1778.

Shelton, K. H., Taylor, P. J., Bonner, A., & van den Bree, M. (2009). Risk factors for homelessness: Evidence from a population-based study. *Psychiatric Services, 60,* 465–471.

Tessler, R., Rosenheck, R., & Gamache, G. (2002). Comparison of homeless veterans with other homeless men in a large clinical outreach program. *Psychiatric Quarterly, 73,* 109–119.

The City of New York. (2004). *Uniting for Solutions beyond Shelter: The Action Plan for New York City.* New York City: The City of New York.

U.S. Department of Health and Human Services. (2003). *Blueprint for change: Ending chronic homelessness for persons with serious mental illnesses and/or co-occurring substance use disorders.* Rockville: U.S. Department of Health and Human Services.

U.S. Department of Housing and Urban Development Office of Community Planning and Development. (2009). *The 2008 Annual Homeless Assessment Report to Congress.*

VA FY 2008 Mental Health Residential Treatment Programs Annual Report. (2009). Department of Veterans Affairs Northeast Program Evaluation Center (NEPEC).

Weissman, E., Covell, N., Kushner, M., Irwin, J., & Essock, S. (2005). Implementing peer-assisted case management to help homeless veterans with mental illness transition to the community. *Community Mental Health Journal, 41,* 267–276.

CHAPTER NINE

Housing for Older Americans

Kenneth A. Knapp and Charlotte Muller

INTRODUCTION

Shelter is a basic universal need and the availability of a safe and sanitary dwelling unit with basic amenities is an assumption upon which most people base all aspects of their life. However, security of tenure in a home is a prerequisite, and as people grow older they face enormous hurdles to retaining that tenure. As people age, they may become overwhelmed by changes in their economic circumstances, by failing health, or by the weakening of support networks as life situations change and family members and neighbors relocate. Older adults often find themselves in a community that has deteriorated and that no longer provides the basic amenities they need to function independently. They may be frail or financially insecure, or so fearful of losing their home through foreclosure or eviction that they avoid making necessary repairs to their dwelling unit. Ironically, by forestalling home repairs they feed into a situation where it becomes difficult for them to remain safely in their home.

In a national survey of housing and home modification conducted by the AARP (formerly, American Association of Retired Persons) in 2000, well over 90% of people age 65 and older responded that they would like to stay in their current domicile for as long as possible. However, the loss of home equity resulting from economic difficulties, the deterioration or outright abandonment of housing stock in a community, midlife unemployment, the price of heating and other necessities, and changing neighborhoods and family situations all play a role in determining whether an older person will remain in the same community and how that person will fare with the passage of time.

This chapter will address the elements that affect home security as people grow older, including changes that occur over time in a built environment where people may have lived for decades and the resulting precarious security of tenure. The pathway that leads older adults into homelessness will be explored, with special emphasis on the circumstances that promote homelessness amongst older women. The chapter will provide information regarding Naturally Occurring Retirement Communities (NORCs), and will discuss aging in place and creative approaches to developing elder-friendly housing that facilitates aging in one's home environment (Bedney, Schimmel, & Goldberg, 2007).

BEYOND THE BUILT ENVIRONMENT

The built environment is a term used to describe human-made surroundings that provide the setting for human activity, including land use, access to public transportation, walking paths, the condition of the sidewalks, access to health care, amenities, and cultural venues. Neighborhoods flourish when the built environment meets many of the needs, common interests, and goals of its residents. Schools, community centers, parks and gardens, common grounds in good repair, and places of worship are some aspects of a built community that contribute to its viability (Jackson, 2003). As people age in place, they have an increased need for community amenities, such as good street lighting and well-maintained sidewalks and access. As age-associated physical limitations force people to stop driving, they require easy access to age-friendly public transportation (such as conveyances with elevators or lifts). Older adults who live in sparsely populated rural areas and small towns fare worse than their counterparts who live in denser geographic areas. An AARP study (2005) showed that more than half of all nondrivers aged 65 and older stay at home on a given day because of limited transportation options, exacerbating their isolation and decreasing mobility.

In addition, it is common for persons over age 70 to have functional physical and mental impairments caused by chronic medical conditions, especially cardiovascular disease, hypertension, diabetes, and chronic obstructive pulmonary disease (COPD) (Fisher & McCabe, 2005). Manipulation, exploitation, and abuses are common among this vulnerable population, and eviction—or its threat—exacerbate the functional impairment (Golant, 2003).

Economic security depends not only on the income, savings, and investments of older people, but also on their ability to meet ongoing housing costs. In 2007, 46% of older persons spent more than one-fourth of their income on their dwelling unit, and in 2008 almost 3.7 million were below the poverty level (AOA, 2009).

As people age, they may find it difficult to pay for health care, pharmaceuticals, groceries, transportation, and other nonhousing goods or services. Although they may have paid off a mortgage or live in affordable (usually rental) housing, if the community is collapsing the amenities upon which they depend will deteriorate or have entirely shut down. Poorly lit streets and abandoned buildings foster crimes, and older persons often find that their home has become a virtual prison, making a trip to the corner grocery store a risky venture.

THE HOMELESS ELDERLY

Living alone is a risk factor for homelessness. Isolation can breed distrust, and older adults often become resistant to help and fail to obtain adequate assistance when they are threatened with eviction proceedings or foreclosure (Cattan, White, Bond, & Learmouth, 2005). According to Milder (2008), an older adult who is evicted from his/her home and has moved to a homeless shelter or nursing home has a life expectancy of less than 6 months (see also Barrow, Herman, Cordova, & Struening, 1999). New York City is an arresting example. Each year, in Manhattan (NY County) alone, more than 600 elderly adults become homeless through eviction— often from apartments where they have lived for decades. The confluence of three factors enables one of the country's most competitive and predatory real-estate markets to victimize these older persons: (1) the individual has developed a functional impairment that may be age related including dementia and deteriorating health and/or mental illness and/or substance abuse (Garibaldi, Conde-Martel, & O'Toole, 2005); (2) they live alone, isolated because of advancing age and frequently become distrustful, resist help, and fail to obtain adequate assistance when eviction proceedings are threatened; and (3) as a result of NYC's rent control/stabilization laws, they live in apartments that can command dramatically higher rents from a new tenant.

Most importantly, eviction forces older persons to live out their lives in desperation and fear, because the social resources to protect them are weak and lack the infrastructure and collaborative capacity to intervene in a timely way. Nationally, many older persons who become homeless sleep on the street, because they distrust the crowds at shelters and clinics. However, they are often ignored by law enforcement, and this in turn makes them vulnerable to victimization. One study from

Detroit found that almost half of older homeless persons had been robbed and one-fourth had been assaulted within the preceding year (Douglass et al., 1988).

Older persons who become homeless are often unaware of their own eligibility for public assistance programs and face difficulties applying for and receiving benefits in that they frequently need help navigating the complex application process (Kendall-Raynor, 2007).

In a survey conducted by Crane et al. (2005), it was reported that of the persons aged 50 and older, half were living alone before losing their homes. Older persons living alone were much more likely to be poor (17.1%) than were older persons living with families (3.0%). Among those 50+ who live alone, the highest poverty rates were found among Hispanic women (43.1%) and black women (34.7%). In 1999, Cohen reported that the elderly homeless are almost twice as likely as younger counterparts persons to have been living alone.

In 1986, Karen Davis and The Commonwealth Fund Commission on the Elderly Living Alone conducted a national telephone survey. It revealed that one-third of older Americans live alone and one-quarter of these persons, typically older women, live in poverty and report poor health. In a testimony to the Committee on Aging, NYC Council in February, 2006, Gusmano and Rodwin (2006) noted that an older person living alone is often a widowed woman in her 80s who struggles alone to make ends meet on a meager income. They point out that being older, she is more likely to be in fair or poor health. She may be either childless or lacks family assistance nearby. Absent social supports, she is at high risk for losing her independent lifestyle (the full testimony can be seen at: www.wagner.nyu.edu/faculty/testimony/rodwinNycCouncil021106.pdf).

Because present-day cohorts of older women spent all or most of their working lives in traditional roles that provided them with limited work experience, and had interrupted work patterns owing to childbearing and childrearing responsibilities (Rogers, 1999), older women have a higher poverty rate (11.9%) than older men (6.7%). As they age, the prospect of continuing or returning to work or gaining income through marriage is often unlikely.

Muller and Volkov (2009) wrote:

> While the gap is narrowing, the specifics of female economic activity are less favorable to acquisition of financial security after 60—large proportions employed in service and clerical jobs with low pay scales and fewer benefits, pay differences within an occupation, and low earnings compared to men. Although for many such women adding to their income through work

could reduce the risk of poverty, at the same time, caregiving responsibilities of midlife and older women for both spouses and aging parents can be expected. In the United States, a study based on the Health and Retirement Survey showed that women who took care of elderly parents incurred a much higher risk of living in poverty later in life compared to non-caregivers.
—*Wakabayashi and Donato, 2006, p. 271*

HELPING THE OLDER HOMELESS POPULATION

In addition to low-income housing and income supports, health-care services are necessary to sustain independent living. For those older adults who have already lost their homes, comprehensive outreach health and social services must be made available as well as special assistance to access existing public assistance program. These would include geriatric social workers experienced in the provision of services to homeless adults; geriatricians to assess and intervene to meet medical, mental health, and/or substance abuse treatment needs; an attorney who specializes in geriatric and housing litigation; supportive services designed to prevent or overcome eviction threats and a network of residential, treatment, and supportive services for the target population of adults over age 60.

Legal Hurdles

There are many legal aspects affecting housing for the elderly. Older persons may be unaware or misinformed regarding their rights, leases, mortgages, deeds, etc. The various agencies that deal with these issues may have different standards and regulations. For example, housing assistance for older people seeking affordable housing varies between cities. Where one lives may affect how easy it is to access legal entitlements. There are many other issues involving the protection of elderly in their right to live where they are living. Elderlaw has grown up, but the challenge of getting affordable services regarding housing remain. The issue is intensified by limitations of immobility (getting to the lawyer's office) as well as losses in hearing, vision, or short-term memory.

A Model for the Disabled Elderly

Beginning in 2004, the National Council on Disability (NCD) developed a model for individuals with disabilities that incorporates not only consumers' preferences for independent living, but also environmental factors that facilitate autonomy (NCD, 2004a, 2004b, 2006, 2007, 2008). Beginning in 2000, the NCD and AARP engaged over 1100 consumers aged 50 and older with disabilities and younger people with disabilities. They used surveys and stakeholder forums to identify elements that stakeholders considered valuable as well as those that presented obstacles to independent living. The investigators found a number of central themes: Consumers feared a loss of independence and control over decision making. They desired continuous social connection and valued routine daily activities and physical exercise. Significantly, stakeholders found their communities unresponsive to individuals with disabilities or health conditions, pointed to the lack of dependable and accessible transportation, and viewed community services as unhelpful in maintaining independence (Gibson et al., 2003 in NCD, 2004a).

Reimagining Housing Design to Meet New Needs

A built community that supports older people as they age in place would have accommodations that run the gamut from altering the length of a stop light to enable persons who walk slowly or require a walker to cross streets in safety, to the development of home-based services and shopping assistance. It would have a backup power system with a generator and emergency supplies in case of an untoward event.

In designing an aging-friendly community, domiciles would be built without steps and easily accessible by ambulettes, with convenient parking and turnaround space. The streets would be paved for age-friendly walking, and the grounds smooth and regular to avoid falls that can occur on hilly or uneven terrain. Domiciles would be clustered to facilitate receipt of visiting services and access to community activities and cultural events.

Life in the City

New York offers prime examples of the strengths and weaknesses of growing old in a large urban environment. On the positive side, the convenience of nearby stores and other amenities, the quality and proximity of public transportation, the existence of cultural and educational events and institutions, and the availability of a large number of excellent health-care facilities as well as supportive services are commonly cited as major advantages of growing older in New York. For those fortunate enough to be financially secure, whose network of family and friends provide a support system, New York is "a great place to grow old" (Finkelstein, 2008, p. 22).

However, Gusmano and Rodwin (2006) note that:

> The combination of population aging and the erosion of the extended family have fractured the assumptions on which municipal services and social welfare programs have been financed and organized. The health and social welfare systems are neither prepared nor preparing for the unprecedented change and the consequences of this situation.
>
> —*Gusmano and Rodwin, 2006, p. 2*

Older New Yorkers live in one of three types of building structures: one- or two-family homes; multiunit buildings with elevators; and "walkups," (multiunit buildings without elevators). Nearly 2 out of 10 older New Yorkers live in walkups, and must use stairs to access their dwellings. While it is not uncommon in many other cities in the country for older people to move to a new home because they can no longer manage the stairs of their previous homes, this option is not available to many older New Yorkers because age-friendly homes are relatively scarce (Finkelstein, 2008).

Older New Yorkers struggle with the same major housing issues that older people faced nationally: affordability, inefficient coordination between housing, health and supportive services, disparities in housing and neighborhood quality, and elder services. A shortage of federal funding, zoning restrictions and limited availability of land, and poor incentives to developers for constructing affordable housing, all are barriers to ensuring an affordable housing stock in New York (Finkelstein, 2008; Gusmano et al., 2002; U.S. Bureau of Census, 2003).

In their report on social isolation among older persons (65+) in NYC, the United Neighborhood Houses (UNH) of New York identified several risk factors that are more pronounced in NYC than they are nationwide: living alone, disability, poverty, linguistic isolation, never having married, and being divorced, separated, or widowed. Based on unpublished work of the NYC Department of Health and Mental Hygiene, this report also identifies 12 Community Districts (out of 59 in NYC) that are "likely the most at risk for senior isolation based on the number of seniors living alone and the level of need among the elderly residents (p. 18)."

Nationally, inefficiencies in the approval process for federal funding construction of subsidized housing for older persons add to the problem. For example, the U.S. Government Accounting Office estimated that as many as 2 million "rent-burdened" older persons might have benefited from the Section 202 Supportive Housing for the Elderly Program were it not for unnecessary bureaucratic hurdles (U.S. Government Accounting Office, 2003).

THE SENIOR COMMISSION ON AFFORDABLE HOUSING

The Senior Commission's 2002 report to Congress, *A Quiet Crisis in America*, documented the immediate and long-term housing and health facility needs for older people. The Senior Commission was mandated by Congress to recommend policy actions that would "increase affordable housing and improve health-related service options for seniors (p. 230)." They reported that:

> Senior individuals who are able to remain in the community should receive the services they need to be as independent as possible. Those who must move from their preferred setting should have viable and affordable alternatives that ensure their well-being. Neither institutionalization nor neglect should be the only alternatives they must accept.
> *—Commission on Affordable Housing and Health, 2002, p. 13*

The Commission focused on the unmet need for greater integration of housing and health services for older people, noting that "The most striking characteristic of seniors' housing and health care in this country is the disconnection between the two fields (p. 16)." It recognized "that appropriate and affordable housing" is an "equal partner" with "accessible, high-quality" health and support services for older people (p. 47). Further, the Commission observed that housing has a central role to play in addressing the nation's long-term care needs.

The Commission recommended that existing housing stock be preserved and that successful housing assistance programs, community-based services, housing production, and models of supportive housing be expanded. They encouraged efforts to explore innovative housing and service programs and models, as well as to promote aging in place through a better coordination of shelter and services. Finally, they noted that federal financing programs need to be reformed in order to greatly improve flexibility and increase production of housing and coverage of health and supportive services.

The Commission pointed out that programs designed to provide housing assistance "are implemented with little reference to health care or supportive service needs."[1] In addition, they noted that Medicare is "centered on acute care and episodic medical interventions"—an orientation not ideally suited to meet the more common chronic care needs of older people. Moreover, Medicaid provides only a "skeleton of a payment system for much-needed home- and community-based care."

NATURALLY OCCURRING RETIREMENT COMMUNITIES

Naturally Occurring Retirement Communities (NORCs) are specific communities or neighborhoods with a large proportion of older persons. An NORC may refer to a specific apartment building, or a street of old single family homes, and it differs from units intended for older people in that it was not originally designed for this purpose. Under Fair Housing laws, a housing complex with 80% of its residents over 55 may become officially age restricted. Services that apply specifically to older persons include scheduled transportation services, meal programs, emergency and preventive health-care programs, and information and counseling, as well as recreational and educational programs (www.seniorresource.com/ageinpl. htm; CRS Report for Congress). (Florence Heller Graduate School at Brandeis University, 1996).

CONCLUSION

Housing affordability in the United States is an issue faced by many residents nationally, but it is especially acute for older people. In addition to affordability, other issues of special relevance include inadequate coordination between housing and health/supportive services; the disparities in housing and neighborhood quality; and, as people grow old, the increased need for a variety of services that help them age in place and avoid being institutionalized or homeless (Schill & Daniels, 2003). Clearly, these issues intersect, such as when a neighborhood in a disadvantaged area contributes to negative health outcomes (Ross & Mirowsky, 2001), or when grandparents who are primary caregivers of grandchildren are denied access to senior housing. And although for the younger population high housing costs relative to income are often "episodic" and the

---

[1]Commission on Affordable Housing and Health, 2002, p. 6.

result of "temporary income shortfalls," older residents often "live for long periods under extreme housing cost pressure" (Braconi, 2003).

The aging of the Baby Boom generation is a significant concern for policy makers, as well as the private sector. The size and longevity of this group has triggered debate about possible modifications to housing. To ensure safe, secure, and affordable housing for Americans as they age, arguably the most effective approach would be greater integration of housing and health-related and other services, as recommended by the Senior Commission. It remains unclear whether policy makers at the local, state, and national level can coordinate their efforts in order to achieve this goal.

REFERENCES

AARP. (2000). *Fixing to stay: A national survey of housing and home modification issues.* Washington, DC: AARP.

AARP. (May 2005). *Beyond 50.05. A report to the nation on livable communities: Creating environments for successful aging.*

Administration on Aging. *A Profile of Older Americans: 2009.* Washington, DC: U.S. Department of Health and Human Services, p. 11. http://www.aoa.gov/AoARoot/Aging_Statistics/Profile/2009/docs/2009profile_508.pdf, accessed on September 15, 2010.

Barrow, S. M., Herman, D. B., Cordova, P., & Struening, E. L. (1999). Mortality among homeless shelter residents in New York City. *American Journal of Public Health, 89*(4), 529–534.

Bedney, B., Schimmel, D., & Goldberg, R. (2007). Rethinking aging in place: Exploring the impact of NORC Supportive Service Programs on older adult participants. 2007 Joint Conference of the American Society on Aging and the National Council on Aging.

Braconi, F. (2003). Heavy burdens. *The Urban Prospect: Housing, Planning and Economic Development in New York. Citizens Housing and Planning Council, 9*(1), March/April, 4.

Cattan, M., White, M., Bond, J., & Learmouth, A. (2005). Preventing social isolation and loneliness among older people: A systemic review of health promotion interventions. *Aging in Society, 25,* 41–67.

Cohen, C. I. (1999). Aging and homelessness. *The Gerontologist, 39*(1), 5–14.

Commission on Affordable Housing and Health Facility Needs for Seniors in the 21st Century. (2002). A quiet crisis in America. A Report to Congress submitted to the Committee on Financial Services, Committee on Appropriations, United States House of Representatives; and the Committee on Banking, Housing and Urban Affairs, Committee on Appropriations, United States Senate. Washington, DC, (June 30). Quotation is from the Preface.

Crane, M., Byrne, K., Fu, R., Lipmann, B., Mirabelli, F., Rota-Bartelink, A. et al. (2005). The causes of homelessness in later life: Findings from a three-nation study, *Journal of Gerontology: Social Sciences, 60B*(3), S152–159.

Davis, K., & The Commonwealth Fund Commission on the Elderly Living Alone. (1986). National Survey of Problems Facing Elderly Americans Living Alone [Computer file]. ICPSR09379-v1. Ann Arbor, MI: Inter-university Consortium for Political and Social Research [distributor], 1991. doi:10.3886/ICPSR09379.

Davis, K., & The Commonwealth Fund Commission on Elderly People Living Alone. (1988). National Survey of Hispanic Elderly People [Computer file]. ICPSR09289-v2. Ann Arbor, MI: Inter-university Consortium for Political and Social Research [distributor], 1997. doi:10.3886/ICPSR09289.

Douglass, R. (2009). *Aged, alone, and adrift*. Detroit, MI: Detroit Area Agency on Aging.

Douglass, R. L., Atchison, B. J., Lofton, W. J., Hodgkins, B. J., Kotowski, K., & Morris, J. (1988). Aged, adrift and alone: Detroit's elderly homeless. Final report to the Detroit Area Agency on Ageing. Ypsilanti (MI): Department of Associated Health Professions.

Finkelstein, R., Garcia, A., Netherland, J., Walker, J. et al.. (2008). Toward an age-friendly New York city: A findings report. New York, NY: The New York Academy of Medicine.

Fisher, H., & McCabe, S. (2005). Managing chronic conditions for elderly adults: The VNS CHOICE model. *Health Care Financing Review, 27*(1), 33–45.

Garibaldi, B., Conde-Martel, A., & O'Toole, T. P. (2005). Comorbidities, perceived needs, and sources for usual care for older and younger homeless adults. *Journal of General Internal Medicine, 20*(8), 726–730.

Gibson, M. J., Freiman, M., Gregory, S. et al. (2003). *A Report to the Nation on Independent Living and Disability*. Washington, DC: AARP. Beyond 50 report series.

Golant, S. M. (2003). Conceptualizing time and behavior in environmental gerontology: A pair of old issues deserving new thought. *The Gerontologist, 43*, 638–648.

Gusmano, M. K., Hodgson, M. G., & Tobier, E. (2002). Old and poor in New York City. International Longevity Center-USA, *Issue Brief* (September/October).

Gusmano, M. K., & Rodwin, V. G.. (2006). Testimony given to the Committee on Aging. New York, NY: NYC Council.

Jackson, R. (2003). The impact of the built environment on health: An emerging field. *American Journal of Public Health, 93*(9), 1382–1383.

Kendall-Raynor, P. (2007). Analysis: Eviction of elderly is "lawful" despite the Human Rights Act. *Nursing Standard, 21*(45), 14–18.

Milder, L. (2008). Morbidity and mortality in a random sample of elderly adults evicted following proceedings in NYC Housing Court. Unpublished manuscript.

Muller, C., & Volkov, O. (2009). Older women: Work and caregiving in conflict? A study of four countries. *Social Work in Health Care, 48*, 665–695.

National Council on Disability (NCD). (2004a). *Livable communities for adults with disabilities*. Washington, DC: National Council on Disability.

National Council on Disability (NCD). (2004b). *Consumer directed health care*. Washington, DC: National Council on Disability.

National Council on Disability (NCD). (2006). *Creating livable communities*. Washington, DC: National Council on Disability.

National Council on Disability (NCD). (2007). *Issues in creating livable communities for adults with disabilities: Proceedings of the Panel.* Washington, DC: National Council on Disability.

National Council on Disability (NCD). (2008). *Inclusive livable communities for adults with disabilities.* Washington, DC: National Council on Disability .

Naturally occurring retirement communities (NORCs) (1996). Offers opportunities for delivering health care and related services. Florence Heller Graduate School for Advanced Studies in Social Welfare at Brandeis University.

Rodwin, V., & Gusmano, M. (Eds.). (2006). *Growing older in world cities: New York, London, Paris and Tokyo.* Nashville, TN: Vanderbilt University Press.

Rogers, C. C. (1999). *Changes in the older population and implications for rural areas. Economic Research Services—Rural Development Research Report No. 90.* Washington, DC: US Department of Agriculture.

Ross, C. E., & Mirowsky, J. (2001). Neighborhood disadvantage, disorder, and health. *Journal of Health and Social Behavior, 42*(3), 258–276.

United Neighborhood Houses. (2005). *Aging in the shadows: Social isolation among seniors in New York City.* UNH Special Report.

U.S. Bureau of the Census. (2003). New York City Housing and Vacancy Survey: 2002. Conducted by the Census Bureau for the New York City Department of Housing Preservation and Development. Washington: The Census Bureau 2003.

U.S. Government Accountability Office. (2003). Elderly housing project funding and other factors delay assistance to needy households, *Report to the Special Committee on Aging,* U.S. Senate. Publication # GAO-03-512.

Wakabayashi, C., & Donato, K. M. (2006). Does caregiving increase poverty among women in later life? Evidence from the Health and Retirement Survey. *Journal of Health and Social Behavior, 47*(3), 258.

FURTHER READING

Schill, M. H., & Daniels, G. (2003). State of New York City's housing and neighborhoods. In *Economic Policy Review: Policies to Promote Affordable Housing,* Proceedings of a Conference Cosponsored by the Federal Reserve Bank of New York and New York University's Furman Center for Real Estate and Urban Policy, *9*(2).

Shapiro, A., & Taylor, M. (2002). Effects of a community-based early intervention Title 42—The Public Health and Welfare, Chapter 35—Programs for Older Americans, Subchapter IV—Activities for Health, Independence, and Longevity (formerly, Training, Research, and Discretionary Programs).

Victor, C., Scambler, S., Bond, J., & Bowling, A. (2000). Being alone in later life: Loneliness, social isolation and living alone. *Reviews in Clinical Gerontology, 10,* 407–417, doi: 10.1017/S0959259800104101.

CHAPTER TEN

Behavioral Health Issues for Older Adults

Substance Abuse and Psychiatric Disability

Frank Guida and Steven A. Estrine

INTRODUCTION

The behavioral health issues of older adults are complex. The high prevalence of medical and cognitive comorbidity in this population, combined with Psychiatric disabilities necessitates a clinical knowledge base that recognizes the complex intermingling of medical and psychiatric disorders. The medical community's relatively poor knowledge base regarding drug interactions, and indeed the extent of psychiatric disabilities of the older patient compromises the quality of care provided. As patients grow older and develop conditions that require prescription and over-the-counter medications, the opportunities for alcohol–drug interactions dramatically increase.

At the same time, as an older person's expectations and beliefs about his or her mental and physical health diminish, they may become reluctant to avail themselves of psychiatric and psychological services since, during their youth, only individuals thought of as "crazy" would be provided with mental health treatment. The current generation of older persons vividly recalls stories of peers who were institutionalized, some against their will, for serious psychiatric disabilities. Many older people fear institutionalization; often hiding the need for treatment from family and friends. The stigma of psychiatric disabilities still exists for some older persons.

Although the current public mental health system and beliefs regarding the acceptance of psychiatric care have changed; older persons are still impressed with what they remember from past years. Therefore, older persons are often wary of seeking mental health intervention even when they may understand its significance in improving their lives. The prevalence of stigma distorts the perception of the level of need, falsely suggesting that older persons do not need the breadth of mental health treatments they require. Moreover, existing mental health services generally are not designed to address the specific needs of the older client requiring psychiatric or psychological care, contributing to their reluctance in availing themselves of necessary treatment.

Many older adults self-medicate to alleviate emotional pain; and alcohol and substance misuse go hand in hand with their depression and mental health issues. The Substance Abuse and Mental Health Services Administration (SAMHSA) estimates that nationwide as many as 17% of older adults are currently affected by alcohol and or prescription/drug misuse (SAMHSA, 1998). However, it is generally recognized that this significant public health problem for older adults tends to be undetected or misdiagnosed, ignored, mistreated, and underreported (Curtis, Geller, & Stokes, 1989; Geller, Levine, & Manon, 1989).

This chapter will discuss drug and alcohol abuse among older persons, including drug interactions between alcohol and medications, comorbidities, and prevalence among women. It will discuss the fiscal impact on the economy of older persons with substance abuse and comorbid conditions. The chapter will also address working with older minority populations. Finally, the chapter will offer several innovative evidence-based treatment interventions. It will conclude with ways to overcome barriers to treatment.

ALCOHOLISM AND SUBSTANCE ABUSE AMONG OLDER ADULTS

At-risk drinking is defined as "alcohol use that is excessive or potentially harmful in combination with select co-morbidities or medications." Approximately 50% of men and more than one-third of women in the United States over the age of 60 are current drinkers (Barnes et al., 2010). They are a population at risk, because physiological changes as well as age-associated morbidity and medication use may increase the effects of alcohol consumption in older adults; and make no mistake for, alcohol is a drug. Psychiatric comorbidities, particularly depressive disorders, also tend to co-occur with alcohol misuse (Guida, Tavolacci, & Provet, 2003). Data from the National Longitudinal Alcohol Epidemiology Survey demonstrate that among persons older than 65, those with alcoholism are approximately three times more likely to exhibit a major depressive disorder than those without alcoholism. Among persons older than 65, moderate and heavy drinkers are 16 times more likely than nondrinkers to die of suicide. (Conwell & Duberstein, 2001)

Morley (2002) reports that in hospital settings, where appropriate screenings are carried out, more than one-fifth of the older patient population have been diagnosed as alcohol abusers; nearly half the residents in nursing homes were found to have medical problems related to recent or previous alcohol abuse and dependence (Weintraub et al., 2002).

Even conservative estimates of increases in the number of older persons needing treatment for substance abuse point to a growing problem. Gfoerer, Penne, Pemberton, and Folsom (2003) determined that nationwide the number of adults aged 50 and older in need of substance abuse treatment will grow from 1.6 million in 2000 to approximately 3 million in 2020, this increase, expected for all gender and race groups among aging adults.

While longitudinal studies (Glynn, Bouchard, LoCastro, & Hermos, 1984; Reich, Cloniger, & Van Eerdewegh, 1988) have provided evidence of stable drinking and drug abuse patterns as a person ages (lifelong users), Gomberg (1982), and Williams (1984) found that subjects may increase their consumption as a response to age-related stresses, such as loss of employment, widowhood, or other bereavement. Hurt, Finlayson, Morse, and Davis (1988) found 41% of people aged 65 and older enrolled at the Mayo Clinic alcoholism treatment program reported late-onset (over the age of 55) symptoms of alcoholism. A study conducted at Odyssey House by Guida, Unterbach, Tavolacci, and Provet (2004) found that 37% of elder clients residing in a residential drug abuse treatment program were late-in-life abusers (defined as over the age of 55).

Medical Comorbidities

A history of alcohol and/or drug abuse in older adult patients is associated with high rates of medical treatment (Moos, Mertens, & Brennan, 1994), and longer hospitalizations (Ingster & Cartwright, 1995). Among older patients admitted to general hospitals, 30% were problem users of alcohol, sedative/hypnotics, antianxiety agents, and/or analgesics (McInnes & Powell, 1994; Whitcup & Miller, 1987). Adams, Barry, and Fleming (1996) found that 70% of hospitalizations for this population were for alcohol/drug-related illnesses and injuries, more than the number admitted for heart disease. In their study of emergency department visits, McIntire et al. (1996) found that one-third of substance abuse-related visits were by adults aged 65 and over. Older substance-abusing inpatients have mortality rates approximately 2.5 times higher than expected for this population (Moos et al., 1994).

Medication Interactions

Changes in the absorption, distribution, and metabolism of alcohol and other illegal drugs in older adults can create deleterious interactions with medications—both prescription and over the counter. Side effects can include extreme blood pressure changes, cardiac arrest, difficult breathing, coma, and death (Barnes and Chappell, 1981). Alcohol can exacerbate or reduce a medicine's therapeutic effects, and interfere with the effectiveness of some medications to treat conditions like hypertension, gastroesophageal reflux, insomnia, and depression (Barnes and Chappell, 1981).

Alcoholism in Older Women

According to a treatment protocol published by SAMHSA (2009), "... women are more sensitive to the consumption and long-term effects of alcohol and drugs than men. From absorption to metabolic processes, women display more difficulty in physically managing the consequences of use. In general, with higher levels of alcohol and drugs in the system for longer periods of time, women are also more susceptible to alcohol- and drug-related diseases and organ damage."

The protocol notes that older women respond to alcohol somewhat differently than do younger women. They have less body water, a heightened sensitivity to and decreased tolerance for alcohol, and a decrease in alcohol metabolism in the gastrointestinal tract.

Financial Impact

The potential interaction between substance abuse and comorbid conditions also has a financial impact on health-care costs for this population. One study found that the mean monthly medical costs increased for persons with alcohol problems prior to the initiation of treatment, with older persons experiencing the highest level of medical cost (Emlet, 2001). A study by the National Center on Addiction and Substance Abuse at Columbia University found that about one out of every $4

Medicare spends on inpatient hospital care, and one out of every five Medicare hospital admissions, can be attributed to substance abuse (Carlson, 1994).

MENTAL DISORDERS AMONG OLDER ADULTS

Mental disorders among older adults are underreported, underdiagnosed, and undertreated. Nationwide, nearly 20% of adults over the age of 55 experience mental disorders, including depression, anxiety, Alzheimer's disease, late-life schizophrenia, alcohol and substance abuse/misuse/ polypharmacy, and other conditions which can result in negative, even fatal consequences, including a surprisingly high rate of suicide.

According to the U.S. Census Bureau, in 2006 there were 50,622,590 adults aged 60 or older living in the United States (US Census, 2007). Estimates from a variety of public and private studies indicate that the prevalence of depression among older Americans is anywhere from 2% to 20% (Waugh, 2006). Several estimates of depression prevalence have placed the rate at 5% for adults aged 60 or older (Steffens et al., 2006). One particular review by Snowden, Steinman, and Frederick (2008) estimated that 5–15% of urban community-dwelling older adults suffer from depression.

Mental health problems, particularly depression, affect a large number of older adults. Both SAMHSA and the Centers for Disease Control and Prevention (CDC) consider depression to be a major area of concern among the elderly, and both have recommended that programs address this problem (CDC, 2008). In a recent Healthy Aging report by the CDC, the authors identified depression as an emerging public health issue that affects older adults. The authors state that treating depression is "critical," and recognize effective treatment of depression as an opportunity to improve older adults' health and quality of life (CDC, 2008).

The health-effects of depression are well studied. Evidence shows that depression is associated with a host of physical and psychological conditions. Depression has been associated with more severe courses of heart disease and diabetes, and has been shown to occur quite frequently with generalized anxiety disorder. In a recent study of data from the National Health and Nutrition Examination Survey, Onitilo and Egeda (2006) states that "the coexistence of cancer and depression is associated with a significantly increased risk of death, and the effect of depression on the risk of death differs by cancer site." In an examination of HMO data for individuals aged 65 and older, the authors found those with clinically significant depressive symptoms at baseline had significantly lower quality of life over the 4-year study period than nondepressed subjects (Unutzer et al., 2000).

A diagnosis of depression is also associated with higher medical costs, with one study finding that total ambulatory and inpatient costs were 47–51% higher in depressed older patients compared with nondepressed older patients, even after adjustment for chronic medical illness (Katon, Lin, Russo, & Unotzer, 2003). Many depressed older adults are not receiving the necessary mental health care, with some studies finding that less than 3% of adults aged 65 and older receive treatment from a mental health professional (Olfson & Pincus, 1996). A report released by the University of Michigan in 2004 stated that "even moderately depressed older adults .... require far more hours of care than those without symptoms of depression, regardless of other health problems they may have." (Langa, Valenstein, Fendrick, Kabito, & Vijan, 2004).

Fewer than 50% of the seven million older adults with a diagnosable mental disorder currently receive treatment (USDHHS, 2001). Suicide rates are highest among this population, with the suicide rate for persons aged 85 years and older twice the overall national rate (Jeste et al., 1999). Older individuals who have experienced trauma—recently or long ago—have suicide rates almost double that of the older population overall.

Mental Health, Depression, and Minorities

Hispanic Americans: Mental health studies in Hispanic American older adults are underrepresented in the scientific literature (Surgeon General, 1999). One study in the Los Angeles area found that Hispanic residents aged 60 and older had rates of major depression and dysphoria near 26% (Kemp, Staple, & Lopez-Aqueres, 1987). Another more recent analysis using data from the National Latino and Asian American Study, which included a nationally representative sample of Latinos, found that lifetime prevalence rates of (one or more) depression, anxiety, and substance abuse to be 28.1% for Latino males and 30.2% for Latinas. Older Hispanic Americans are also less likely to seek treatment for depression, and the treatment that is received by those that seek care is less likely to follow evidence-based guidelines (Young et al., 2001). The same study found that fewer Hispanics receive appropriate mental health care (24%) than do whites (34%). Another study found the rates of depression in middle-aged and older Puerto Rican primary care patients to be anywhere from 34% to 61%, with 12% meeting the DSM-IV criteria for major depression (Robison, Gruman, Gaztambide, & Black, 2002).

Mental health workers and other direct service staff must be able to communicate with the client in his/her native language, and they should be culturally competent and sensitive to the values, norms, beliefs, and diversity of the various cultural subgroups that exist. For example, among Caribbean Latinos one expression of distress is termed "ataque de nervios" and includes symptoms which may also be associated with anxiety and depression such as crying, trembling, and suicidal gestures (Liebowitz et al., 1994). When confronted with these distressing symptoms, many Caribbean Latinos turn to traditional forms of healing that reflect blended Afro-Christian belief systems expressed through practices such as Santeria. The staff needs to acknowledge and integrate complementary sources of care provided through the traditional healing practices of the Santero or Espiritista and integrate culturally significant beliefs, symbols, and practices with cognitive behavioral interventions when appropriate and desired.

African Americans: Psychiatric disabilities retain considerable stigma, and African-American cultural attitudes toward psychiatric disabilities are a barrier to seeking mental health care. Seeking treatment is not always encouraged. Even if care is sought, it is often not equivalent to the care white Americans receive. African Americans seeking care for depression have been found to be less likely prescribed an antidepressant medication at first diagnosis, compared to whites (27% versus 44%) (Melfi, Croghan, Hanna, & Robinson, 2000). A study by Blazer (2003) in older community-based individuals found that whites were four times as likely to use an antidepressant as were African Americans.

In a recent survey, older African Americans exhibited a higher rate of cognitive impairment than other groups, even after controlling for demographic factors and socioeconomic status. Studies also suggested that many older African Americans living in nursing homes and public housing require mental health services. Program strategies which include outreach to nursing homes and the capacity to deliver services to older African Americans living in public housing are congruent with need for this population. There is also recent evidence that suggests that pharmacotherapy protocols for treatment of some mental health disorders among African Americans must be adjusted to compensate for differences in metabolism.

African Americans and Hispanics individuals who have been diagnosed with depression have been found to be less likely to obtain counseling and drug therapy to treat their depression than are white patients. Factors contributing to this disparity may include financial and insurance barriers to obtaining treatment, a belief by more African-American and

Hispanic persons than white persons that antidepressant therapy is unacceptable or ineffective, or a preference for other types of therapy (Miranda & Cooper, 2004).

EVIDENCE-BASED PRACTICES FOR OLDER ADULTS

Home-Based Treatments

Evidence has shown that clinic and home-based treatments for depression in older persons are very effective. To determine the effectiveness of a home-based program of detecting and managing minor depression or dysthymia among older adults, (Ciechanowski et al., 2004) compared the home-based program with treatment as usual and found patients receiving the home-based intervention were more likely to have at least a 50% reduction in depressive symptoms (43% vs 15%), to achieve complete remission from depression (36% vs 12%;), and to have greater health-related quality-of-life improvements in functional well-being and emotional well-being.

Cognitive Behavioral Therapy (CBT) for Late-Life Depression

Depression is one of the mental health disorders most prevalent among older adults (Cole, 2005). CBT for late-life depression is a highly appropriate evidence-based practice. It is time limited, well structured with clear practices proscribed by complementary therapist and consumer manuals. This practice has been shown to be effective in a variety of studies conducted with older adults with depression. CBT has also been shown effective with chronic anxiety disorders (Wetherell, Lenze, & Stanley, 2005).

CBT for late-life depression is an active, directive, time-limited, and structured problem-solving approach that includes strategies to facilitate learning, such as repeated presentation of material using different modalities, slower rates of presentation, and greater use of practice, structure, and modeling behavior than other similarly oriented cognitive–behavioral approaches. Clients are taught to identify, monitor, and ultimately challenge negative thoughts about themselves or their situation, and develop more adaptive and flexible thoughts where appropriate emphasis is also placed on teaching patients to monitor and increase pleasant events in their daily lives using behavioral treatment procedures. Intervention consists of up to twenty, 50–60 minute sessions following a structured manual. This intervention is evidence based, and appears on SAMHSA's

National Registry for Evidence-Based Programs and Practices (SAMHSA, 2006—NREPP CBT).

A key active ingredient with CBT for late-life depression is the concept that isolation and loneliness exacerbate and sometimes is a cause for depression among older persons. CBT for late-life depression helps the client to recognize the situations in which they are most likely to feel isolation, avoid those situations, and cope more effectively with the range of problems associated with isolation and loneliness. CBT emphasizes the fostering of motivation to become more social, teaching of coping skills to overcome isolation, change reinforcement contingencies to make social overtures more satisfying than isolation behaviors. CBT assists in fostering management of painful effects associated with isolation such as depression and anxiety, improve interpersonal functioning, and enhance social supports. The use of brief cognitive behavioral or life review interventions for older, bereaved, and disabled older adults is a proven evidence-based practice for treatment of depression. Three of the five identified risk factors are potentially modifiable (bereavement, sleep disturbance, and chronic illness and disability); previous depression and female gender are the other two risk factors for geriatric depression (Cole & Dendukuri, 2003).

A 2007 report found that those given CBT treatment had significant improvement in their depression symptoms after less than one year. The expert panel went on to recommend CBT as a primary treatment for late-life depression in older adults (Snowden et al., 2008).

Motivational Enhancement Therapy (MET)

Motivational Enhancement Therapy (MET) is a systematic intervention approach for evoking positive behavior change and appropriate decision-making in individuals. Based on the principals of Motivational Psychology, MET is designed to produce rapid, internally motivated change. MET has been implemented and replicated over the course of many years. It is a deceptively simple and rational intervention to change behavior. MET seems effective, because by design it addresses ambivalence to change that is often presented by older adults in general and especially apparent as a clinical feature of depression among depressed older adults.

MET employs motivational strategies to mobilize the client's own change resources. Although it was originally designed to be offered in an outpatient setting, Miller (1995) states that the application of MET in a residential or home-bound setting is also feasible. MET is derived from the transtheoretical model of behavior change first posited by Prochaska and

DiClemente (1983). MET is also listed as an evidence-based practice in SAMHSA's National Registry for Evidence-Based Programs and Practices (SAMHSA, 2006).

The Principles of MET (Miller, 1995) are: (1) express empathy—much of MET is "listening" instead of "telling." A therapist must remain gentle, subtle, and maintain the perspective that change is entirely up to the client. (2) Develop discrepancy—MET seeks to focus a client's attention on a discrepancy between where they are and where they want to be. In mental health treatment, it may be necessary to first develop such a discrepancy by raising awareness of the adverse consequences of untreated psychiatric disabilities. (3) Avoid argumentation—MET avoids direct argumentation. (4) Roll with resistance—MET strategies do not meet resistance head-on, rather, "roll with" the momentum of the treatment process, with the goal of shifting client perceptions in the process. (5) Support self-efficacy—the client must be persuaded that it is possible to change his/her negative behavior and thus, reduce the related problems. If an individual has hope that things can change, there is more motivation to face the problem.

MET is designed for use with every population in need of behavior change; however, evidence exists that the therapy may be particularly effective for older adults, individuals who tend to be more motivated to engage in substance abuse/mental health treatment.

CBT for late-life depression is developed specifically to decrease depression in the targeted population (NREPP, 2006). MET is designed specifically to prompt change. CBT can also be used to treat generalized anxiety disorder in this older population. The combination of CBT and MET is helpful in enabling the older adult to examine and/or re-examine his/her life, and hopefully change the conception of generativity, or the level of satisfaction of personal and familial needs supplemented by the development of interest and welfare of others and ego-integrity or recognizing and adjusting to aging with a sense of satisfaction about the past and an acceptance of the future (Erikson, 1974).

Assertive Community Treatment (ACT)

It is common for older adults with lifelong or late-onset severe psychiatric disabilities with residual impairment to experience external stresses in everyday living that lead to specific clinical states such as anxiety, depression, substance abuse, grief, and transient paranoid state—emotional disorders that may stem from a long physical illness or chronic discomfort, from despair and loneliness and from an invariably lowered self-esteem that comes from diminished social, physical, and personal status. The Assertive Community Treatment (ACT) team is a "best practices" approach that can be tailored to meet the needs of this population.

The ACT team is a collaborative care model encompassing both medical and mental health services with a multidisciplinary staff to be a bridge between ongoing outreach services and specialized psychiatric care. An ACT team working with a highly vulnerable population of older mentally ill would focus on the principles of rehabilitation, recovery, and the goal of movement toward independent living. A multidisciplinary staff with a commitment (indeed a passion) to work with and serve older persons with psychiatric disabilities must be culturally competent to work with specific populations. ACT teams working with older adults must have a substantive knowledge base about the unique treatment needs of older persons, with an ability to provide timely barrier-free access to care that is flexible and community based (including flexible hours of operation).

CONCLUSION

Older persons are a population at risk, with the combination of substance abuse and depressive symptoms associated with high risk for suicidal ideation and poor physical well-being.

Barriers to successful outreach to older adults with mental health issues include stigmatizing attitudes and antiquated notions about older persons that prevent physicians from correctly diagnosing and treating older persons with depression and/or alcohol and drug misuse. Overcoming this barrier requires that physicians and health-care workers at all levels become sensitized to indications of alcohol and substance abuse, and that they provide appropriate intervention and referral.

Another barrier is cultural. Older people whose native language is not English may be self-conscious about their fluency and may feel embarrassed with talking to a physician or case manager. Under the strain of an illness, mental and/or physical, communicating in English may become more difficult. Strong extended families typically care for the elders and may play an important role in the patient's treatment. There is also a need to understand how unique cultural norms and beliefs influence the role of alternative modalities and to work with the family to integrate traditional cultural mores with Western approaches to behavioral health.

Overcoming barriers of stigma requires that social workers be trained to provide carefully delivered outreach efforts that include nonjudgmental presentation of factual information. Presentations must avoid labeling or categorizing mental health problems or service recipients. Rather, the outreach approach should use the techniques of MET, CBT, and ACT to deliver information, which allows for each consumer to self-evaluate his/her own services needs with support of an outreach worker, who uses language that destigmatizes and normalizes the symptoms of late-life and lifelong depression for consumers and for staff members at organizations that host outreach activities.

REFERENCES

Adams, W. L., Barry, K. L., & Fleming, M. F. (1996). Screening for problem drinking in older primary care patients. *Journal of the American Medical Association, 276,* 1964–1967.

Barnes, A. J., Moore, A. A., Xu, H., Ang, A., Tallen, L., Mirkin, M., et al. (2010). Prevalence and correlates of at-risk drinking among older adults: The Project SHARE study. *Journal of General Internal Medicine.* (Open access: http://www.Springerlink.com) (Accessed 7/01/10).

Barnes, G. E., & Chappell, N. L. (1981). Pharmacists' knowledge in the area of alcohol, and alcohol/drug interactions. *Social Science and Medicine. Part A: Medical Sociology, 15,* 649–657.

Blazer, D. G. (2003). Depression in late life: Review and commentary. *Journal of Gerontology. A Biological Sciences and Medical Sciences, 58*(3): M249–M265.

Carlson, K. (1994). *The prevention of substance abuse and misuse among the elderly: Review of literature.* University of Washington, Alcohol and Drug Abuse Institute.

Ciechanowski, P., Wagner, E., Schmaling, K., Schwartz, S., Williams, B., Diehr, P., et al. (2004) Community-integrated home-based depression treatment in older adults: A randomized controlled trial. *Journal of American Medical Association, 291*(13), 1569–1577.

Cole, M. G., & Dendukuri, N. (2003). Risk factors for depression among elderly community subjects: A systematic review and meta-analysis. *American Journal of Psychiatry, 160,* 1147–1156.

Cole, M. G. (2005). Evidence-based review of risk factors for geriatric depression and brief preventive interventions. *Psychiatric Clinics of North America, 28,* 785–803.

Conwell, Y., & Duberstein, P. R. (2001). Suicide in elderly. *Annals of New York Academy of Science, 932,* 132–147.

Curtis, J. R., Geller, G., & Stokes, E. J. (1989). Characteristics, diagnosis, and treatment of alcoholism in elderly patients. *Journal of the American Geriatric Society, 37,* 310–316.

Emlet, C. (2001). Alcohol use and abuse in a population of community-dwelling, frail older adults. *Journal of Gerontological Social Work, 35,* 21–33.

Erikson, E. H. (1974). *Dimensions of a New Identity.* New York, NY: Norton Publishing.

Geller, G., Levine, D. M., & Manon, J. A. (1989). Knowledge, attitudes, and reported practices of medical students and house staff regarding the diagnosis of alcoholism. *Journal of the American Medical Association, 261,* 3115–3120.

Gfoerer, J., Penne, M., Pemberton, M., & Folsom, R. (2003). Substance abuse treatment need among older adults in 2020: The impact of the aging baby-boom cohort. *Drug and Alcohol Dependence, 69,* 127–135.

Glynn, R., Bouchard, G., LoCastro, J., & Hermos, J. (1984). Changes in alcohol consumption behaviors among men in the normative aging study. NIAAA Research Monograph 14. Washington, DC: US Government Printing Office.

Gomberg, E. S. L. (1982). Alcohol use and problems among the elderly. *National Institute on Alcohol Abuse and Alcoholism, Special Population Issues: Alcohol and Health Monograph, 4,* 262–290.

Guida, F., Tavolacci, J., & Provet, P. (2003). An Elder Care exploratory study: Lifelong versus late-in-life. The American Psychological Association convention, Toronto.

Guida, F., Unterbach, A., Tavolacci, J., & Provet, P. (2004). Residential substance abuse treatment for older adults: An enhanced therapeutic community model. *Journal of Gerontological Social Work, 44,* 95–109.

Hurt, R., Finlayson, R., Morse, R., & Davis, L. (1988). Alcoholism in elderly persons: Medical aspects and prognosis of 216 inpatients. *Mayo Clinical Proceedings, 64,* 753–760.

Ingster, L. M., & Cartwright, W. S. (1995). Drug disorders and cardiovascular disease: The impact on annual hospital length of stay for the Medicare population. *American Journal of Drug and Alcohol Abuse, 21,* 93–110.

Jeste, D. V., Alexppoubs, G. S., Bartels, S. J., Cummings, J. L., et al. (1999). Consensus statement on the upcoming crisis in geriatric mental health. *Archives of General Psychiatry, 56,* 848–853.

Katon, W. J., Lin, E., Russo, J., & Unotzer, J. (2003). Increased medical costs of a population-based sample of depressed elderly patients. *Archives of General Psychiatry, 60*(9), 897–903.

Kemp, B. J., Staple, F., & Lopez-Aqueres, W. (1987). Epidemiology of depression and dysphoria in an elderly Hispanic population prevalence. *Journal of the American Geriatrics Society, 35,* 920–926.

Langa, K. M., Valenstein, M. A., Fendrick, A. M., Kabito, M. U., & Vijan, S. (2004). Extent and cost of informal caregiving for older Americans with symptoms of depression. *American Journal of Psychiatry, 161,* 857–863.

Liebowitz, M. R., Salmen, E., Jusino, C. M., Garfinkel, R., Street, L., Cardenas, D. L., et al. (1994). Ataque de nervios and panic disorder. *American Journal of Psychiatry, 151,* 871–875.

McInnes, E., & Powell, J. (1994). Drug and alcohol referrals: Are elderly substance abuse diagnoses and referrals being missed? *British Medical Journal, 308,* 444–446.

McIntire, O., Farnen, T. A., Gordon, N., et al. (1996). Medication misadventures resulting in emergency department visits at an HMO medical center. *American Journal of Health System Pharmacology, 53,* 1416–1422.

Melfi, C. A., Croghan, T. W., Hanna, M. P., & Robinson, R. L. (2000). Racial variation in antidepressant treatment in Medicaid population. *Journal of Clinical Psychiatry, 61*(1), 16–21.

Miller, W. R. (1995). *Motivational enhancement therapy with drug abusers: A therapist manual.* Center on Alcoholism, Substance Abuse, and Addictions, The University of New Mexico, Albuquerque.

Miranda, J., & Cooper, L. A. (2004). Disparities in care for depression among primary care patients. *Journal of General Internal Medicine, 19*(2), 120–126.

Moos, R. H., Mertens, J. R., & Brennan, P. L. (1994). Rates and predictors of four-year readmission among late-middle-aged and older substance abuse patients. *Journal of Studies on Alcohol, 55,* 561–570.

Morley, C. (2002). *Alcohol and other drug problems.* The Future of Aging in New York State, Project 2015. New York State Department for the Aging.

Olfson, M., & Pincus, H. A. (1996). Outpatient mental health care in nonhospital settings: Distribution of patients across provider groups. *American Journal of Psychiatry, 153,* 1353–1356.

Onitilo, A. A., & Egeda, L. E. (2006). Effect of depression on all-cause mortality in adults with cancer and differential effects by cancer site. *General Hospital Psychiatry, 28*(5), 296–402.

Prochaska, J. O., & Diclemente, C. C. (1983). *Journal of Consulting and Clinical Psychology, 51*(3), 390–395.

Reich, T., Cloniger, R., & Van Eerdewegh (1988). Secular trend in the familial transmission of alcoholism. *Alcoholism: Clinical and Experimental Research, 12,* 458–464.

Robison, J., Gruman, C., Gaztambide, R., & Black, K. (2002). Screening for depression in middle aged and older Puerto Rican primary care patients. *Journal of Gerontology A, 57*(5), M308–M314.

Snowden, M., Steinman, L., & Frederick, J. (2008). Treating depression in older adults: Challenges to implementing the recommendations of an expert panel. *Preventing Chronic Disease, 5*(1), http://www.cdc.gov/pcd/issues/2008/jan/07_0154.htm. (Accessed 7/01/10).

Steffens, D. C., Otey, E., Alexopoulos, G. S., Butters, M. A., Cuthbert, B., et al. (2006). Perspectives on depression, mild cognitive impairment, and cognitive decline. *Archives of General Psychiatry, 63,* 130–138.

Substance Abuse and Mental Health Services Administration (SAMHSA). (1998). Substance abuse among older adults: National Household Survey on Drug Abuse. Bethesda, MD.

Substance Abuse and Mental Health Services Administration (SAMHSA). (2006). National registry of evidence-based practices protocols. Bethesda, MD.

Substance Abuse and Mental Health Services Administration (SAMHSA). (2009). Substance use among women during pregnancy and following childbirth. National Survey on Drug Use and Health. Bethesda, MD.

Surgeon General. (1999) Mental health: A report of the Surgeon General. Washington, D.C: U.S. Department of Health ad Human Services. http://www.surgeongeneral.gov/library/mentalhealth/chapter1/sec4.html#chap5 (Accessed July 1, 2010).

U.S. Census Bureau (2007). Income, Earnings and Poverty Data for the 2006 American Community Survey, U.S. Department of Commerce, Washington, D.C.

U.S. Department of Health and Human Services (2001). Mental health: Culture, race and ethnicity — A supplement to mental health: A report of the surgeon general. Rockville, MD: U.S. Department of Health and Human Services, Substance Abuse and Mental Health Services Administration. Center for Mental Health Services, National Institutes of Health, National Institute of Mental Health.

Unutzer, J., Patrick, D. L., Diehr, P., Simon, G., Grembowski, D., & Katon, W. (2000). Quality adjusted life years in older adults with depressive symptoms and chronic medical disorders. *International Psychogeriatrics, 12*(1), 15–33.

Waugh, A. (2006). Depression and older people. *Nursing Older People, 18*(8), 27–30.

Wetherell, J., Lenze, E. J., & Stanley, M. A. (2005). Evidence-based treatment of geriatric anxiety disorders. *Psychiatric Clinics of North America, 28,* 871–896.

Weintraub, E., Weintraub, D., Dixon, L., Delahanty, J., Gandhi, D., Cohen, A., et al. (2002). Geriatric patients on a substance abuse consultation service. *American Journal of Geriatric Psychiatry, 10,* 337–342.

Whitcup, S. M., & Miller, F. (1987). Unrecognized drug dependence in psychiatrically hospitalized elderly patients. *Journal of the American Geriatric Society, 35,* 297–301.

Williams, M. (1984). Alcohol and the elderly: An overview. *Alcohol and Health Research World, 8,* 3–9.

Young, A. S., Klap, R., Sherbourne, C. D., & Wells, K. B. (2001). The quality of care for depressive and anxiety disorders in the United States. *Archives of General Psychiatry, 58,* 55–61.

CHAPTER ELEVEN

Elder Abuse

The Hidden Epidemic

Nora O'Brien-Suric and Judith Estrine

INTRODUCTION

The mistreatment of older Americans cuts across ethnic, racial, and class boundaries. According to the National Center on Elder Abuse at American Public Human Services Association, elder abuse may be broadly defined as any act that has the potential to harm the patient emotionally, physically, or financially. It can take many forms, from intimidation and name calling to physical harm and sexual coercion. Evidence suggests that there are over 1 million victims of elder abuse annually; however, estimates vary, because there are no official national statistics. The most common and difficult to identify cases often involve subtle issues that are not easily identifiable and go unreported to the authorities (Stoukides Holtzer, Ritzau, & Burbank, 2006).

Abuse can be as specific as withholding proper nutrition or medical care, or as subjective as failing to provide a loving home environment. Data on elder abuse in domestic settings suggest that only 1 in 14 incidents (excluding incidents of self-neglect) come to the attention of authorities (Pillemer & Finkelhor, 1988).

Aged persons who are systematically denied the companionship of friendly, caring people may be as victimized as older individuals who are malnourished, but they may remain under the radar. According to the best available estimates, between 1 and 2 million Americans aged 65 or older have been injured, exploited, or otherwise mistreated by someone on whom they depended for care or protection (Bonnie & Wallace, 2002).

Estimates of the frequency of elder abuse range from 2% to 10% based on various sampling, survey methods, and case definitions (Lachs & Pillemer, 2004).

Women are victims of three-fourths of the incidents of psychological abuse and 92% of financial abuse cases. However, as will be discussed further, older adults of both sexes are victims of physical abuse by their spouse.

In October 1998, the National Elder Abuse Incidence Study, sponsored by the Administration on Aging, estimated that for every case of elder abuse, neglect, exploitation, or self-neglect reported to the authorities, about five more go unreported. Other estimates suggest that 1 out of 10 persons living with a family member is subject to abuse—~2.5 million a year (Griffin & Williams, 1992, p. 20) and 1 in 25 older adults are victimized annually (Heisler, 1991).

This chapter will provide an overview of this hidden epidemic. It will describe in detail what constitutes elder abuse, observations regarding reasons for its prevalence, and the challenges society faces in identification and prevention. Finally, it will describe an innovative program that has spearheaded community support and provided respite and resources for older persons who are victims of elder abuse.

THE EMERGENCE OF ELDER ABUSE AS A SOCIAL CONCERN

In 1978, Dr. Suzanne Steinmetz, *an expert on issues involving family violence, social policy, and the aged and aging,* brought mistreatment of older persons to the attention of Congress when she presented her research to the Congressional Subcommittee hearings on domestic violence. One of the primary researchers on the National Family Violence Survey funded by the National Institutes of Mental Health in 1975, Dr. Steinmetz published extensively on her findings, including her most controversial finding that older male spouses were as likely to become victims of abuse as their female counterparts (Steinmetz, 1978).

Her testimony prompted the House Select Committee on Aging, chaired by the late U.S. Representative Claude Pepper, to examine the issue. The "Pepper Committee" subsequently introduced the term "elder abuse," and alerted the nation to the widespread severity of this problem. The National Council on Elder Abuse (NCEA) was created to promote understanding, knowledge sharing, and action on elder abuse, neglect, and exploitation. It continues to serve as a national resource for elder rights advocates, adult protective services, law enforcement and legal professionals, medical and mental health providers, public policy leaders, educators, researchers, and concerned citizens.

RISE IN INCIDENTS OF ELDER ABUSE

At the same time as medical advances and the implementation of a variety of protective measures, notably Social Security and Medicare, have greatly increased the length of life for many Americans, other societal changes may contribute to some individuals becoming abusive toward older persons. Extended families that shared the responsibilities of caring for their aging relations have given way to a society with smaller nuclear families with limited resources. For a variety of reasons, families are more likely to be scattered, so that when the time comes for an aging family member to need care, the responsibility typically falls on one family member, a paid caregiver, or on a nursing home (Griffin & Williams, 1992).

CATEGORIES OF ELDER ABUSE

Most researchers agree that the abuse of the elderly fall within the five following categories: physical abuse, sexual abuse, psychological abuse, financial abuse, and neglect.

Physical Abuse

Physical abuse is defined as "Non-accidental physical force that results in injury" (Commonwealth of Pennsylvania, 1988). Physical frailty, decreased physical ability, and vision and audio impairments make older persons especially susceptible to physical abuse (NOVA, 1985).

Indicators of physical abuse may include the following:

- Fractures and dislocations;
- Lacerations and abrasions;
- Burns;
- Injuries to the head, scalp, face; and/or
- Bruises on upper arms (from shaking), around wrists, or ankles (from being tied down), in shapes similar to objects, inside of thighs or arms (Bloom, Pamela, & Matthew, 1989, p. 41).

Sexual Abuse

Sexual abuse is defined as "Non-consensual sexual contact" (Commonwealth of Pennsylvania, 1988). As aged victims are less physically able, often all that is needed to subdue them during a sexual assault is intimidation by physical force (Muram, Miller, & Cutler, 1992).

Indicators of sexual abuse may include the following:

- Sexually transmitted diseases; and/or
- Pain, itching, bleeding, or bruising in the genital area.

Psychological Abuse

Psychological abuse is defined as "Infliction of mental anguish by threat, intimidation, humiliation, or other such conduct" (Commonwealth of Pennsylvania, 1988). A diminished ability to cope with stress, termed a "decrease in homeostatic capacity," as well as the state of "chronic loss" that often accompanies aging (i.e., loss of one's home, peers, spouse, etc.), renders elders susceptible for psychological abuse (NOVA, 1985).

Indicators of psychological abuse may include the following:

- Low self-esteem;
- Overly anxious or withdrawn;
- Extreme changes in mood;
- Depression;
- Suicidal behavior; and/or
- Confusion or disorientation (Bloom et al., 1989, p. 41).

Financial Abuse

Financial abuse is defined as "Unauthorized use of funds or property" (Commonwealth of Pennsylvania, 1988). Financial abuse or exploitation involves the theft or conversion of money or property belonging to an elder, accomplished by force, misrepresentation, or other illegal means often by taking advantage of the elder's partial or total lack of legal competency (Hyman, 1990, p. 6).

In "The Fleecing of America's Elderly," John Wasik reported that current estimates put the overall reporting of financial exploitation at only 1 in 25 cases, suggesting that there may be at least 5 million financial abuse victims each year.

(Wasik, 2000. "The Fleecing of America's Elderly," *Consumers Digest,* March/April.)

Indicators of financial abuse may include the following:

- Unexplainable change in financial situation, with an inability to pay for food, medication, or housing.

Neglect

Neglect is defined as "Failure to fulfill a caretaking obligation" (Commonwealth of Pennsylvania, 1988).

Indicators of neglect may include the following:

- Poor personal hygiene;
- Signs of overmedication or undermedication, and/or misuse of medication (Bloom et al., 1989, p. 42);
- Incontinent and dressed in soiled clothing;
- Left alone and deprived of stimulation and affection (Skeates & Douglas, 1990), and/or
- Malnutrition (Bloom et al., 1989, p. 42).

Neglect can be active and occurs when a caregiver willfully fails to provide care. It can also be passive, resulting from inadequate knowledge or infirmity on the part of the caregiver. Additionally, *self-neglect* is a failure of an older person to care for herself or himself (Commonwealth of Pennsylvania, 1988).

CRIMINAL VICTIMIZATION

In addition to the abuse to which older people are subject by relatives and/or caretakers in their homes or in institutions, they may become targets for criminal victimization. Older persons are subject to severe crimes and because they are often physically frail with concurrent visual and hearing impairments, they are more fearful of crime than are younger adults; thus the consequences of victimization are often psychological as well as physical (Burgess & Hanrahan, 2006).

Although physical limitations and lifestyle choices often determine the time spent outside their homes, older Americans are particularly vulnerable to being victims of personal larceny, which includes assault by pickpockets and purse snatchers outside the home as well as robbers in their homes. Older adults are twice as likely as younger persons to be victimized in or near their homes, and to be victimized by offenders with weapons, including firearms. They are more easily injured, heal more slowly, are less resilient emotionally, and are less financially stable than younger victims recover from these assaults to their person (Commonwealth of Pennsylvania, 1988).

TREATING VICTIMS OF ELDER ABUSE: AN INNOVATIVE COMMUNITY-BASED PROGRAM

The Harry & Jeanette Weinberg Center for Elder Abuse Prevention, Intervention and Research is a comprehensive regional prevention and intervention program for victims of elder abuse living in the community. It is the nation's first *long-term care-based shelter* dedicated to elderly victims of emotional, physical, and financial abuse. Its mission is to prevent elder abuse, intervene to stop abuse when it is discovered, conduct research to document elder abuse, and serve as a resource for those interested in replicating the Weinberg Center model (http://www.elderserve.org/details.asp?ID=10).

The Center provides emergency shelter and legal services to older adults whose lives have been disrupted by mistreatment and abuse, utilizing an existing long-term care facility model to ensure that each recipient is offered a coordinated system of crisis intervention services; medical, psychiatric, and rehabilitative care as indicated; housing placement assistance; individual and family counseling, as indicated; and a full-range of community-based services.

The Weinberg Center enhances and extends its direct intervention in the lives of abused seniors through programs that promote professional and public awareness and information about elder abuse, building collaborative service networks, and facilitating successful replication of the Weinberg Center shelter model in the United States and abroad.

The Harry & Jeanette Weinberg Center for Elder Abuse Prevention was founded in 2004. It is the first comprehensive regional long-term care-based shelter dedicated exclusively to caring for victims of elder abuse in the United States. The Center serves older people who are victims of physical, emotional, and sexual abuse or financial exploitation, regardless of ability to pay. The Center and its toll-free phone line are available 24 hours a day, 7 days a week. The location of emergency shelter services for seniors within a well-established, non-profit, geriatric long-term care facility offers a cost-effective paradigm for providing victims with a safe environment and the full range of support services required to respond to their health-care and psychosocial needs.

The original program, located on the grounds of the Hebrew Home at Riverdale, is designed to be easily replicable by other long-term care facilities. Noteworthy features include the use of existing (but unused) long-term care beds permits rapid start-up with minimal capital investment. Like the Hebrew Home, many long-term care facilities have on-site access to a wide range of diagnostic, medical, and psychosocial treatment, and rehabilitative services. (It is noteworthy that older adults admitted to a stand-alone shelter face extensive barriers if they require access to these services.) The Home has continuity with the communities, their services, and support systems in which they (the Weinberg model shelters) are based. To date, sites in Connecticut, New Jersey, Rhode Island, the District of Columbia, Maryland, Illinois, Minnesota, Texas, California, Florida, Canada, and Israel have replicated the Weinberg Center or are in the process of replicating some of its most important facets.

The Weinberg Center staff includes a staff attorney to provide legal advocacy and representation for such matters as obtaining guardianships, orders of protection, divorce, banking and housing issues; and designated social workers and nurses trained to meet the complex needs of victims of elder abuse, in order to provide the substantial emotional support and psychological counseling they require. Clients are encouraged to make full use of all of the Home's social, recreational, and educational programs, and to enjoy the facilities as a sanctuary from their previous environments. An interdisciplinary plan of care is developed with each client, which incorporates discharge planning that begins at admission. The Center seeks ways to *safely* return clients back home—if possible and indicated—and utilizes its network of collaborating community-based providers to arrange placements in alternate housing when returning home is not feasible.

The Center developed an outreach program to those most at risk. The staff began by visiting senior centers, retirement communities, and shopping centers to disseminate information about available resources. The Weinberg team established ties with local district attorneys, developed programs that train pharmacists, doormen, and others in the community to recognize and respond to abused older persons.

The Center collaborates with police and prosecutors, hospitals, and domestic violence shelters, having established a panel of pro bono and reduced rate attorneys who provide help with civil legal remedies for victims and with presenting training sessions for professional and community groups. The Center uses members of the nursing home's volunteer program to help shelter residents with assistance for such activities as wheelchair transportation, accompaniment to recreational activities, and health-care appointments. In addition, volunteer attorneys provide legal advocacy and representation for victims. The Weinberg Center uses its position in the community to raise awareness of the extent of the problem of elder abuse and to help influence local, state, and federal policies.

The Center's leadership actively supported landmark urban legislation to protect older persons from elder abuse by mandating all employees of city-run senior centers and any other entities that contract with the Department for the Aging to undergo training in elder abuse prevention, detection, and counseling every 3 years. They have presented expert testimony on elder abuse for the United States Senate Special Committee on Aging, published numerous articles, and presented at annual professional meetings

Outreach teams train health-care personnel, legal, law enforcement, as well as clergy, home care workers, postal workers, and numerous other community groups and individuals who have frequent contact with older persons and may not otherwise have been aware of the phenomenon of elder abuse.

CONCLUSION

Physical frailty and cognitive deficits make older persons a population at risk for abuse. Shelters designed specifically for older adults who experience violence or other types of abuse at home do not exist as yet. Elder abuse in the community is difficult to detect, and when it is suspected, it is difficult to address, in part because existing domestic violence shelters are rarely equipped to deal with either the concrete needs of aging persons, or to cope with their cognitive and physical disabilities, frailty, and lack of financial resources. Elder abuse must be brought out of the shadows. Nationwide, communities must work to identify the problem and address the growing epidemic for older people, to create a safe harbor for emotional support, psychological counseling, health care, legal advocacy, and representation, to ensure their safe return to their own homes or alternative housing in the community.

REFERENCES

Administration on Aging (AOA). (2000). *Profile of older Americans*: 2000. Washington, DC: U.S. Department of Health and Human Services.

Bloom, J. S., Pamela, A., & Matthew, N. B. (1989). Detecting elder abuse: A guide for physicians. *Geriatrics, 44*(6), 40–4, 56.

Bonnie, R. J., & Wallace, R. B. (Eds). (2002). Panel to Review Risk and Prevalence of Elder Abuse and Neglect, National Research Council. Washington, DC: National Academies Press.

Bureau of Justice Statistics. (2001). *Criminal victimization 2000.* Washington, DC: U.S. Department of Justice.

Burgess, A., & Hanrahan, N. (2006). *Identifying forensic markers in elderly sexual abuse.* Washington, DC: National Institute of Justice.

Commonwealth of Pennsylvania. (September, 1988). Attorney General's family violence task force: Violence against elders.

Griffin, L. W., & Williams, O. J. (1992). Abuse among African–American elderly. *Journal of Family Violence, 7*(1), 19–35.

Heisler, C. (1991). The role of the criminal justice system in elder abuse cases. *Journal of Elder Abuse and Neglect, 3*(1), 5–33.

Hyman, J. A. (1990). From the frontlines: Financial abuse and legal assistance. *NARCEA Exchange, 2*(4).

Lachs, M. S., & Pillemer, K. (2004). Elder abuse. *The Lancet, 364,* 1192–1263.

Muram, D., Miller, K., & Cutler, A. (March, 1992). Sexual assault of the elderly victim. *Journal of Interpersonal Violence, 7*(1), 70–76.

National Center on Elder Abuse. (September, 1998). National elder abuse incident study; Final report. Washington, DC: Administration for Children and Families, Administration on Aging, U.S. Department of Health and Human Services.

National Center on Elder Abuse. (2004). Survey of state adult protective services: Abuse of adults 60 years of age and older, prepared for the National Center on Elder Abuse, 2006.

NOVA. (1985). The elderly crime victim. *Network Information Bulletin, 2*(2)

Pillemer, K., & Finkelhor, D. (1988). The prevalence of elder abuse: A random sample survey. *The Gerontologist, 28*(1), 51–57.

Skeates, E., & Douglas, I. (1990). Abuse of elderly people. *Nursing (Lond), 4*(6), 6–8.

Steinmetz, S. K. (1978). The battered husband syndrome. *Victimology, 2,* 499–509.

Stoukides, J., Holtzer, C., Ritzau, J., & Burbank, P. (2006). Health care strategies. In C. B. Patricia (Ed.), *Vulnerable older adults: Health care needs and innovations* (pp. 38–40). New York: Springer Publishing Company.

Wasik, J. F. (2000). The fleecing of America's elderly. A special report. *Consumer Digest,* 77–83.

FURTHER READING

McCoy, K., & Hansen, B. (May 25, 2004). Special report: Havens for elderly may expose them to deadly risks. *USA Today.*

CHAPTER TWELVE

Understanding the Refugee Experience of Trauma

Andrea K. Blanch

INTRODUCTION

This chapter presents an introduction and overview of the issues faced by refugees in the United States and a public health framework for working with them. Perhaps the most fundamental principle of a public health model is to focus on wellness rather than illness. This credo is particularly applicable when working with refugees. As Muecke (1992) states: "Refugees present perhaps the maximum example of the human capacity to survive despite the greatest losses and assaults on human identity and dignity." The majority of refugees do, in fact, overcome significant challenges, get jobs, raise families, and adapt well to life in their new country. They deserve our respect as well as our assistance. However, all refugees have experienced life-threatening situations. Public mental health systems can play a key role in supporting their resettlement and in helping to heal the consequences of trauma. The development of trauma-informed services is one promising strategy for assisting refugees without pathologizing them.

BACKGROUND: THE INTERNATIONAL CONTEXT

While people often use the term "refugee" to refer to anyone who has fled his or her home, the term has a precise legal definition. Understanding the basic differences between refugees and other newcomers (see below) can help sensitize caregivers to unique aspects of the refugee experience.

According to the United Nations, there are currently 9.9 million refugees displaced from their home countries across the globe (United Nations

High Commission on Refugees, UNHCR, 2007). An additional 25 million people are internally displaced (Eschenbächer, 2005), about half of whom (12.8 million) are receiving assistance from UNHCR. The vast majority of refugees come from developing countries: an estimated 8 out of every 10 refugees flee from one poor country to another, often the country next door. Although gender and age ratios vary widely according to the nature of the refugee situation, region of asylum, and other factors, approximately 50% of all refugees are women, and 45% are children under the age of 18. Together, women, and children comprise about 75% of the world's refugee population. Women are also overrepresented in the older age category (60 years and older).

Distinctions Between Refugees and Other Newcomers

The experience of refugees often differs significantly from that of other displaced persons or newcomers to the United States. According to the UN, a *refugee* is a person outside of his or her country of nationality who is unable or unwilling to return because of persecution or a well-founded fear of persecution on account of race, religion, nationality, membership in a particular social group, or political opinion. With rare exceptions, refugee status is determined while the individual is still outside the United States, and whether or not a person is granted refugee status depends on why he or she fled the home country. Table 12.1 summarizes the differences in terminology.

Internally displaced persons are persons or groups of persons who have been forced or obliged to flee or to leave their homes or places of habitual residence, in particular as a result of or in order to avoid the effects of armed conflict, situations of generalized violence, violations of human rights or natural or human-made disasters, and who have not crossed an internationally recognized State border.

Asylees are individuals who, on their own, travel to the United States and apply for/receive a grant of asylum, a status that acknowledges that they meet the definition of a refugee, allows them to remain in the United States, and makes them eligible for refugee assistance and services. Persons admitted through the resettlement system or granted asylum may change to permanent resident status after one year, which puts them on the road to citizenship.

Sources of trauma for refugees may include war, rape, or atrocities during conflict or repressive regimes, or "disappearance" of friends and family. Trauma may also result from previous experiences within the

TABLE 12.1
Definitions for Categories of Displaced People

Category	Definition
Refugee	Forced to flee home; is outside of country of origin; has well-founded fear of persecution
Asylum seeker	Makes a claim that he/she is a refugee
Migrant	Moves to a foreign country for a variety of reasons (e.g., work) and for a certain length of time (usually a minimum of one year)
Immigrant	Takes up permanent residence in a country other than original
Economic migrant	Leaves country of origin for economic reasons
Internally displaced person	Like refugees, forced to move, but remains in own country
Stateless person	Not considered a national by any country or does not enjoy fundamental rights enjoyed by others in their home state

country of origin—domestic violence, rape, honor killings, racism, state-sanctioned violence, experience in combat, terrorism. While other groups, such as disaster victims, may also experience severe trauma, there are major legal and psychological differences between fleeing persecution as a refugee and fleeing disasters as an evacuee. The trauma experienced by refugees is likely to have been prolonged and repeated, consciously caused by other human beings, and exacerbated by forced exile (Brune et al., 2002).

Resettlement Programs for Refugees

Local resettlement programs are state funded; the only state without a refugee program is Wyoming. States contract with nine private organizations (called "voluntary agencies" or "volags") that help the newly arrived refugees settle into local communities. The volags also have a network of over 400 affiliates (ethnic, self-help, and community organizations) that assist with refugee resettlement (Ranard, 1990). The nine voluntary agencies are:

- U.S. Conference of Catholic Bishops/Migration and Refugee Services,
- Lutheran Immigration and Refugee Service,
- Episcopal Migration Ministries,
- Hebrew Immigrant Aid Society,
- Church World Service/Immigration and Refugee Program,

- International Rescue Committee,
- U.S. Committee for Refugees and Immigrants,
- World Relief, and
- Ethiopian Community Development Center.

The Office of Refugee Resettlement (ORR) is the main coordinating body for resettlement services, working closely with State Refugee Coordinators and Refugee Health Coordinators. Through its Division on Refugee Assistance, ORR oversees numerous state-administered programs for refugees, including cash and medical assistance and targeted preventive health grants. Through its Divisions on Community Resettlement and Unaccompanied Children's Services, ORR provides economic and social integration assistance and ensures the safety of unaccompanied alien children.

Assisting in the coordination of mental health services to refugees is SAMHSA's Center for Mental Health Services (CMHS) Refugee Mental Health Program (RMHP). Founded in 1980, RMHP provides technical assistance, consultation, mental health and community assessments, treatment, and training for resettlement staff and mental health personnel. Particularly relevant to the issue of trauma is the Torture Victims Relief Act of 1998. Under this act, services are provided to torture survivors in all immigration categories—citizens, undocumented individuals, refugees, asylum seekers, and asylees. The majority served are asylum seekers. Services include treatment of the physical and psychological effects of torture, social and legal support, and research and training for health-care providers. ORR supports a national consortium of torture treatment providers as well as capacity building projects to expand the availability of services to torture survivors, within both specialized treatment settings and mainstream provider organizations.

STAGES OF THE REFUGEE EXPERIENCE

There are three major stages of refugee experience: the premigratory period, migration or period of flight, and resettlement. Each stage has unique risks and stressors. Caregivers need to be aware that refugees have been through a long process even to get to the point of resettlement, and that there have likely been significant life stresses and losses along the way. This is particularly important from a trauma perspective, since the impact of trauma is cumulative.

In the *premigratory period*, refugees flee conditions in their home countries and find temporary shelter in refugee camps or communities in neighboring countries. The experience of refugees varies widely. Depending on their situation, they may be fleeing from violence, have prolonged experience with harsh conditions in refugee camps, be exposed to infectious and parasitic diseases, experience malnutrition and exposure to the elements, or be victimized by pirates, border guards, army and resistance units, and others with whom they come in contact.

UNHCR interviews individuals while they are in refugee camps or other temporary shelter to determine whether they should be granted refugee status and to determine the best course of action — voluntary repatriation, integration into the country of asylum, or resettlement into a third country. If resettlement is the best solution, they may be referred to the U.S. Citizenship and Immigration Services (CIS) for determination of eligibility for resettlement in the United States. If they are deemed eligible, nongovernmental agencies known as "overseas processing entities" do much of the groundwork for *migration* — interviewing, preparing paperwork, arranging medical examinations and background security checks, and gathering information about the refugee's work history and job skills, family situation, and special needs. The International Organization for Migration generally arranges and covers the costs of transportation, which the refugee must repay after resettlement. Before departing for the United States, refugees receive a cultural orientation to life in the United States.

During *resettlement* in the United States, refugees may face significant challenges in finding employment and housing, overcoming racial discrimination and language barriers, and navigating an unfamiliar service system. They may also experience chronic situational stressors such as fear of being repatriated (Sinnerbrink et al., 1997). The resettlement experience differs from state to state and community to community and can vary widely for different refugee groups. For example, some refugee groups come to the United States without a strong "receiving community" — established communities of earlier immigrants who can help the newcomers adjust. Under these circumstances, it is easy for refugees to remain both linguistically and socially isolated. They may end-up living in communities without a strong economic base or with high crime rates. In contrast, some refugees move directly into well-established communities that can assist with resettlement. For example, Dearborn, Michigan is currently home to the largest group of Arabs outside of the Middle East, and provides significant support to Arab refugees resettling in that area.

Research has identified four major factors that together account for 62% of resettlement stress: social and economic strain, alienation, discrimination and status loss, and violence and threats (Lindencrona et al., 2008). During resettlement, refugees continue to be at risk for chronic diseases, trauma-related symptoms, and other consequences of their experience during premigration and flight.

DEFINING AND RESPONDING TO VIOLENCE: ADOPTING A PUBLIC HEALTH FRAMEWORK

Within the field of refugee services, there is a strong push to adopt a holistic, public health model and to focus on wellness rather than illness. Given the risk factors that refugees are exposed to, classic concepts of secondary prevention (population-based interventions) and tertiary prevention (case finding and referral) are clearly relevant. Similarly, health promotion and strengths-based approaches support the natural resilience displayed by many refugees. SAMHSA's toolkit *Refugee Well-Being: Partnering for Refugee Health and Well-Being* provides an excellent introduction to this approach.

The seminal work of Aaron Antonovsky (1979) on "sense of coherence" is particularly helpful in framing refugee mental health and trauma services. Antonovsky conceptualizes health as a continuum, and argues that we need to shift our attention from factors that are "pathogenic" (disease producing) to factors that are "salutogenic" (health producing). He also suggests that people's ability to create positive health depends on their "sense of coherence"—a combination of the ability to assess and understand their situation, to find meaning in their circumstances, and to move in a health-promoting direction (Lindstrom & Eriksson, 2005).

Research on the refugee experience supports this framework. For example, there is evidence that a strong belief system—whether grounded in faith or in a political ideology—is a protective factor for refugees and assists in coping with trauma (Brune et al., 2002). Similarly, it is clear that relocation to a new country may challenge an individual's sense of coherence. Mental health or trauma services should work to support refugees' resilience by helping them to understand and find meaning in their experience and to adopt health-promotion behaviors. It is also essential not to pathologize the suffering of refugees or to over-generalize their experience. Thus, while it is safe to assume that all refugees have undergone a challenging journey, and that all may benefit from some forms of assistance, it is inaccurate to assume that all are traumatized or require trauma treatment.

Focus on the Individual versus the Community

The public health model addresses the health of entire populations, and promotes the use of community-level interventions whenever appropriate. Within the refugee service system, there is reason for concern that an overemphasis on individual trauma healing may divert attention from important social, economic, and political issues. Internationally, the adoption of a clinical trauma model has sometimes resulted in a shift away from an economic approach to solving community problems. For example, following a wave of interest in Post Traumatic Stress Disorder (PTSD), crisis centers in Indonesia that previously focused on a range of community development needs were renamed and retooled as "trauma clinics," and a long-standing concern for human rights, women's rights and democratization dissolved (Dwyer & Santikarma, 2007). Similarly, the introduction of trauma programs for survivors of a terrorist bombing in Bali diverted attention from long-term structural inequalities and state repression that had resulted in the mass killing of 5–8% of the island's population (Dwyer & Santikarma, 2007). Some worry that a focus on trauma may be used as a substitute for effective international political action. As Silove notes, "there is much to be said for the argument that peace and security provide the best immediate therapy for the majority of populations exposed to mass violence and displacement" (Silove, 2007, p. 255). The public health focus on community-level interventions is supported by evidence that refugees are more concerned with social and economic issues than with psychological problems. In a study of the major concerns of people tortured for political reasons in South Africa, somatic health problems were identified most often, followed by economic concerns, dissatisfaction with the current political situation, and finally, symptoms of posttraumatic stress (Kagee, 2004). Consistent with this finding, Blackwell (2005) asserts that people whose lives have been con-strained or damaged by political violence do not see themselves as sick or as victims. Treating them as such depoliticizes their experience and is inherently problematic, if not retraumatizing. He and others propose wider use of community interventions such as human rights and truth and reconciliation commissions, which they believe are more respectful, simultaneously providing emotional healing and supporting collective resilience (Tummala-Nara, 2007). Some international groups have moved to implement trauma programs that work collectively with all community members, including both "victims" and "perpetrators" (see, e.g., www.FriendsPeaceTeams.org).

While the implementation of trauma treatment for refugees in the United States may not reflect such stark polarities, the concern about focusing on individual pathology versus social factors is still salient, and care providers need to be aware of the social and political concerns of the specific refugee populations they are working with.

Relevance of the PTSD Model

There is also ongoing debate about how well the PTSD model applies to the experience of violence in non-western countries. PTSD, first recognized in soldiers returning from Vietnam, results from exposure to a life-threatening event that produces a sense of current threat. Symptoms fall into three clusters: intrusive symptoms, avoidance symptoms, and symptoms of hyper arousal (Johnson & Thompson, 2007). PTSD was introduced into the *Diagnostic and Statistical Manual-III* to address the need for a common diagnostic category covering the wide range of clinical syndromes associated with a traumatic experience (Fischman, 1998). The rapid growth in the use of the PTSD diagnosis has been criticized as spawning a "self-sustaining trauma counseling industry" and encouraging a culture of victimization, in some cases undermining traditional, nonprofessional support mechanisms and natural recovery processes (Silove, 2007).

Some argue that the PTSD model is irrelevant to the experience of many refugees, since the model presumes that trauma is an aberration—an unexpected, isolated, or infrequent event that occurs outside the norms of society. In contrast, in war-torn societies violence is an ongoing, routine part of people's everyday experience, even after "peace accords" have been signed (Radan, 2007), and for most refugees traumatic stress is a continuing condition even upon resettlement (van Willigen, 1992). Although some theoretical models of trauma, such as "complex PTSD" and "DESNOS" (disorders of extreme stress not otherwise specified) focus attention on chronic or repeated exposure, few clinical models reflect the complexities of conflict and postconflict life: situations where perpetrators live alongside victims as neighbors, or where victims are also forced to commit acts of violence against others (Lemelson, Kirmayer, & Barad, 2007). Others note that symptoms of trauma are largely culturally determined, and evidence of refugee trauma may be missed altogether if clinicians are looking for symptoms that are normative in western populations. Both the construct itself and the assessment instruments designed to measure it may not accurately reflect non-western cultures (Johnson & Thompson, 2007).

Concerns have also been raised about studies that report PTSD to be at epidemic levels in refugee and post-conflict populations—commonly reported at levels of 20–35% and sometimes as high as 99% (deJong et al., 2007). Although PTSD symptoms are ubiquitous after mass exposure to trauma, in situations of extreme stress symptoms may represent a normal rather than pathological reaction, and "diagnosing" entire populations may be misleading. Moreover, most people exposed to extreme trauma do *not* go on to develop chronic, disabling PTSD. Meta-analyses show that on average only 20% of those who experience traumatic events develop PTSD (Rousseau & Measham, 2007), and an even smaller percentage come for treatment (Chow, Jaffee, & Choi, 1999). Advocates concerned about the over-diagnosis of PTSD suggest that when entire populations are affected by violence, clinical treatment should be seen as an intervention of last resort. Rather than providing trauma treatment to everyone, they argue, it makes more sense to support and enhance indigenous supports and natural recovery processes for all who can benefit, and make more intensive interventions available for those *most* in need. This approach has been borne out in communities such as East Timor, where there has been remarkable recovery from mass trauma—even though very few people received PTSD counseling—but where a sizable minority continue to suffer severe and disabling symptoms (Silove, 2007).

Understanding Cultural Perspectives

One of the major challenges in providing services to refugees in the United States is recognizing the degree to which our understanding of violence and safety, and our responses to trauma, are culturally determined. In relatively "peaceful" Euro-American societies, violence is seen as something both perpetrated and experienced by individuals (Rousseau & Measham, 2007). Governments, armies, police, and other forms of organized authority are generally considered to be instruments of maintaining safety, not imposing terror. We have little experience in dealing with state-sanctioned violence, and may make inaccurate assumptions about what constitutes safety for a refugee.

Our western assumptions also lead us to believe that violence is something "other than ourselves," and to maintain a sharp dichotomy between victim and aggressor. Thus, we may unconsciously categorize people from violent societies as either "barbaric and uncivilized aggressors" or "defenseless victims dependent on our help" (Rousseau & Measham, 2007). In reality, identities are complex, and often combine several aspects of the experiences of violence. For example, women refugees from Kosovo (many of whom had been raped and tortured) were unlikely to describe themselves as traumatized women, rape survivors, or torture victims. Rather, they defined their identity in terms of their role in the armed struggle—that is, as wives and sisters of the Kosovar Liberation Army (KLA) fighters, political dissidents, and as Muslims whose right to practice religion was violated (Gozdziak, 2002; Gozdziak & Tuskan, 2000). Effective treatment programs work within the frame of reference adopted by the refugees themselves (Trix, 2000).

A similar dilemma may result from conflicting social and personal narratives. Under normal situations, we all hold multiple identities and construct multiple narratives about our experiences. When the narratives conflict, we find ways to resolve the contradictions between them. However, extreme circumstances may violate or change the construction of identity narratives in ways that are irreconcilable. For example, for women who survived rape and violence in Bosnia, both their ethnic identity and their gender identity were involved. As ethnic victims, elements of their stories created a "survivor plot" characterized by absence of guilt, family support, and political action. However, as women, the violence they experienced created a "victim plot," characterized by feelings of guilt and shame, hiding their experiences from family, and trauma symptoms (Skjelsbaek, 2006). During recovery, both of these narratives may play a critical role.

It is also not uncommon for violence and extreme hardship to become a critical part of collective cultural, ethnic, or religious narratives. BenEzer describes how this process has occurred with the Ethiopian Jews who immigrated to Israel through Sudan during the 1980s (BenEzer, 2007). Along with their Jewish identity, the Ethiopians understood *physical and emotional suffering* and *bravery and inner strength* as the central themes of their journey and of their identity as a people. The collective narrative about their journey, which is quickly assuming mythic proportions, has created group cohesion and a sense of direction for the future of Ethiopians in Israel. This social narrative may have helped people to cope with the extreme hardships they experienced along the way and may serve as a "protective shield" against future trauma (BenEzer, 2007). However, this social identity could also come into conflict with the personal identity narrative of an individual who has experienced extreme stress and needs assistance. Balancing individual and collective identities may be the key in assisting some refugee populations.

A further complication may occur over time, as a particular experience of violence or trauma becomes part of large-group identity (Rousseau,

2005; Volkan, 2001; Young, 2007). For most refugees, violence is a recent or ongoing issue. However, historical trauma may also be relevant for some refugee groups. Often, as an ethnic, religious, or national group incorporates a massive trauma into their collective narrative, the experience may come to play a key role in defining their cultural identity (Young, 2007). When an external threat arises, the old trauma may be reactivated. While this may have negative psychological consequences, it may also provide positive support for the threatened identity. Similarly, in times of stress, individual identity often fades into the background and issues of group identity predominate (Volkan, 2001). Clearly, anyone working with refugees needs to be aware of how different situational contexts are likely to affect the meaning ascribed to their experiences.

Finally, understanding the experience of the refugee means constantly staying open to unexpected emotions and interpretations. While we may be trained to focus on healing trauma symptoms, for some refugees the restoration of dignity may be more important than the alleviation of fear and anxiety. Others may choose to focus on an issue that might not even occur to us—for example, the loss of one's youth in a refugee camp may be perceived as a more grievous wound than the experience of violence itself.

Trauma Informed Care as a Framework for Refugee Services

The distinction between *trauma-specific* and *trauma-informed* services is extremely helpful for developing refugee services in a public health model (Fallot & Harris, 2008). *Trauma specific* services are those that directly address the impact of trauma and facilitate healing and recovery—for example, therapies that focus on PTSD. In contrast, in a *trauma-informed* culture, everyone involved has a good understanding of trauma, and trauma is taken into account in all aspects of the program. In trauma-informed services, each contact, relationship, activity, and aspect of the physical environment reflects knowledge of trauma. In refugee services, to be trauma informed requires a thorough understanding of the refugee experience. Any service or program or setting can be trauma informed— mental health programs, medical care settings, job training, education, the criminal justice system, legal aid, law enforcement, etc.

The benefits of trauma-informed care are substantial. First, programs and services are more effective: Whether teaching literacy, providing primary health care, or counseling refugees on issues of resettlement, services that are fully trauma informed are sensitive to factors that can undermine success. Second, a trauma-informed culture benefits staff as well as clients. Staff may have their own trauma histories, and are vulnerable to secondary traumatization from working with people who have experienced extreme violence. Third, in a trauma-informed environment, trauma is everyone's responsibility rather than the exclusive territory of the mental health clinician. And finally, when services are *not* trauma informed, they can be inadvertently retraumatizing—that is, they may unintentionally recreate the interpersonal patterns or situational context in which the original violence occurred. Without a commitment to becoming trauma informed, helping services may end-up hurting the very people they are designed to help.

To be trauma informed, all services and programs for refugees should be aware of the pervasiveness of trauma, its impact, and its self-perpetuating nature. They should be familiar with the multiple and complex paths to healing and recovery; and they should thoroughly incorporate this knowledge into all aspects of service delivery. Fallot and Harris (2008) have identified five critical values in creating a trauma-informed culture: safety, trustworthiness, choice, collaboration, and empowerment. These are the antidotes to the toxic effects of traumatic violence in people's lives. Implementing these values requires organizational change at all levels, with all staff, and requires a fundamental reframe of the typical human service relationship. Implementing the values of trauma-informed care requires seeing things from the perspective of the refugee, whose survival may have depended on being attuned to the slightest sign of danger. Unless our service environments are trauma informed, even the best trauma treatment may be ineffective.

Developing a Public Mental Health Response to Refugee Trauma

In general, refugees in the United States are few in number, have little political support, and face significant discrimination. They are widely dispersed across the country, and tend to be isolated within their own communities. As a result, it is difficult to garner significant public policy attention to their issues or adequate funds to meet their needs.

Although the public mental health system is theoretically available to all in need, it is based on a diagnostic system that is not relevant or helpful to many refugees. Moreover, mental health services are organized and financed as part of the overall health care system, which favors professionally oriented inpatient and clinic-based services rather than the flexible and informal outreach services needed by refugees. In general, the mental health workforce is not trained to respond to refugees, and recruitment of culturally and/or linguistically competent professionals is difficult, especially in rural areas. Moreover, the mainstream mental health system is chronically underfunded and is not designed to meet the many non-mental health needs of refugees—including housing, legal services, adult education and ESL, vocational services, etc.—needs which may far overshadow the need for mental health services. Given this situation, it is not surprising that refugee mental health has not become a priority issue for public mental health systems.

However, our knowledge about the violence experienced by many refugees should give us pause. Childhood trauma can have severe and long-lasting health and mental health consequences, even in adulthood, and leads to increased utilization of social services across the lifespan (Felitti et al., 1998). Children who experience or witness violence are at risk for becoming violent in adulthood. For adults, untreated trauma from a wide variety of sources may affect people's ability to perform the tasks of daily living (Jennings, 2003). There is every reason to assume that the violence experienced by refugees will have similar effects. Common sense suggests that an investment in addressing refugee trauma will prevent significant disabling and costly problems in the future.

CONCLUSION

Refugees are "normal" people exposed to extremely stressful events. Understanding their experiences in their home country, in flight, and during resettlement is the key to providing effective services and supports. Being aware of our own western biases about culture and violence is also essential. A public health model, with its emphasis on wellness and population-based interventions, provides a framework that respects the unique experiences and natural resilience of refugees. The adoption of principles of trauma-informed care is one way to ensure that services and supports are knowledgeable about the refugee experience and sensitive to the possible impacts of trauma on all aspects of refugees' lives.

ACKNOWLEDGMENTS

An earlier version of this chapter was prepared for Abt Associates Inc., National Center of Trauma Informed Care, under SAMHSA contract #280-03-2905. Helpful assistance was provided by Elzbieta Gozdziak, Susan Martin, John Tuscan, Marta Brenden, Susan Salasin, Gail Robinson,

Blanca Gurolla, Helga West, Luc Nya, Lorna Hines-Cunningham, Leslie Brower, Arabella Perez, Claire Harrison, Noel Bonam, Colleen Clark, and Carole Warshaw.

REFERENCES

Antonovsky, A. (1979). *Health, stress and coping*. San Francisco, CA: Jossey-Bass.
BenEzer, G. (2007). Trauma, culture, and myth: Narratives of the Ethiopian Jewish exodus. In L. J. Kirmayer, R. Lemelson, & M. Barad (Eds.), *Understanding trauma: Integrating biological, clinical and cultural perspectives*. New York, NY: Cambridge University Press.
Blackwell, D. (2005). Psychotherapy, politics and trauma: Working with survivors of torture and organized violence. *Group Analysis. 38*, 307–323.
Brune, M., Haasen, C., Krausz, M., Yagdiran, O., Bustos, E., & Eisenman, D. (2002). Belief systems as coping factors for traumatized refugees: A pilot study. *European Psychiatry, 17*, 451–458.
Chow, J., Jaffee, K. D., & Choi, Y. (1999). Use of public mental health services by Russian refugees. *Psychiatric Services, 50*, 936–940.
deJong, K., Mulhern, M., Ford, N., van de Kam, S., & Kleber, R. (2007). The trauma of war in Sierra Leone. *Lancet, 355*, 2067–2068.
Dwyer, L., & Santikarma, D. (2007). Posttraumatic politics: Violence, memory, and biomedical discourse in Bali. In L. J. Kirmayer, R. Lemelson, & M. Barad (Eds.), *Understanding trauma: Integrating biological, clinical and cultural perspectives*. New York, NY: Cambridge University Press.
Eschenbächer, J. (Ed.). (2005). *Internal displacement. Global overview of trends and developments in 2004*. Global IDP Project. Norwegian Refugee Council: Geneva, Switzerland. http://www.idpproject.org/global_overview.htm
Fallot, R. D., & Harris, M. (2008). Trauma-informed services. In G. Reyes, J. D. Elhai, & J. D. Ford (Eds.), *The encyclopedia of psychological trauma*. Hoboken, NJ: John Wiley and Sons.
Felitti, V., Anda, R., Nordenberg, D., Williamson, D., Spitz, A., Edwards, V., et al. (1998). Relationship of childhood abuse and household dysfunction to many of the leading causes of death in adults: The adverse childhood experiences (ACE) study. *American Journal of Preventive Medicine, 14*, 245–258.
Fischman, Y. (1998). Metaclinical issues in the treatment of psycho political trauma. *American Journal of Orthopsychiatry, 68*, 27–38.
Gozdziak, E. M. (2002). Spiritual emergency room: The role of spirituality and religion in the resettlement of Kosovar Albanians. In E. M. Gozdziak & D. J. Shandy (Eds.), *Special Issue: Religion and Forced Migration. Journal of Refugee Studies, 15*(2), 136–152.
Gozdziak, E. M., & Tuskan, J. J., Jr. (2000). Operation provide refuge: The challenge of integrating behavioral science and indigenous approaches to human suffering. In E. M. Gozdziak, & D. J. Shandy (Eds.), *Rethinking refugee and displacement. Selected papers on refugees and immigrants*, Vol. VIII (pp. 194–222). Fairfax, VA: American Anthropological Association.

Jennings, A. (2003). The damaging consequences of violence: Facts, discussion points, and recommendations for the behavioral health system. SAMHSA's Center for Mental Health Services.

Johnson, H., & Thompson, A. (2008). Development and maintenance of post-traumatic stress disorder in civilian adult survivors of war trauma and torture: A review. *Clinical Psychology Review, 28*(1), 36–47.

Kagee, A. (2004). Present concerns of survivors of human rights violations in South Africa. *Social Science and Medicine, 59*, 625–635.

Lemelson, R., Kirmayer, L. J., & Barad, M. (2007). Trauma in context: Integrating biological, clinical, and cultural perspectives. In L. J. Kirmayer, R. Lemelson, & M. Barad (Eds.), *Understanding trauma: Integrating biological, clinical and cultural perspectives*. New York, NY: Cambridge University Press.

Lindencrona, F., Ekblad, S., & Hauff, E. (2008). Mental health of recently resettled refugees from the Middle East in Sweden: The impact of pre-resettlement trauma, resettlement stress and capacity to handle stress. *Social Psychiatry Psychiatric Epidemiology, 43*, 121–131.

Lindstrom, B., & Eriksson, M. (2005). Salutogenesis. *Journal of Epidemiology and Community Health, 59*, 440–442.

Muecke, M. A. (1992). New paradigms for refugee health problems. *Social Science and Medicine, 35*(4), 515–523.

Radan, A. (2007). Exposure to violence and expressions of resilience in Central American women survivors of war. *Journal of Aggression, Maltreatment and Trauma, 14*, 147–164.

Ranard, D. (1990). Mutual assistance associations: Refugee self-help groups play key role. *America: Perspectives on Refugees, 8*, 10.

Rousseau, C. (2005). Diving into complexity: John Sigal's work on the long-term consequences of the holocaust. *Clinical Child Psychology and Psychiatry, 10*, 262–265.

Rousseau, C., & Measham, T. (2007). Posttraumatic suffering as a source of transformation: A clinical perspective. In L. J. Kirmayer, R. Lemelson, & M. Barad (Eds.), *Understanding trauma: Integrating biological, clinical and cultural perspectives*. New York, NY: Cambridge University Press.

Silove, D. (2007). Adaptation, ecosocial safety signals, and the trajectory of PTSD. In L. J. Kirmayer, R. Lemelson, & M. Barad (Eds.), *Understanding trauma: Integrating biological, clinical and cultural perspectives* (255p.). New York, NY: Cambridge University Press.

Sinnerbrink, I., Silove, D., Field, A., Steel, Z., & Manicavasagar, V. (1997). Compounding of preimmigration trauma and postimmigration stress in asylum seekers. *Journal of Psychology: Interdisciplinary and Applied, 131*, 463–470.

Skjelsbaek, I. (2006). Victim and survivor: Narrated social identities of women who experienced rape during the war in Bosnia–Herzegovina. *Feminism and Psychology, 16*, 373–403.

Trix, F. (2000). Reframing the forced migration and rapid return of Kosovar Albanians. In E. M. Goździak, & D. J. Shandy (Eds.), *Rethinking refuge and displacement. Selected papers on refugees and immigrants* (Vol. VIII). Fairfax, VA: American Anthropological Association.

Tummala-Narra, P. (2007). Conceptualizing trauma and resilience across diverse contexts: A multicultural perspective. *Journal of Aggression, Maltreatment and Trauma, 14*(1–2), 33–53.

UNHCR. (2007). *2006 Global trends: Refugees, asylum-seekers, returnees, internally displaced and stateless persons*. Division of Operational Services.

van Willigen, L. H. M. (1992). Organization of care and rehabilitation services for victims of torture and other forms of organized violence: A review of current issues. In M. Başoğlu (Ed.), *Torture and its consequences: Current treatment approaches*. Cambridge: Cambridge University Press.

Volkan, V. D. (2001). Transgenerational transmissions and chosen traumas: An aspect of large-group identity. *Group Analysis, 34*, 79–97.

Young, A. (2007). Bruno and the Holy Fool: Myth, mimesis, and the transmission of traumatic memories. In L. J. Kirmayer, R. Lemelson, & M. Barad (Eds.), *Understanding trauma: Integrating biological, clinical and cultural perspectives*. New York, NY: Cambridge University Press.

CHAPTER THIRTEEN

Innovative Program Approaches to Refugee Trauma

Andrea K. Blanch

INTRODUCTION

This chapter is an introduction and overview of innovative models for trauma treatment for refugees in the United States. It is based on international and US-based research and practice demonstrating that for refugees who have experienced longstanding, complex, or repetitive trauma, clinical treatment alone is not sufficient. To be effective, treatment services must respect the unique circumstances and culture of the refugee, attend to other pressing needs and issues in the refugee's life, and be delivered in the context of a trauma-informed environment. The previous chapter detailed issues in the refugee experience. This chapter focuses primarily on trauma interventions, including the application of current trauma treatment models to refugees and new approaches to trauma healing emerging from direct experience with refugee communities. It also includes a discussion of gender issues, since the needs of women refugees are often unique. Finally, it provides suggestions for how mental health providers can develop a trauma-informed clinical culture and trauma-informed partnerships with other agencies.

BACKGROUND: THE INTERNATIONAL CONTEXT

Recent years have seen an increase in the number of international programs addressing refugee trauma, as well as concerns about their relevance and effectiveness (Bracken, Giller, & Summerfield, 1997; Watters, 2001). In one review, a majority of refugee aid projects offered direct psychological services (63%) or psychologically oriented groups (54%), mostly self-help.

Thirty-three percent of the projects provided psychiatric services and 63% had staff training programs focusing on trauma (Summerfield, 1999). These programs are serving large numbers of children and adults. For example, a trauma center established in Rwanda in the mid-1990s had, by 1996, trained over 6000 "trauma advisors" in basic trauma alleviation methods, and had assisted an estimated 144,000 children. Similar efforts to train mental health staff and to deliver trauma services have been undertaken in other parts of the world by the United Nations High Commission on Refugees (UNHCR) and the World Health Organization (Summerfield, 1999).While few of these programs have been carefully evaluated, many have been described in the literature, and several important lessons have been learned.

First, there is a complex interplay between the stresses experienced during different phases of relocation. While exposure to severe traumatic events is often assumed to explain mental health symptoms in refugees, postmigration stressors may also contribute. In one study, resettlement stressors and personal capacity to handle stress accounted for 50% of the variance in mental health symptoms, with preresettlement trauma accounting for only 5.5% (Lindencrona, Ekblad, & Hauff, 2008). Similarly, a recent meta-analysis found that economic opportunities and permanent private housing were highly associated with better mental health outcomes (Porter & Haslam, 2005). These findings suggest that meeting basic needs for refugees may be as important as providing trauma treatment.

Diagnostically, refugees may suffer from a complex mix of trauma-related problems, including depression, complicated grief, PTSD, psychotic disorders, somatic complaints, and health problems (Ferrada-Noli, 1998; Kirmayer, Lemelson, & Barad, 2007; Momartin, Silove, Manicavasagar, & Steel, 2004). Groups that have experienced colonization or have been the targets of ethnic cleansing may internalize their rage and show no signs of post-traumatic stress disorder (PTSD), yet have high rates of substance abuse, suicide, and violence (Sanchez-Hucles & Gamble, 2006). Severe trauma can also alter an individual's worldview and capacity to handle stressful situations (Lindencrona et al., 2008).

Our diagnostic lens must be wide enough to see all of these conditions as trauma related. As Richard Mollica (2006) points out, in many conventional mental health settings symptoms of refugee trauma may be misdiagnosed as a psychotic illness. As a result, the individual may end up involuntarily committed to a mental hospital and strongly advised (or forced) to take psychotropic drugs without being given appropriate counseling or social rehabilitation. Mental health programs working with refugees need to be aware of the many ways in which trauma can affect mental health.

Finally, practitioners working with refugees may need to abandon common assumptions, including the belief that people who have experienced extreme violence will never recover, and that severely traumatized people do not want to talk about their experiences (Mollica, 2006). Practitioners will certainly need to take into account local "idioms of distress," that is, specific ways in which people from different cultures experience and communicate pain and suffering, as well as traditional ways of coping. The task may seem overwhelming, especially since there is far more literature documenting the problem of violence and trauma among refugees than describing effective ways to treat it (Miller, Kulkami, & Kushner, 2006). However, research is beginning to identify ways in which trauma treatment can be modified for refugee populations, and new clinical models are being developed and tested.

APPLICATION OF CURRENT TRAUMA TREATMENT MODELS TO REFUGEE POPULATIONS

Over the past 10 years, there has been an explosion of research and theory on trauma (Kirmayer et al., 2007). There is a wide and growing repertoire of therapies for dealing with trauma-related disorders, including psychopharmacology, trauma counseling, psychodynamic approaches, cognitive–behavioral treatments (exposure therapy, flooding, systematic desensitization, eye-movement desensitization and reprocessing (EMDR)), psychodrama and body-based therapies, Eastern-based interventions (acupuncture, meditation), and a host of others (Pedersen, 2002). Approaches that have been developed and proven effective with general mental health populations, such as therapeutic communities, are also being applied to trauma survivors (Tziotziou et al., 2006).

Over a dozen treatment models for trauma have been designated as "evidenced-based practices" on the Substance Abuse and Mental Health Services (SAMHSA) National Registry of Evidence-Based Programs and Practices (http://www.nrepp.samhsa.gov/index.asp). Several models focus specifically on the symptoms of PTSD, while others are designed to work primarily with substance abuse or with complex diagnostic pictures. While these models have been widely implemented and shown to be effective with western populations, it is important to remember that they have not been tested or normed with refugees. Outcome studies on trauma treatment with refugees are scarce and show varying levels of improvement over time (Carlsson, Mortenson, & Kastrup, 2005; Carlsson, Olsen, Mortensen et al., 2006), and research on the comparative efficacy of different therapies with refugee populations is in its infancy.

For trauma providers seeking to apply or adapt existing clinical treatment models to refugees, evidence of effectiveness on western populations should be only one factor in making a decision. It is equally important to consider how the clinical treatment model will be implemented. Any program serving refugees needs to support natural resilience, acknowledge and respect cultural norms, and prioritize people with the most severe symptoms for treatment.

Supporting Resilience

Trauma interventions for refugees need to be especially vigilant about not undermining natural recovery, resilience, and self-healing processes. The impact of trauma is real and sometimes debilitating, but there is a great deal of variability in the way people react to even very severe trauma. While refugees have by definition undergone extremely stressful events, many show enormous resilience.

The most typical response to acute psychological trauma is recovery over time (Konner, 2007), and believing that recovery is possible has long been considered an essential element of trauma healing (Herman, 1992). More recently, the concept of resilience has emerged as a distinct factor in understanding trauma and loss (Bonnano, 2004). Unlike the term recovery, which connotes overcoming a temporary loss of normal functioning, resilience implies an ability to maintain a steady level of functioning despite significant trauma. While resilient individuals may experience brief and transitory symptoms, they generally maintain healthy functioning and retain their capacity for generating positive emotional experiences. There is substantial evidence that many individuals are able to endure traumatic events remarkably well, with little or no apparent disruption in psychological or physical functioning. Some theorists estimate, based on available research, that the vast majority of individuals exposed to violence do not exhibit chronic symptom profiles, and that the majority show the type of healthy functioning that would imply resilience (Bonnano, 2004).

The concept of resilience as a separate and distinct trajectory from recovery has important implications for intervention. First, it implies that an absence of pronounced distress may be normal for some people: such an absence does not necessarily reflect a delayed PTSD response. Second, it suggests that not all people who experience severe trauma will benefit from treatment, and in fact, treatment may undermine natural resilience for some (Bonnano, 2004). Third, it implies that clinical interventions aimed at entire populations may be misguided. Mollica (2006) suggests that our current orientation to violence and trauma focuses too heavily on the negative consequences of traumatic events, and may inadvertently be short-circuiting natural resilience, creating dependency, and creating real disease and illness. He concludes that we need a revolution in our thinking, making the engagement of survivors in their own recovery the "mantra of social recovery" (p. 236).

While research on resilience is in its early stages, it appears to be a multidimensional phenomenon. In many cases, trauma survivors may be "simultaneously suffering and surviving" (Harvey, 2007, p. 15). In addition, resilience is not a static trait, but an unfolding process in which strengths and vulnerabilities emerge over time (Tummala-Narra, 2007). Clinical interventions therefore need to recognize that people who display severe and recurrent trauma symptoms in some areas of functioning may be resilient in others, and that resilience may take time to unfold. Finally, providers need to be aware that what is seen as promoting resilience in one culture may be seen as a liability in another (Tummala-Narra, 2007).

Respecting Cultural Norms

Some common trauma treatment models may be culturally inappropriate for some refugee groups. The very notion of confronting trauma directly reflects a western bias that we need to face our problems to overcome them, and may not be relevant to all cultures (Kinzie, 2007). Moreover, some trauma is so existentially profound and disturbing that bringing up memories may be unnecessarily cruel. For individuals who have endured massive or repeated violence, or who have lost their sense of trust or meaning, other forms of intervention may be called for. Bonds of social support, reconnections with loved ones, and narratives of hope for the future may all be critical for recovery (Kirmayer et al., 2007). Some of the emerging program models that emphasize narrative and storytelling, community empowerment, and psychosocial supports described in the next section respond to these needs.

Treating Severe Symptoms

Despite the above cautions, there are some refugees who display severe and persistent trauma symptoms who can benefit from intensive trauma treatment. Once a fear response is learned, it persists, being incorporated in the molecular structure of the brain (Barad & Cain, 2007). The original fear response remains available, ready to re-emerge, even after an alternative "safety" response is learned. Since learned fears generalize more readily to new contexts than learned safety does—and since even the passage of time may constitute a new context—there is a biological basis for the phenomenon of chronically relapsing PTSD (Bouton & Waddell, 2007). For those with severe and persistent symptoms, cognitive–behavioral therapies, such as exposure therapy or EMDR, may be especially helpful. Prolonged exposure therapy, which incorporates breathing retraining, prolonged and repeatedly titrated reliving of trauma memories, and repeated *in vivo* exposure to trauma-related situations and objects, appears to assist in generalizing the safety response to more situations (Yadin & Foa, 2007). In some cases, especially for people who have suffered for long periods of time, relief of symptoms through psychopharmacology may be a high priority (Kinzie, 2007).

EMERGING CLINICAL MODELS AND APPROACHES FOR REFUGEE POPULATIONS

While not as widely researched as evidence-based practices, a number of new clinical approaches have shown promising results with refugee populations. Many of these emerging clinical models emphasize self-care, traditional healing modalities, storytelling and narratives, psychosocial needs, and religion and spirituality.

Self-Care and Self-Healing

Self-healing is part of the body's natural biological response to injuries of all types: biological healing has been shown to occur naturally following all forms of violence (Charney, 2004). The importance of self-care and self-healing for refugees is being championed by Richard Mollica, among others. As a psychiatrist, he was trained to diagnose and treat, primarily with medications. However, after 30 years of clinical work with Cambodian refugees, he has come to the conclusion that the key to healing the wounds of even the most severe forms of violence lies within the individual (Mollica, 2006), and that our clinical treatment models must shift significantly to embrace this truth.

Refugee communities naturally understand and support their own self-healing and empowerment; self-help groups and advocacy are often among the first responses of refugee communities upon resettlement

(Light, 1992; Ranard, 1990). However, professionals are sometimes unclear about what their role is in a self-help model. Supporting self-help does not mean political abandonment (Puggioni, 2005), nor does it mean there is no role for professional help. As Mollica states: "Traumatized people throughout the world voice the same request for help with self-healing" (Mollica, 2006, p. 26). Supporting self-healing involves recognizing that each individual's experience of violence and recovery is unique and cannot be understood without understanding the person's own history and personality. It also involves the development and maintenance of trust, despite uneven power relationships and a host country that views refugees with considerable suspicion (Rousseau & Measham, 2007). Other practices that support self-healing include placing oneself as close as possible to the pain and suffering of the individual in order to hear their truth; helping them tell their story in a healing manner; helping them to take a conscious inventory of their own self-healing efforts; learning about and supporting cultural healing practices; and reinforcing the individual's self-healing efforts in every way possible (Mollica, 2006). Social behaviors such as humor, friendship, and physical exercise can also contribute to self-healing (Southwick, Vythilingam, & Charney, 2005).

Traditional Healing

Many authors have written about the importance of understanding the ways in which suffering is experienced, understood, and expressed within the refugee's culture. It is particularly important to become aware of culturally specific symptoms, to understand local patterns of help-seeking, and to support cultural healing resources whenever possible (Miller et al., 2006). The cultural specificity of trauma symptoms has obvious clinical significance. It may be crucial for practitioners to know, for instance, that somatic complaints are particularly prominent among Southeast Asian refugees with trauma histories (Hinton & Otto, 2006), that sleep paralysis is a common occurrence for Cambodian refugees with PTSD (Hinton et al., 2005), or that for Afghans, intrusive memories of trauma are not particularly troubling because they fade quickly, while long-term feelings of depression and hopelessness (called "jigar khun") are a major concern (Miller et al., 2006). Understanding the associations of specific symptom patterns to trauma experiences can also be important. For example, dizziness is a very common symptom for Cambodian refugees. There is evidence that Asian groups are particularly susceptible to some forms of dizziness, and in Cambodian ethno-physiology, dizziness is greatly feared. Dizziness may also have critical trauma associations, since it was a common experience during the Pol Pot regime due to overwork, starvation, and malaria (Hinton & Otto, 2006). Obviously, attending to this particular symptom may be far more important to trauma healing for Cambodian refugees than might be assumed from a western perspective.

Effective refugee trauma interventions also incorporate cultural traditions. For example, Stepakoff and colleagues used indigenous healing practices (including songs, cultural stories, dance/movement, and rituals) in their work with Sierra Leonean and Liberian refugees (Stepakoff, 2007). Working in partnership with traditional healers may at times be indicated. In one case reported by Miller and colleagues (2006), a deeply religious Bosnian Serb refugee made more progress after one meeting with the head of the Greek Orthodox Church, who was sympathetic to her loss and her bereavement, than she had made after months of psychotherapy and medication. It is not always necessary to bring traditional healers into clinical practice—in some cases, the community trauma may be so severe that it exceeds the coping resources or knowledge and skills of local healers (Miller et al., 2006). However, being knowledgeable about indigenous healing practices and willing to incorporate them may be crucial to forming an effective clinical alliance and to developing a set of interventions that maximizes the chances of recovery.

Storytelling and Narratives

The value placed on "telling one's story" varies significantly between cultures. Some cultures place great value on a sense of coherence, and will seek persistently to find meaning in their experience, retelling and reshaping the story until it acquires a satisfactory form (Ying, 1997). Other cultures value concealment as one of the key indicators of psychological well-being (Whittaker, Hardy, Lewish, & Buchan, 2005). For refugees, telling their story has additional complications. Refugee status depends on meeting the criteria of a "well founded fear of being persecuted," and to be credible, a refugee's official personal story must fit with some larger socially accepted account of what is happening to people of a certain background from a certain part of the world. The refugee's story is thus not just his or her own, but necessarily "invokes the voices of others," and has very real implications for the person's future (Kirmayer et al., 2007). Refugees may also have had to tell their stories repeated to migration officials, family members, employers, clinicians, and other social service workers, and the very telling may have become retraumatizing.

Practitioners in the field have begun to address these concerns by developing guidelines and models for clinically effective and culturally sensitive storytelling. Rousseau and Measham (2007) propose a model of "modulated disclosure" which focuses on the appropriate timing for disclosure of particular aspects of the traumatic experience. This process recognizes that avoidance and disclosure may represent equally important responses to trauma, and introduces a dialectic between approaching the past and moving away from it. Others, concerned about pathologizing political violence, have developed techniques based on clients giving "testimony" about what happened to them, then providing a written copy to the client for use in pursuit of justice. In this approach, attention to emotional issues occurs in a political context, the client is provided with a form of potential positive action, and the therapist becomes an ally in the struggle for social justice (Blackwell, 2005). Finally, there may be times when it is critical to ask: "When does remembering have worse consequences than forgetting for survivors of extreme trauma?" (Rousseau, 2005). If the desire to forget is strong, it may be essential to explore other mechanisms of repairing trauma (Rousseau & Measham, 2007).

Despite these cautions, Mollica (2006) concludes that one of the deepest fears for trauma survivors is that they will be unable to reconnect with the normal world—that those closest to them will remain indifferent and turn away from hearing their truth. Providing an opportunity to tell one's story and to be heard is thus critical. The important thing, according to Mollica, is *how* the story is told. Mollica suggests that there are four components in an effective trauma narrative, each contributing to healing. First, a factual accounting of the events occurs. Trauma survivors can often clearly state the exact date and even hour when the violence began, the motivation of the perpetrators, and extensive details about the violence. Telling the facts of the story invokes conscious memories, which are stored in the hippocampus. In contrast, emotional memories— the memories that encode unconscious fear associations, and that can become intrusive and repetitive—are stored in the amygdala. If the facts of the story are told in such a way as to avoid triggering the emotional memories, biological extinction of the traumatic emotional memories will be enhanced (Mollica, 2006). Second, every trauma story reveals the survivor's culture, history, traditions, and values. Stories are therefore an important source of information about the survivor's cultural framework. Mollica suggests that mental health professionals and others working with refugees would benefit from training in how to listen, not as a clinician or professional, but as a learner. Classes which put the trauma survivor in the role of teacher and the healing professional in the role of learner have been quite successful.

Third, the trauma story can be a stage on which meaning and transformation may be constructed. How the trauma story is told can make a crucial difference. Trauma stories that focus on the brutal facts of the violence are likely to retraumatize the teller and possibly turn the listener away. However, if the story focuses on the survival skills and resiliency demonstrated by the survivor, he or she may come to deep new insights about themselves. Finally, the listener–storyteller relationship is key. Helping refugees to tell their trauma stories in a healing fashion is difficult and takes practice. The listener must be prepared to hear what the survivor needs to reveal, and to empathize with the experience, no matter how painful. This requires visualizing and experiencing what the person actually endured without becoming overwhelmed. At the same time, the survivor must learn to tell their story in a sensitive way in order not to overload the listener. Mollica suggests that the clinician can assist in this process by acting as a "storytelling coach," teaching the survivor to tell the entire story, including the context of their lives and their self-healing capacities, to use symbols and metaphors, and to modulate the expression of emotions.

Psychosocial Approaches

Refugee mental health concerns also need to be addressed in the context of psychosocial needs such as housing, employment, language skills, and other essential support services. For mental health practitioners, this approach is consistent with the community support and rehabilitation model developed in the 1980s and 1990s as a comprehensive approach to meeting the needs of people with severe mental illnesses (Saraceno, 1997; Turner, 1978).

Approaches that provide a full array of psychosocial needs in addition to clinical treatment are gaining currency with ethnic community-based organizations and others, particularly in developing countries (Loughery & Eybar, 2003; Silove, 2007). One survey identified 185 such projects within Bosnia and Croatia alone (Makinson, 1999). Psychosocial programs address the physical and mental health of a person, their knowledge and skills, the social connections they share, and the specific context of their communities. They often include specialized mental health services, recreational and social support groups, housing and legal assistance, and income generation (employment) activities. One model designed for responding to mass violence proposes five broad psychosocial pillars: security; social bonds and family networks; justice and human rights; roles and identity; and meaning—institutions that both individuals and society attempt to defend and to rebuild if they are destroyed (Silove, 1999).

In developing countries, programs that address economic empowerment are often seen as more responsive to local conditions than typical trauma relief programs (Weyermann, 2007). Psychosocial programs are also more likely to incorporate local cultural practices. One program in Guinea for Liberian and Sierra Leonean refugees incorporated African cultural and healing activities and advocacy to prevent future torture along with other psychosocial modalities. Follow-up assessments found significant reductions in trauma symptoms and increased daily functioning and social support (Stepakoff et al., 2006). In the United States, psychosocial approaches for refugees are also being developed. Community services designed and run by refugee communities almost always follow a psychosocial framework, and mainstream mental health providers are moving in this direction. For example, Khamphakdy-Brown and colleagues (2006) added psychoeducational home visits to supplement clinic-based counseling in their program for refugee and immigrant women, and Goodkind (2006) describes a "mutual learning" program that emphasizes advocacy and resource development for Hmong refugees.

There is little evidence to date about the effectiveness of psychosocial programs for refugees (Makinson, 1999). Many programs use concepts, measurement instruments, and approaches that have not been validated and tested in the settings in which they are being applied, and few of the practitioners who devise and implement the programs have adequate training. Outcome evaluations are rare. Nonetheless, these programs have intuitive appeal, largely because they respond to basic human needs in addition to psychological trauma. Mollica (2006) stresses that unlike many refugee relief systems that create and sustain dependency and unemployment, psychosocial programs emphasize the critical importance of work and of having a chance to help others rather than merely being the recipient of help.

Religion and Spirituality

The role of religion/spirituality in recovery from trauma and from serious mental health problems is receiving increased attention in the mental health literature (Blanch & Russanova, 2007). This is new terrain for many mental health workers. In the United States, mental health practitioners are accustomed to a fundamental separation of church and state, and many are uncomfortable with discussions about the divine. However, religion and spirituality may be particularly important to refugees, who often come from cultures where religion is not segregated from other aspects of life, and who have recently encountered ultimate questions of life and death. To understand the refugee experience and to support their recovery from trauma therefore requires at least a basic understanding of religion and a willingness to address matters of spirit and faith.

Much has been written about the impact of violence on faith. Intense trauma may constitute a moral crisis, or even be the individual's first encounter with evil. This may destroy the belief in one's own invulnerability or in the world as understandable, and may ultimately result in a collapse of faith (Boehnlein, 2007). On the other hand, faith and prayer may help an individual survive the most horrible conditions, and surviving violence can strengthen the relationship between survivors and their sources of spiritual succor (Mollica, 2006). Researchers who have begun to examine these issues have found relationships between measures of religious coping, severity of trauma symptoms, and post-trauma growth (Ai, Peterson, & Huang, 2003; Ai & Peterson, 2005; Ai et al., 2005; Ai et al., 2007).

Violence may also affect the individual's relationship to organized religion. At various times in history, organized religions have been complicit in mass violence, either as active or passive participants. In contrast, there have been times when organized religion has played a significant role in opposing oppression and violence and/or helped to heal the collective wounds of society. In the United States, religious leaders played a critical role in the fight for civil rights. In a more recent example, a highly regarded Bosnian Muslim cleric issued a decree that Muslim women who had been sexually abused during the ethnic violence should be given the status of martyrs and supported both morally and materially (Mollica, 2006). Without the cleric's action, these women might well have been considered unclean and ostracized from family and society.

There are many ways in which spiritual or religious practices can assist in the recovery process. The relationship with a clergy person or spiritual guide may help to build a renewed sense of trust and healing; the connection with a faith community may be essential to combating isolation; religious practices and prayer can help contain and modulate emotions that might otherwise run out of control; the practice of forgiveness can fundamentally shift the meaning given to the experience (Blanch, 2007).

Gender Issues: The Need for a Focus on Women

The refugee field has struggled for years with the issue of incorporating gender into theory and practice. In the past decade, the United Nations has emphasized both the special vulnerabilities and strengths of women refugees and the need to address sexual and gender-based violence. In 1995, the U.S. Office of Refugee Resettlement established the Refugee Women's Network, a national nonprofit organization dedicated to empowering refugee and immigrant women through leadership training, education, and advocacy.

In general, women who suffer from a traumatic event are significantly more likely than men to develop mental health problems (Sanchez-Hucles & Gamble, 2006). Within refugee populations, women have been shown to have higher levels of PTSD severity and more depressive and anxiety symptoms than men (Ai & Peterson, 2005; Keller et al., 2006). In one study, women had twice the risk of experiencing PTSD as men, a difference that persisted after adjusting for age, marital status, being a parent, loss of family members, amount of social support, education level, and level of depression (Ranasinghe & Levy, 2007). Women's vulnerability may also be exacerbated by other gender-related factors. For example, in one study, women with large families and those who were less educated or did not speak English reported statistically higher counts of trauma and torture as well as more associated problems (Robertson et al., 2006).

There are many reasons why the circumstances and needs of refugee women require special attention. Women and girls are often exposed to higher levels of violence than men. Women and children now comprise 80% of international war casualties, and increasingly serve as combatants (Sanchez-Hucle & Gamble, 2006). They are at special risk for torture because of their smaller size, the fact that they are less likely to be considered credible reporters of their experience, in retaliation for actions of their family members, or in order to intimidate their male partners (Pope, 2001).

Women refugees are also at high risk for rape and other forms of gender-based violence. While rape has always been a consequence of war, the systematic and widespread use of sexual violence during recent genocides in Bosnia-Herzegovina (Schultz, 2006; Skjelsbaek, 2006) and Darfur (Wagner, 2005) have led to the recognition that rape during wartime may be a conscious tool of terrorism and genocide. In these situations, mass rapes were apparently carried out under orders, with multiple assailants, and were often committed on girls as young as seven and in the presence of the victim's family. The apparent intention was to humiliate or destroy the identity of the victim; in particular, to impregnate and destroy ethnic purity (Skjelsbaek, 2006). Rape was thus used strategically for the purposes of destabilizing populations, destroying bonds within communities and families, advancing ethnic cleansing, expressing hatred for the enemy, or supplying combatants with sexual services. The consequences of state-sponsored rape and terror include not just the terror and trauma of the violence itself, but rage at the impunity of the perpetrators and at the silencing of both individual and community (Radan, 2007).

Women and girls are also extremely vulnerable during migration and in refugee settings, where violence is sometimes perpetrated by male refugees or by the very people charged with protecting them, including peacekeepers, camp authorities, and relief workers (Vasquez Han, & De Las Fuentes, 2006). Often, refugee camps are controlled by men, and unaccompanied women are particularly at risk. The abuse may be as flagrant as outright rape and abduction or as subtle as an offer of protection, documents, or assistance in exchange for sexual favors. In 2003, the U.S. General Accounting Office reported that "sexual abuse of refugee women and girls is pervasive and present in almost all refugee settings" (US GAO, 2003, p. 1).

Violence against women does not necessarily end upon resettlement. Women refugees continue to be vulnerable to gender-based violence, discrimination and exploitation in their adopted homeland (Bhuyan, 2005; Radan, 2007). Struggling to find security in a strange land with different customs, women may easily fall prey to sexism, racism, or gender-based violence in new and unfamiliar forms (Casimiro, 2007). Often, refugees come from male-dominated societies where men are the sole breadwinners and decision makers, and violence may continue in patterns already established in the home county. In other cases, women relocated in the United States may find it easier to get a job, decreasing their male partner's traditional power and respect, and increasing the woman's vulnerability (Vasquez et al., 2006). In still other cases, refugee men who have suffered their own trauma during war or who believe they have failed to protect themselves or their families may become perpetrators (Radan, 2007).

Gender-based refugee trauma programs need to respect these vulnerabilities, creating environments that foster safety first. They also need to view all services in a family context (Vasquez et al., 2006), and to address women's health issues (Harris Humphries, & Nabb, 2006). Gender-based programs generally advocate an empowerment model and a multi-sectoral approach that takes into account prevention of abuse, the physical and psychological consequences of violence, the potential need of the victim for a safe haven, economic needs, legal rights, and community awareness

(Rees, 2007). As an example, Medica Zenica in Bosnia-Herzegovina began addressing war-related violence but quickly expanded its programming to include a counseling center, medical services, a hotline, and two safe houses with education, training, and microenterprise activities. Its research unit collects and analyzes data on gender-based violence to be used in prevention and advocacy programs (Vann, 2002).

In a second example, women in Burundian refugee camps in Tanzania undertook a needs assessment that showed an increased incidence of violence against women. Resulting programs included a drop-in center at which women's health and protection needs were addressed; community awareness activities that reached out to men as well as women; social forums for women to discuss issues affecting their lives; and training for staff in the camps to alert them to gender-based violence (Martin, 2004).

Gender-based trauma programs also need to recognize that women refugees often survive multiple and extreme forms of violence with incredible resilience. In one study of Central American women refugees, a majority of women who had endured extreme poverty, physical and/or sexual abuse, and war-related trauma had survived and built satisfying lives in their new homeland (Radan, 2007). Programs that build on women's strengths and capacity for self-healing, while also addressing the needs of those with persistent problems, will be most effective.

DEVELOPING A TRAUMA-INFORMED CLINICAL ENVIRONMENT

To be effective, trauma-specific treatment interventions must be delivered in a trauma-informed clinical environment—an environment where all staff, programs, and policies reflect an understanding of trauma and recovery. This model of "trauma integrated services" was originally developed in the public mental health system specifically for people with complicated needs who were not being well served by traditional mental health and substance abuse programs (Salasin, 2004). While not designed specifically with refugees in mind, the trauma-integrated model is based on acknowledging the pervasive impact of violence, building on people's natural strengths and capacities, and empowering individuals to define their own problems—principles that are consistent with the basic needs of refugees reviewed above.

In a trauma-informed organization, people are not automatically assumed to have a biological mental illness or to need psychiatric services. Because staff are sensitive to trauma dynamics people are not inadvertently retraumatized by policies or procedures that recreate or resemble previous traumatic events. People are always given an opportunity to talk about what happened to them. Staffs realize that they must earn the trust of their clients, and that their clients are the experts in their own healing. Trauma-specific clinical services are available for those who need and want them, but they are not seen as a substitute for other needed services. Everyone who walks in the door benefits, whether or not they choose to identify themselves as a trauma survivor, and opportunities are provided for staff as well as client healing.

Trauma-informed care is not a stand-alone clinical intervention. Rather, the principles of trauma-informed care are meant to be applied across an entire organization—whether a mental health agency, a school, or a social service provider. Fallot and Harris (2006) have identified five essential values for trauma informed care—safety, trustworthiness, choice, collaboration and empowerment—and have developed an organizational self-assessment protocol. These values, which apply to staff as well as clients, provide a basis on which effective trauma interventions can be constructed.

BUILDING TRAUMA-INFORMED PARTNERSHIPS

The construct of trauma-informed care can also assist in building effective partnerships between mental health providers and other refugee services and supports. Many refugee groups have developed strong national and local "Mutual Assistance Associations" (MAAs) that provide a whole range of social support, self-help, and advocacy services (see, for instance: www.cdss.ca.gov/refugeeprogram or www.searac.org/maa). Linking with and supporting these organizations can provide the mental health partner with a strong grounding in the culture and values of refugees, while simultaneously providing the refugee partner with needed services and technology. Principles of trauma-informed care, based on values of consumer empowerment and choice, make a natural bridge between mental health providers and MAAs.

Partnering with refugee providers and their social service networks can also be beneficial to all parties. Refugee service providers often recognize that many of their clients need mental health services, but they may also be acutely aware that traditional psychiatric care is not indicated. They may not know that other forms of mental health treatment, such as trauma-informed services, are even available. Relationships built over time, with both agencies working together to become trauma informed, would create the foundation for ongoing consultation and community-level responses. Trauma-informed social services would be a tremendous support for most refugees. Ongoing partnerships could also facilitate better linkages between arriving refugees and state social services and health care, since refugees are eligible for Temporary Assistance for Needy Families (TANF), medical assistance, etc. (with actual eligibility requirements varying from state to state)

Finally, partnering with primary health-care providers is essential since critical health problems may be misdiagnosed as psychosomatic trauma. For example, it is well known that Vitamin D deficiency may be a serious problem, especially for dark-skinned people and/or veiled women who are relocated to a northern climate (Benson & Smith, 2007). Vitamin D deficiency may also cause PTSD-like symptoms. A trauma-informed partnership between primary health providers, mental health providers, and the refugee community could be a powerful stimulus to the development of a holistic, public-health approach to refugee health, trauma recovery, and well-being.

CONCLUSION

Refugees are "normal" people exposed to extremely stressful events, and transitory resettlement and adjustment problems are common. In addition to stresses and/or traumas in the country of origin or during flight, negative experiences during resettlement may increase the risk of mental health problems. While many current trauma treatments may be useful, the selection of a treatment modality should consider three factors: (1) Does the modality support natural resilience? (2) Does it respect cultural experience? and (3) Does it focus on treating those who have the most severe symptoms? In addition, because of the unique experience and the cultural disorientation experienced by some refugees, nonconventional interventions and solutions need to be considered. Self-help, psychosocial approaches, traditional healing, narratives and storytelling, and religion and spirituality are some of the most promising emerging models. Gender-based approaches may also be important, especially for some refugee groups.

Adaptation to a new country is a long-term process that may continue over the lifetime of the refugee. Special supports may be needed at vulnerable points in time, even long after the refugee has mastered a new language and found a comfortable social and professional niche. The development of trauma-informed partnerships between refugee groups and services, social service providers, and mental health and health-care providers is one way to begin building a truly trauma-informed community support system for refugees.

ACKNOWLEDGMENTS

An earlier version of this chapter was prepared for Abt Associates Inc., National Center of Trauma Informed Care, under SAMHSA contract #280-03-2905. Helpful assistance was provided by Elzbieta Gozdziak, Susan Martin, John Tuscan, Marta Brenden, Susan Salasin, Gail Robinson, Blanca Gurolla, Helga West, Luc Nya, Lorna Hines-Cunningham, Leslie Brower, Arabella Perez, Claire Harrison, Noel Bonam, Colleen Clark, and Carole Warshaw.

REFERENCES

Ai, A. L., & Peterson, C. (2005). *Symptoms, religious coping, and positive attitudes of refugees from Kosovar war*. In T. A Corales (Ed.), *Focus on posttraumatic stress disorder research.* Hauppauge, NY: Nova Science Publishers.

Ai, A. L., Peterson, C., & Huang, B. (2003). The effect of religious–spiritual coping on positive attitudes of adult Muslim refugees from Kosovo and Bosnia. *International Journal for the Psychology of Religion, 13,* 29–47.

Ai, A. L., Tice, T. M., Huang, B., & Ishisaka, A. (2005). Wartime faith-based reactions among traumatized Kosovar and Bosnian refugees in the United States. *Mental Health, Religion and Culture, 8,* 291–308.

Ai, A. L., Tice, T. M., Whitsett, D. D., Ishisaka, A., & Chim, M. (2007). Posttraumatic symptoms and growth of Kosovar war refugees: The influence of hope and cognitive coping. *The Journal of Positive Psychology, 2,* 55–65.

Barad, M., & Cain, C. K. (2007). *Mechanisms of fear extinction: Toward improved treatment for anxiety.* In L. J. Kirmayer, R. Lemelson, & M. Barad (Eds.), *Understanding trauma: Integrating biological, clinical and cultural perspectives.* New York, NY: Cambridge University Press.

Benson, J., & Smith, M. M. (2007). Early health assessment of refugees. *Australian Family Physician, 36*(1/2), 41–43.

Bhuyan, R., Mell, M., Senturia, K., Sullivan, M., & Shiu-Thornton, S. (2005). Women must endure according to their karma: Cambodian immigrant women talk about domestic violence. *Journal of Interpersonal Violence, 20*(8), 902–921.

Blackwell, D. (2005). Psychotherapy, politics and trauma: Working with survivors of torture and organized violence. *Group Analysis, 38,* 307–323.

Blanch, A. (2007). Integrating religion and spirituality in mental health: The promise and the challenge. *Psychiatric Rehabilitation Journal, 30,* 251–260.

Blanch, A., & Russanova, Z. (2007). Special issue on spirituality and recovery. *Psychiatric Rehabilitation Journal, 30,* 247–325.

Boehnlein, J. K. (2007). *Religion and spirituality after trauma.* In L. J. Kirmayer, R. Lemelson, & M. Barad (Eds.), *Understanding trauma: Integrating biological, clinical and cultural perspectives.* New York, NY: Cambridge University Press.

Bonnano, G. A. (2004). Loss, trauma and human resilience. Have we underestimated the human capacity thrive after extremely aversive events? *American Psychologist, 59*(1), 20–28.

Bouton, M. E., & Waddell, J. (2007). Some biobehavioral insights into persistent effects of emotional trauma. In L. J. Kirmayer, R. Lemelson, & M. Barad (Eds.), *Understanding trauma: Integrating biological, clinical and cultural perspectives.* New York, NY: Cambridge University Press.

Bracken, P. J., Giller, J. E., & Summerfield, D. (1997). Rethinking mental health work with survivors of wartime violence and refugees. *Journal of Refugee Studies, 10,* 431–442.

Carlsson, J. M., Mortenson, E. L., & Kastrup, M. (2005). A follow-up study of mental health and health-related quality of life in tortured refugees in multidisciplinary treatment. *Journal of Nervous and Mental Disease, 193,* 651–657.

Carlsson, J. M., Olsen, D. R., Mortensen, E. L., & Kastrup, M. (2006). Mental health and health-related quality of life: A 10-year follow-up of tortured refugees. *Journal of Nervous and Mental Disease, 194,* 725–731.

Casimiro, S. (2007). Isolation and insecurity: Resettlement issues among Muslim refugee women in Perth, Western Australia. *Australian Journal of Social Issues, 42,* 55–69.

Charney, D. S. (2004). Psychobiological mechanism of resilience and vulnerability: Implications for successful adaptation to extreme stress. *American Journal of Psychiatry, 161,* 195–216.

Fallot, R. D., & Harris, M. (2006). Trauma-*informed services: A self-assessment and Planning protocol.* Unpublished manuscript.

Ferrada-Noli, M. (1998). Suicidal behavior after severe trauma. Part 1: PTSD diagnoses, psychiatric comorbidity and assessments of suicidal behavior. *Journal of Traumatic Stress, 11,* 103–112.

Goodkind, J. R. (2006). Promoting Hmong refugees' well-being through mutual learning: Valuing knowledge, culture and experience. *American Journal of Community Psychology, 37*(1–2), 77–93.

Harris, M., Humphries, K., & Nabb, J. (2006). Delivering care for women seeking refuge. *RCM Midwives, 9,* 190–192.

Harvey, M. R. (2007). Towards an ecological understanding of resilience in trauma survivors: Implications for theory, research and practice. *Journal of Aggression, Maltreatment and Trauma, 14*(1–2), 9–32.

Herman, J. (1992). *Trauma and recovery.* New York, NY: Basic Books.

Hinton, D. E., Otto, M. W., & Pollack, M. (2006). Symptom presentation and symptom meaning among traumatized Cambodian refugees: Relevance to a somatically focused cognitive-behavioral therapy. *Cognitive and Behavioral Practice, 13,* 249–260.

Hinton, D. E., Pich, V., Chhean, D., et al. (2005). The ghost pushes you down: Sleep paralysis-type panic attacks in a Khmer refugee population. *Transcultural Psychiatry, 42,* 46–77.

Keller, A., Lhewa, D., Rosenfeld, B., Sachs, E., Alladjem, A., Cohen, I., Smith, H., & Porterfield, K. (2006). Traumatic experiences and psychological distress in an urban refugee population seeking treatment. *Journal of Nervous and Mental Disease, 194,* 188–194.

Khamphakdy-Brown, S., Jones, L. N., Nilsson, J. E., Russell, E. B., & Klevan, C. L. (2006). The empowerment program: An application of an outreach program for refugee and immigrant women. *Journal of Mental Health Counseling, 28,* 38–48.

Kinzie, J. D. (2007). *PTSD among traumatized refugees.* In L. J. Kirmayer, R. Lemelson, & M. Barad (Eds.), *Understanding trauma: Integrating biological, clinical and cultural perspectives.* New York, NY: Cambridge University Press.

Kirmayer, L. R., Lemelson, R., & Barad, M. (Eds.). (2007). *Understanding trauma: Integrating biological, clinical and cultural perspectives.* New York, NY: Cambridge University Press.

Konner, M. (2007). Trauma, adaptation and resilience: A cross-cultural and evolutionary perspective. In L. J. Kirmayer, R. Lemelson, & M. Barad (Eds.), *Understanding trauma: Integrating biological, clinical and cultural perspectives.* New York, NY: Cambridge University Press.

Light, D. (1992). Healing their wounds: Guatemalan refugee women as political activists. *Women and Therapy, 13,* 297–308.

Lindencrona, F., Ekblad, S., & Hauff, E. (2008). Mental health of recently resettled refugees from the Middle East in Sweden: The impact of pre-resettlement trauma, resettlement stress and capacity to handle stress. *Social Psychiatry Psychiatric Epidemiology, 43,* 121–131.

Loughery, G., & Eyber, C. (2003). *Psychosocial concepts in humanitarian work with children: A review of the concepts and related literature.* Washington, DC: National Academies Press.

Makinson, C. (1999). Program on refugees and forced migration 1999 annual report. Andrew W. Mellen Foundation.

Martin, S. F. (2004). *Refugee women* (2nd ed.). Lanham, MD: Lexington Books.

Miller, K. E., Kulkami, M., & Kushner, H. (2006). Beyond trauma-focused psychiatric epidemiology: Bridging research and practice with war-affected populations. *American Journal of Orthopsychiatry, 76,* 409–422.

Mollica, R. F. (2006). *Healing invisible wounds.* New York, NY: Harcourt, Inc.

Momartin, S., Silove, D., Manicavasagar, V., & Steel, Z. (2004). Complicated grief in Bosnian refugees: Associations with posttraumatic stress disorder and depression. *Comprehensive Psychiatry, 45,* 475–482.

Pedersen, D. (2002). Political violence, ethnic conflict, and contemporary wars: Broad implications for health and social well-being. *Social Science and Medicine, 55,* 175–190.

Pope, K. (2001). Torture. In J. Worell (Ed.), *Encyclopedia of women and gender: Sex similarities and differences and the impact of society on gender* (pp. 1141–1150). San Diego, CA: Academic Press.

Porter, M., & Haslam, N. (2005). Predisplacement and postdisplacement factors associated with mental health of refugees and internally displaced persons. *Journal of the American Medical Association, 294*(5), 602–612.

Puggioni, R. (2005). Refugees, institutional invisibility, and self-help strategies: Evaluating the Kurdish experience in Rome. *Journal of Refugee Studies, 18,* 319–339.

Radan, A. (2007). Exposure to violence and expressions of resilience in Central American women survivors of war. *Journal of Aggression, Maltreatment and Trauma, 14,* 147–164.

Ranard, D. (1990). Mutual assistance associations: Refugee self-help groups play key role. *America: Perspectives on Refugees, 8,* 10.

Ranasinghe, P. D., & Levy, B. R. (2007). Prevalence of and sex disparities in post-traumatic stress disorder in an internally displaced Sri Lankan population 6 months after the 2004 tsunami. *Disaster Medicine and Public Health Preparedness, 1*(1), 34–41

Rees, S. (2007). Domestic violence in refugee families in Australia: Rethinking settlement policy and practice. *Journal of Immigrant and Refugee Studies, 5,* 1–19.

Robertson, C. L., Halcon, L., Savik, K., Johnson, D., Spring, M., Butcher, J., Westermeyer, J., & Jaranson, J. (2006). Somali and Oromo refugee women: Trauma and associated factors. *Journal of Advanced Nursing, 56,* 577–587.

Rousseau, C. (2005). Diving into complexity: John Sigal's work on the long-term consequences of the holocaust. *Clinical Child Psychology and Psychiatry, 10,* 262–265.

Rousseau, C., & Measham, T. (2007). *Posttraumatic suffering as a source of transformation: A clinical perspective.* In L. J. Kirmayer, R. Lemelson, & M. Barad (Eds.), *Understanding trauma: Integrating biological, clinical and cultural perspectives* (p. 263). New York, NY: Cambridge University Press.

Salasin, S. E. (2004). Evolution of women's trauma integrated services at the Substance Abuse and Mental Health Services Administration (SAMHSA).

Sanchez-Hucles, J., & Gamble, K. (2006). *Trauma in the lives of girls and women.* In J. Worell, & C. D. Goodheart (Eds.), *Handbook of girls' and women's psychological health* (pp. 103–112). Oxford: Oxford University Press.

Saraceno, B. (1997). Psychosocial rehabilitation as a public health strategy. *Psychiatric Rehabilitation Journal, 20,* 10–15.

Schultz, P. M. (2006). Cognitive-behavioral treatment of rape- and war-related post-traumatic stress disorder with a female Bosnian refugee. *Clinical Case Studies, 5,* 191–208.

Silove, D. (1999). The psychosocial effects of torture, mass human rights violations and refugee trauma. Toward an integrated conceptual framework. *Journal of Nervous Mental Disorders, 187,* 200–207.

Silove, D. (2007). *Adaptation, ecosocial safety signals, and the trajectory of PTSD.* In L. J. Kirmayer, R. Lemelson, & M. Barad (Eds.), *Understanding trauma: Integrating biological, clinical and cultural perspectives.* New York, NY: Cambridge University Press.

Skjelsbaek, I. (2006). Victim and survivor: Narrated social identities of women who experienced rape during the war in Bosnia-Herzegovina. *Feminism and Psychology, 16,* 373–403.

Southwick, S. M., Vythilingam, M., & Charney, D. S. (2005). The psychobiology of depression and resilience to stress: Implications for prevention and treatment. *Annual Review of Clinical Psychology, 1,* 255–291.

Stepakoff, S. (2007). The healing power of symbolization in the aftermath of massive war atrocities: Examples from Liberian and Sierra Leonean survivors. *Journal of Humanistic Psychology, 47,* 400–412.

Stepakoff, S., Hubbard, J., Katoh, M., Falk, E., Mikulu, J. B., Nkhoma, P., & Omagwa, Y. (2006). Trauma healing in refugee camps in Guinea: A psychosocial program for Liberian and Sierra Leonean survivors of torture and war. *American Psychologist, 61*, 921–932.

Summerfield, D. (1999). A critique of seven assumptions behind psychological trauma programmes in war-affected areas. *Social Science and Medicine, 48*, 1449–1462.

Tummala-Narra, P. (2007). Conceptualizing trauma and resilience across diverse contexts: A multicultural perspective. *Journal of Aggression, Maltreatment and Trauma, 14*(1–2), 33–53.

Turner, J. E. (1978). Defining a community support system. *Hospital and Community Psychiatry, 29*, 31–32.

Tziotziou, A., Livas, D., Karapostolic, N., & Tsegos, I. K. (2006). Coping with traumatic experiences in a communal setting. Therapeutic communities. *International Journal for Therapeutic and Supportive Organizations, 27*, 589–599.

U.S. General Accounting Office. (2003). Humanitarian assistance: Protecting refugee women and girls remains a significant challenge. GAO-03-663, released May 23, 2003. Information retrieved from http://www.gao.gov/. Accessed 10/07/10.

Vann, B. (2002). Gender-based violence: Emerging issues in programs serving displaced populations, GBV Global Technical Support Project, JSI Research and Training Institute on Behalf of the Reproductive Health for Refugees Consortium.

Vasquez, M., Han, A., & De Las Fuentes, C. (2006). Adaptation of immigrant girls and women. In J. Worell & C. D. Goodheart (Eds.), *Handbook of girls' and women's psychological health: Gender and well-being across the lifespan* (pp. 439–446). New York, NY: Oxford University Press.

Wagner, J. (2005). The systematic use of rape as a tool of war in Darfur: A blueprint for international war crimes prosecutions. *Georgetown Journal of International Law, 37*, 193–244.

Watters, C. (2001). Emerging paradigms in the mental health care of refugees. *Social Science and Medicine, 52*, 1709–1718.

Weyermann, B. (2007). Linking economics and emotions: Towards a more integrated understanding of empowerment in conflict areas. *Intervention, 5*, 83–96.

Whittaker, S., Hardy, G., Lewish, K., & Buchan, L. (2005). An exploration of psychological wellbeing with young Somali refugee and asylum-seeking women. *Clinical Child Psychology and Psychiatry, 10*, 177–196.

Yadin, E., & Foa, E. B. (2007). *Cognitive behavioral treatments for posttraumatic stress disorder*. In L. J. Kirmayer, R. Lemelson, & M. Barad (Eds.), *Understanding trauma: Integrating biological, clinical and cultural perspectives*. New York, NY: Cambridge University Press.

Ying, Y. (1997). Psychological adjustment of Southeast Asian refugees: The contribution of sense of coherence. *Journal of Community Psychology, 25*, 125–139.

CHAPTER FOURTEEN

Intellectual and Developmental Disabilities

Jan L. Roth

INTRODUCTION

This chapter will give the reader a general overview of the field of intellectual and developmental disabilities. Among the topics discussed will be a brief historic background, socio-demographic risk factors, current problems that face this population and a description of conventional modes of prevention, treatment, and management. It will conclude with innovative strategies being implemented around the country. It points out the ways in which this devalued and hidden population (Lennox, 2002) has suffered deficits in health, health care, health promotion, and disease prevention (Lennox, 2002), education (Schreibman, 2005), psychiatric care (Baxter & Kerr, 2002), and opportunities for quality of life and healthy aging (Lennox, 2002). We will discuss how institutional care for people with intellectual and developmental disabilities has given way to community care and family support services, with varying degrees of success. The emergence of an epidemic of autism (Lathe, 2006; Schreibman, 2005) will be discussed as well as the ways in which early intervention, educational programs, and person-centered planning have addressed the problem (Schreibman, 2005).

DEFINITION OF INTELLECTUAL AND DEVELOPMENTAL DISABILITIES

A major problem in conceptualizing intellectual disabilities and dealing with people who are intellectually disabled is the failure of government at all levels to make a distinction between mental illness and intellectual disabilities. They are distinctly different from each other, as are mentally retarded persons and those with various other developmental disabilities. The definition of mental retardation, or *intellectual disability*, as it is commonly referred to in the 21st century, is unfortunately not standardized, limiting the validity of epidemiological research.

However, regardless of how the disorders are defined, there are substantial barriers to good-quality care for people with this diagnosis.

What is a Developmental Disability?

It is unfortunate that developmental disability is defined differently by each state and has been subsumed by the general term intellectual disability. For example, Section 1.03(22) of the New York State Mental Hygiene Law, which is the legal base for eligibility determination, defines Developmental Disability as: A disability of a person that: (a) (1) Is attributable to mental retardation, cerebral palsy, epilepsy, neurological impairment, or autism; (2) Is attributable to any other condition of a person found to be closely related to mental retardation because such condition results in similar impairment of general intellectual functioning or adaptive behavior to that of mentally retarded persons or requires treatment and services similar to those required for such persons; or (3) Is attributable to dyslexia resulting from a disability described in (1) or (2); (b) Originates before such person attains the age of 22; (c) Has continued or can be expected to continue indefinitely; and (d) Constitutes a substantial handicap to such person's ability to function normally in society.

For purposes of determination of eligibility to receive services from the New York State Office for People with Developmental Disabilities (formerly Office of Mental Retardation and Developmental Disabilities), a psychological assessment must address the key element of the diagnosis of a developmental disability. These elements are: (a) date of onset (prior to 22 years of age), (b) a disorder that is *neurologically based* (i.e., affects brain and/or spinal cord), (c) a disorder that produces significant adaptive behavior deficits currently and prior to the age of 22, and (d) the condition will last indefinitely.

How Are Mental Retardation and Mental Illness Different?

The American Association of Mental Retardation (AAMR) (renamed the American Association on Intellectual and Developmental Disabilities in 2007) refers to mental retardation as comprising substantial functional limitations. AAIDD defines mental retardation as: (1) significantly subaverage intellectual functioning ("intelligence quotient," or IQ below 70) existing concurrently with (2) related limitations in two or more of the following applicable adaptive skills areas: communication, self-care, home living, social skills, community use, self-direction, health and safety, functional academics, leisure, and work; and (3) manifesting before the age of 18.

In contrast, mentally ill persons may have superior intellectual functioning, shifting adaptive skills, and may become better or worse at any time during their lives (Herr, Gostin, & Koh, 2003).

What is an Intellectual Disability?

According to the International Classification of Disease (ICD-10; World Health Organization, 1992), intellectual disability (or mental retardation) is defined as "a condition of arrested and incomplete development of the mind," which is notably characterized by impairment of skills during the developmental phase that contribute to the overall intellectual level of functioning (i.e., cognitive, language, motor, and social abilities). Intelligence tests and scales assessing adaptive behavior estimate the range of intellectual disability. The levels are: mild (IQ 50-69), moderate (IQ 35-49), severe (IQ 20-34), profound (IQ less than 20), other and level unspecified.

The American Association on Intellectual and Developmental Disabilities (AAIDD, 2009a) (http://www.aaidd.org/content_100.cfm?navID=21) defines an intellectual disability as a disability characterized by significant limitations both in intellectual functioning and in adaptive behavior, which covers many everyday social and practical skills. This disability originates before the age of 18. Intellectual functioning, also called "intelligence," refers to general mental capacity (i.e., learning, reasoning, problem solving, and other cognitive skills). One criterion used to measure intellectual functioning is an IQ test. Generally an IQ test score of around 70 or sometimes as high as 75 indicates a limitation in intellectual functioning. A standardized test can also determine limitations in adaptive behavior, which comprises three skill types: Conceptual skills (i.e., language and literacy, money, time and number concepts, and self-direction); social skills (i.e., interpersonal skills, social responsibility, self-esteem, gullibility, naiveté or wariness, social problem solving, and the ability to follow rules/obey laws and avoid being victimized); and practical skills (i.e., activities of daily living including personal care, occupational skills, health care, travel/transportation, schedules/routines, safety, use of money, and use of telephone).

Once a multifaceted evaluation has been completed, a professional can determine whether an individual has an intellectual disability and can establish and modify an individual support plan. Yet, AAIDD stresses that in defining and assessing intellectual disability professionals must also take into account additional factors, such as the community environment typical of the individual's peers and culture. It points out that professionals should also consider linguistic diversity and cultural differences in the way people communicate, move, and behave. Assessments must recognize that strengths and limitations often coexist and a person's level of life functioning can improve if appropriate personalized supports are provided over a sustained period.

A BRIEF HISTORICAL BACKGROUND: INSTITUTIONALIZATION VS. DEINSTITUTIONALIZATION

Historically, society has segregated individuals with intellectual disabilities in large residential facilities that are far away from their communities, and with no focus on integration into the larger society (Thorn, Pittman, Myers, & Slaughter, 2009). The Willowbrook Consent Decree of 1975 effectively began the era of deinstitutionalization of mentally retarded citizens in New York State.

According to *Mental Retardation and the Law: A Report on Status of Current Court Cases* (Health and Human Services, 1980) in June 1980, 11 states (Alabama, Arizona, Florida, Kentucky, Maine, Massachusetts, Michigan, New Jersey, New York, Pennsylvania, and Vermont) had court cases relevant to institutions and deinstitutionalization. In addition, several more states, including the District of Columbia, had court cases covering other issues relevant to mental retardation. They included commitment (California, Colorado, District of Columbia, Florida, Illinois, Kansas, Maryland, and New York); community living and services (California, Florida, Kentucky, Michigan, New York, and Vermont); criminal law (California and Louisiana); discrimination (West Virginia); guardianship (Pennsylvania); medical/legal issues (California, Illinois, Massachusetts, and New Jersey); parental rights and sexuality (Alabama, California, Delaware, Nebraska, New Jersey, New York, Ohio, Texas, Utah, and Washington); and special education (California, Colorado, Connecticut, District of Columbia, Florida, Hawaii, Kentucky, Maryland, Massachusetts, Michigan, Minnesota, Montana, New Hampshire, New Mexico, New York, Ohio, Oklahoma, Pennsylvania, South Carolina, Tennessee, Texas, and Vermont).

After abysmal conditions at Willowbrook State School in Staten Island, New York were exposed by eminent politicians, lawmakers, community activists, and journalists. On March 17, 1972, a class action lawsuit was filed against the State of New York by the families and advocates of children and adults who lived there. After losing the suit, New York State began to gradually close Willowbrook and return its residents to their communities of origin. In 1987 the decision was made to close several more institutions in New York State.

On June 22, 1999, the United States Supreme Court ruled in the landmark case of *Olmstead v. L. C.* and *E. W.* The case reached the Supreme Court when the Georgia Department of Human Resources appealed a decision made by the 11th Circuit that it had violated the ADA's "integration mandate" when it segregated two women with mental disabilities in a state psychiatric hospital for over 20 years. Each woman had a history of being periodically discharged to inappropriate settings, among them a homeless shelter, before being returned to the hospital. In delivering the opinion of the court, Justice Ruth Bader Ginsburg noted that under Title II of the federal Americans with Disabilities Act, "States are required to place persons with mental disabilities in community settings rather than in institutions when the State's treatment professionals have determined that community placement is appropriate, the transfer from institutional care to a less restrictive setting is not opposed by the affected individual, and the placement can be reasonably accommodated, taking into account the resources available to the State and the needs of others with mental disabilities."

Problems facing the state in closing its institutions for people with mental retardation and developmental disabilities include: (a) the increasing importance of developmental centers in the state's economy; (b) the fiscal advantage of shifting state's cost to the federal government; and (c) the role of institutions as a nexus of conflict resolution among unionized workers, parents of the developmentally disabled, and advocates.

Willowbrook and many other large developmental centers closed. However, by the end of 1994, there were still 3611 individuals residing in the remaining eleven New York State facilities serving those with intellectual disability in large congregate care. Almost all of them were frail elderly, behaviorally problematic, or criminally involved. The institutions endured but changed and now served "special populations" (Castellani, 2005). In spite of these problems, the situation for many former residents of Willowbrook improved dramatically in the last 40 years. Small community residences in ethnically relevant neighborhoods and staffed by culturally competent caregivers proliferated. Deinstitutionalization was one aspect of the ongoing movement to include people with developmental disabilities in mainstream society.

As people with developmental disabilities have become more visible in mainstream society, they have had to confront some of the social problems of the day. Substance use, HIV/AIDS, homelessness, and psychiatric illness are suffered by people with intellectual and developmental disabilities, yet services are not always available to them at hospitals and clinics, shelters, and treatment programs serving the community at large.

REVIEW OF THE LITERATURE

Human Rights and Social Justice

Social injustice may be defined as the active denial or violation of rights based on the perception of the inferiority of a specific group (Levy & Sidel, 2006). In the past 25 years there has been a change in focus of the international human rights movement from concern about traditional and visible minorities to concern for the rights of underprotected and hidden minorities (Herr, Gostin, & Koh, 2003). In the first group are people of color, ethnic and religious minorities, women, children, and refugees. In the second category are persons living with human immunodeficiency virus/acquired immunodeficiency syndrome (HIV/AIDS), gays and lesbians, and persons with physical or mental disabilities. Recognition of existing human rights for those who are invisible in mainstream society is documented and further development of instruments to protect a broader range of rights for people with mental disabilities is a priority (Rosenthan & Sundram, 2003).

Law and Politics

Castellani (2005) summarizes several relevant laws pertaining to the treatment of people with mental disabilities. In 1972, *Wyatt v. Stickney* ruled that custodial care was not adequate for people with mental retardation and that they required "active treatment." The right to treatment, specific, and measurable objectives, time limitation, sanctions, and an alternative to administrative and legislative inaction were features of *Wyatt v. Stickney* that lit a fire under advocates around the United States. This was the beginning of federal courts stepping into the mental retardation arena. *Baxstrom v. Herold* (382U.S.107) and *Rouse v. Cameron* (387F.

2d241: DC Cir) pertain to mental illness and uphold the rights of people with mental disabilities.

President John F. Kennedy appointed a President's Panel on Mental Retardation. It opened the way for an expanded role of the federal government in issues of concern to people with intellectual disabilities, their families, and advocates.

PREVALENCE OF INTELLECTUAL AND DEVELOPMENTAL DISABILITIES

According to the Arc of the United States (formerly Association for Retarded Citizens), the largest community-based organization advocating for and serving people with intellectual disabilities and their families, there are 7.2 million people living with intellectual and developmental disabilities (www.thearc.org). This represents 2.4% of the population of the United States.

Autism and Asperger's Syndrome

According to the *Diagnostic and Statistical Manual of Mental Disorders*, 4th Edn., Text Revision (DSM-IV-TR) (American Psychiatric Association, 2000) the diagnostic features of autistic disorder are essentially the presence of markedly abnormal or impaired development in social interaction and communication, and a markedly restricted repertoire of activity and interests. The disturbance must be manifest by delays or abnormal functioning in at least one, and often several of the following areas prior to the age of 3 years: social interaction, language used in social communication, or symbolic or imaginary play. The essential features of Asperger's disorder are severe and sustained impairment in social interaction; restricted repetitive and stereotyped patterns of behavior, interests, and activities; and clinically significant impairment in social, occupational, or other important areas of functioning. In contrast to autistic disorder, there are no clinically significant delays in language acquisition (e.g., single nonechoed words are used communicatively by the age of 2 years, and spontaneous communicative phrases are used by the age of 3 years). However, more subtle aspects of social communication (e.g., typical give-and-take in conversation) may be affected. In addition, during the first three years of life, there are no clinically significant delays in cognitive development. In contrast to autistic disorder, intellectual disability is not usually observed in Asperger's disorder, although occasional cases in which mild intellectual disability is present, have been noted (e.g., when the intellectual disability becomes apparent only in the school years with no apparent cognitive or language delay in the first three years of life).

The term autistic spectrum disorder (ASD) is used to refer to a larger group. Each of the disorders on the spectrum has unique symptoms that vary in severity and scope. ASD may include autistic disorder; Asperger's disorder; Rett's disorder; pervasive developmental disorder not otherwise specified; and childhood disintegrative disorder. Together these conditions had grown to represent more than 20% of the total caseload served by the California Department of Developmental Services in June, 1987 (California Department of Developmental Services, 2007) (http://www.dds.ca.gov/AutismReport_2007.pdf).

The *Diagnostic and Statistical Manual of Mental Disorders*, 4th Edn., Text Revision (DSM-IV-TR) (American Psychiatric Association, 2000), which is based on a unique multinational field trial (Volkmar, 2005) reports that the median rate of autistic disorder is five cases per 10,000 individuals with reported rates ranging from 2 to 20 cases per 10,000 individuals. Prevalence data regarding the definitive rates of Asperger's disorder are lacking in the DSM-IV-TR. Prevalence rate of mental retardation has been estimated at approximately 1%. However, different studies have reported different rates depending on the definition used, the methods of ascertainment, and the populations studied. Schreibman (2005) states the California State Department of Developmental Services reported that between 1988 and 1998 there was a 610% increase in autism cases (Schreibman, 2005). The California Department of Developmental Services revealed that the state saw a 12-fold increase during the past two decades in the number of people with ASD receiving services through regional centers (AAIDD, 2009b) (http://www.aaidd.org/content_2159.cfm). The DSM-IV-TR states that "It remains unclear whether the higher reported rates reflect differences in methodology or an increased frequency of the disorder" (American Psychiatric Association, 2000).

SOCIODEMOGRAPHIC RISK FACTORS

Some of the residential settings in which individuals with intellectual and developmental disabilities reside are institutions for 16 or more persons, intermediate care facilities for individuals with mental retardation (ICFs/MR) for 15 or fewer persons, and supported living/personal assistance arrangements. Increasingly, the trend in many states is away from funding small ICFs/MR for 15 or fewer persons (e.g., Alaska, Delaware,

Georgia, Maryland, Massachusetts, Michigan, Montana, New Hampshire, New Jersey, Oregon, South Dakota, and Wyoming). When there is strong parental advocacy community integrated residential services for adults (e.g., with autistic disorder) can be successful, as in Huntington, West Virginia (Sullivan, 2005).

Residential environments can pose a risk of ill-health (Beange, 2002). For example, children in the foster care face significant health risks. *Physical health problems* affect 30–40% of children in the child welfare system and include delayed growth and development, HIV infection, neurological disabilities, malnutrition, and asthma. Vision, hearing, and dental problems are also prevalent. Children in out-of-home care check into hospitals more frequently and stay for longer periods of time than other low-income children. *Developmental disabilities* affect approximately 20% of children in out-of-home care including, mental retardation, cerebral palsy, and learning disabilities, as well as speech, hearing, and sight impairments (Child Welfare League).

CONVENTIONAL MODES OF PREVENTION, TREATMENT, AND MANAGEMENT

Often, behavioral problems in psychiatrically ill persons with developmental disabilities have hindered the diagnosis of conditions. The behaviors themselves may be difficult to interpret (Baxter & Kerr, 2002).

A study of a city jail in New York (Sundram, Platt, & Cashen, 1991) revealed that observations of inmates by reception center staff and corrections officers were better than psychometric tests in making the determination of whom among the inmates had developmental disabilities.

Typically, individuals with developmental disabilities who do not live with their families have been housed in large or small institutions. This includes those with forensic backgrounds. In New York State, the deinstitutionalization movement has been stymied by economic exigencies (i.e., to maximize Medicaid) resulting in slowing down of the process to close the institutions forever. The concept of "special populations" came to be used as justification for building new institutions.

On September 28, 1998, one month after he announced the New York State—Creating Alternatives in Residential Environments and Services (NYS-CARES) Initiative (Office of Mental Retardation and Developmental Disabilities, 2005) (http://www.omr.state.ny.us/nyscares/hpnycares.jsp) to virtually eliminate the waiting list for out-of-home beds, Governor George

Pataki announced plans to build the Center for Intensive Treatment to provide specialized secure services for individuals with serious criminal involvement (Castellani, 2005).

For a thorough and comprehensive discussion of public spending trends for intellectual and developmental disabilities in the 50 states and the District of Columbia during the years 1977–2006, the reader is referred to the excellent book, *The State of the States in Developmental Disabilities*, 7th Edn. (Braddock, Hemp, & Rizzolo, 2008). From their book, three states were chosen at random by this writer as examples of how public spending has evolved. The three states are New York, California, and Mississippi.

Trends in spending show that from 1977 to 2006, New York State has increasingly spent money on community services and individual and family support (IFS) and decreasingly spent money on institutional settings for people with intellectual and developmental disabilities. When fiscal effort is measured across the same span of years in terms of dollars spent per $1000 personal income, $3.05 was spent on institutional settings in 1977 compared with $0.93 in 2006. In contrast, $0.57 was spent on community services and IFS in 1977 compared with $7.00 in 2006. When looking at the medicaid component of public intellectual/developmental disability spending in billions of 2006 dollars; the trend started from 37% (of $1.69 billion) in 1977, 79% (of $2.84 billion) in 1986, 100% (of $4.96 billion) in 1996, 100% (of $6.07 billion) in 2004, and 100% (of $6.40 billion) in 2006. Clearly, the trend is toward spending on the Home and Community-Based Waiver, Intermediate Care Facilities for the Mentally Retarded, and Related Medicaid services. Nonmedicaid spending on this population has consistently been at 0% since 1993.

In the state of California, spending has drastically increased for community services from 1977 to 2006. When fiscal effort is measured in terms of dollars spent per $1000 personal income, $1.01 was spent on institutional settings in 1977 compared to $0.55 in 2006. In contrast, $0.82 was spent on community services and IFS in 1977 compared to $2.93 in 2006. When looking at the Medicaid component of public I/DD spending in billions of 2006 dollars the trend is from 29% (of $1.13 billion) in 1977, 43% (of $1.96 billion) in 1986, 51% (of $3.13 billion) in 1996, 57% (of $4.87) in 2004, and 54% (of $4.86 billion) in 2006. Non-Medicaid spending in California has decreased from approximately 71–46% of all spending on I/DD from 1977 to 2006.

In the state of Mississippi, spending has increased between 1977 and 2006 for both community services and IFS, and institutional setting with 16 or more beds. When fiscal effort is measured in terms of dollars spent per $1000 personal income $1.46 was spent on institutional settings in

1977 in comparison with $2.72 in 2006. Spending on community services and IFS has expanded at a much greater rate from $0.12 per $1000 personal income in 1977 to $1.59 in 2006. When looking at the Medicaid component of public I/DD spending in billions of 2006 dollars, the trend is from 16% (of $65.7 billion) in 1977, to 34% (of $118.2 billion) in 1986, to 76% (of $194.3 billion) in 1996, to 82% (of $309.3 billion) in 2004, to 85% (of 327.3 billion) in 2006. Nonmedicaid spending represented an increasingly small portion during the years 1977–2006.

INNOVATIVE STRATEGIES FROM AROUND THE COUNTRY

Innovative Policy

One aspect of the problem facing nonprofit groups is that when worthy innovative model programs are identified they cannot obtain the funds to grow and be tested for effectiveness in other communities (*The New York Times* Editorial Page, June 2, 2009). The Obama administration has created a Social Innovation Fund housed at the Corporation for National and Community Service. Congress has authorized the fund and President Barack Obama's 2010 budget allots $50 million for it to start. The fund is supposed to identify successful high-impact programs prime for further development and expansion, and then use government dollars as a catalyst to raise sustainable financing from foundations, businesses, and individual donors. According to the Times editorial, the Domestic Policy Council views the innovation fund as "part of a larger push by the administration to tap the expertise of nonprofits working effectively on social problems, to channel new help their way and to use lessons from the field about what works to shape government policies."

Individuals with Disabilities Education Act (IDEA), formerly Education for All Handicapped Act, Public Law 94-142, stipulates special education services that children with developmental disabilities may qualify for (McGee & Morrier, 2005). The United States Department of Education has defined six main principles of IDEA as: (1) the provision of a free appropriate public education; (2) completion of an appropriate evaluation; (3) development and implementation of an individualized education program (IEP); (4) placement in the least restrictive learning environment; (5) parent and student participation in decision making; and (6) provision and reinforcement of procedural safeguards (Mandlawitz, 2005).

Theoretical Innovation

Theories, findings, and approaches used in work with nonintellectually disabled children have been applied to work with several types of intellectually disabled individuals (Hodapp, Burack, & Zigler, 1990). In their innovative book, child development in nonintellectually disabled children is posited in terms of similar sequences of development, cross-domain relations, the environment, and motivation, as several etiologically different groups of intellectually disabled children.

Practical Innovation

Autistic Disorder

Treatment and Education of Autistic and Related Communication Handicapped Children (TEACCH) Program for autistic children is one of the innovative educational programs offered to children with Autistic Spectrum Disorder (Schopler, 2005; Schreibman, 2005). The state of North Carolina's TEACCH is the first university-based statewide program mandated by law to provide service, research, and multidisciplinary training on behalf of autism and related developmental disorders (Schopler, 2005). In addition, early intervention often includes speech, occupational, and physical therapies, as well as special instructions. Behavioral strategies (e.g., Applied Behavior Analysis), which grew out of B. F. Skinner's operant conditioning, have been widely used in early intervention with children diagnosed with autistic disorder. Comprehensive, relationship-based floor time (Greenspan & Wieder, 1997) has also been advocated for people with autism. Controversies swirl around many issues in the field (i.e., causes, prevention, and best treatment of autistic disorder). While almost all strategies focus on early diagnosis and treatment, the plight of adults with autistic disorder is less well addressed. Some of the best programs for adults (i.e., Job Path) provide person-centered planning, inclusion, one-to-one staffing, and flexible schedules. State-operated and voluntary residential options are the choices made by some families who can no longer care for their relatives at home. Sometimes the placement of an adult can occur in an abrupt somewhat traumatic manner even though the placement is a logical next step in the move toward independent living (Marcus, Kunce, & Schopler, 2005). Parental involvement is a key concept in developing and operating high-quality services for adults with autistic disorder (Sullivan, 2005).

Gay, Lesbian, Bisexual, and Transgender People

Rainbow Support Group for gay, lesbian, bisexual, and transgender people with intellectual and developmental disabilities in New Haven, Connecticut is a successful inclusion program (Allen, 2003).

Co-occurring Mental Illness and Developmental Disability

For services to people with dual diagnoses of intellectual disability and mental illness, programs that are noteworthy include Wrentham, Massachusetts, University of California at Los Angeles (UCLA), Children's Hospital in Boston, and Eastern Nebraska Community Office of Retardation (ENCOR) in Omaha (Bouras, 1994). The three organizing principles that underlie these successful initiatives are: (1) normalization, (2) application of the developmental model, and (3) cost–benefit considerations. Mobile mental health services to provide outreach programs in group homes or sheltered places of employment are predicted to be the wave of the future (Bouras, 1994) and will increasingly focus on training personnel to a proficient level of skill in mental health treatment techniques.

Davidson and O'Hara (2007) advocate overcoming the barriers to comprehensive care for people with co-occurring mental illness and developmental disabilities. Their methods include consensus building among providers, individuals, and funders to establish a comprehensive service network for individuals with intellectual disabilities and mental health problems.

McGuire and Chicoine (2006) write about the person who has Down's syndrome (DS). The unique preventive and treatment strategies for mental well-being of the person with DS are outlined.

Substance Use and Addiction

The Center for Substance Abuse Treatment (CSAT) recommends some specific accommodations to the screening and treatment of people with cognitive disabilities in its Treatment Intervention Protocol (TIP) 29: Substance Use Disorder Treatment for People with Physical and Cognitive Disabilities. TIP29 states that people with physical and cognitive disabilities are more likely to have substance use disorders and less likely to get effective treatment for it than their peers without such a coexisting disability. Specific accommodations in screening, treatment planning and counseling, and staff training, funding mechanisms, marketing, and demonstrating an organizational commitment to working with people who have coexisting disabilities are covered in the TIP. Providers must first examine their programs and eliminate the four major barriers to effective treatment: (1) attitudinal barriers; (2) discriminatory policies, practices, and procedures; (3) communication barriers; and (4) architectural barriers. In working with those individuals who have cognitive impairments, the questions should be phrased concretely rather than abstractly. Use of verbal and nonverbal cues is helpful. Those with cognitive disabilities may often benefit from techniques such as expressive therapy or role-playing. Lack of employment may be a particularly serious problem for those with severe disabilities, including those with intellectual/developmental disabilities (Braddock et al., 2008) and may contribute to the likelihood of a substance use problem. Flexible treatment schedules should be implemented to accommodate the transportation and vocational needs of this special population.

HIV/AIDS

Prevention of HIV infection and treatment of sex abusers with developmental disabilities and HIV infection are two of the many issues facing service providers and planners in the field of developmental disabilities (Crocker, Cohen, & Kastner, 1992; Shannon, 2000). As women have become more and more entrapped in the HIV/AIDS epidemic, the result is a growing population of developmentally affected infants (Crocker et al., 1992). The biomedical front is seeing important gains in controlling HIV infection. Yet, in the areas of developmental services, there is much room for improvement in identification of need to provide the supports and linkages to services for the young child. These would always include supports to the mothers and potential mothers. Treatment for drug addiction in women is the key, and must be done with sensitivity to the special personal needs of women with developmental disabilities.

The importance of examining issues such as the treatment of sex abusers with developmental disabilities and HIV infection is courageously addressed by Garwick and Swanson (1992). Typically those individuals with developmental disabilities are more likely than their cognitively normal peers to be caught in sexual abuse incidents. This is due to their frequently being in supervised residential settings. On the other hand, reporting or admitting high-risk behavior may be inhibited in the person with developmental disabilities due to fear of discussing his or her sexuality. The protection of confidentiality is an essential right that must be protected, with the understanding that the interdisciplinary team developing a coordinated approach to meet service needs for an individual necessitates a fully informed, well-trained group of people.

Inmates with Developmental Disabilities

In the population held at a New York City jail, an estimated 1–3% of inmates have developmental disabilities (Sundram et al., 1991). While the need for preliminary screening and identification of the population of intellectually and developmentally disabled people was identified, for many years no systematic program existed. A bold proposal for an Assertive Community Treatment (ACT) Team at Riker's Island city jail was met with interest by OMRDD (now known as OPWDD) at the Deputy Director level but was not funded. The proposal addressed the need for the services of the ACT team to establish who meets the state criteria for classification as developmentally disabled, assistance in appropriate assessment and outcome. If so determined an inmate could go with the ACT team after leaving Riker's as an alternative to serving a prison sentence. Primarily, people incarcerated in the city jail need vocational, educational, rehabilitative, and clinical services. The purpose of the ACT team would be to provide a structure, support, and an alternative to incarceration. An ample staffing ratio of 1:10 would ensure that services are provided to each individual on the ACT team caseload.

Person-Centered Planning (PCP) (Cornell University, 2009; O'Brien, 1989; Mount, 2000), a promising practice, has been used with a target population of developmentally disabled inmates being released from state prison into the community (http://www.ilr.cornell.edu/edi/pcp/). Some of their issues include emotional problems, substance abuse, sex offender status, housing, and employment needs. They may face other challenges as well upon release.

The offender with intellectual disability and antisocial behavior presents a major problem for integration into the community. The key to success has been the provision of adequate supervision as well as the awareness that certain individuals will need lifelong support and supervision (Bouras, 1994). Movement of the ex-inmate to less restrictive environments should be based more on antisocial tendencies than on cognitive and adaptive levels of functioning.

Aging and Wellness

Adults with intellectual disabilities are especially at risk of a range of health problems, including seizures, polypharmacy, and gastrointestinal disorders (Lennox, 2002) that can limit the quality and length of their lives. Proper management of these conditions is crucial in minimizing secondary disabilities and associated deficits that can occur. An innovative approach is needed to correct the substantial deficits in health, health care, and health promotion/disease prevention for adults with intellectual deficits so that they can enjoy healthy aging. But first, there must be awareness of the problem. Only then can appropriate goals be established, goals that support the message of health promotion. The methodologies for achieving goals should be tailored to this population, that is: (1) they must derive from person-centered assessment, (2) the health promoting services should be accessible, and (3) they should be implemented at the individual and organizational levels.

SPECIAL CULTURAL CONSIDERATIONS

The Person-Centered Approach and the use of personal futures planning (Mount, 2000) takes into account the unique strengths and weaknesses, needs, likes, and dislikes of individuals. Cultural considerations are the norm when individual differences rather than institutional exigencies are the priority. Nevertheless, sometimes the inclusion mandate becomes an inappropriate regulation. For example, some elders with intellectual disabilities may not be able to tolerate 5 days a week in day program plus three inclusion activities per week. They may prefer to have only one inclusion activity per week. Individuals with profound intellectual and multiple disabilities may also do better with a modified inclusion schedule (Pawlyn & Carnaby, 2009).

Many of the cultural considerations for other special populations are relevant to the families of individuals with developmental disabilities. Language, religion, attitudes toward professionals, and ethnic pride are all factors to be considered in any evaluation and treatment strategy. The particular history of devaluation and maltreatment of individuals with intellectual and developmental disabilities should be viewed with sensitivity by those who seek to help.

According to a 1991 study on prisoners by the New York State Commission on Quality of Care for the Mentally Disabled, the largest-growing group of inmates in New York City is Spanish speaking (Sundram et al., 1991). Any program serving this population should include ACT team members who are fluent in Spanish. In addition, the team should reflect the multicultural aspects of the city.

CONCLUSION

To be an effective human services professional in the field of developmental disabilities is to make a commitment to tireless work. It takes time, political commitment and willingness to reflect on and put into practice values centered on community integration (Bouras, 1994).

Finally, nothing can replace hands-on work with people who have developmental disabilities. No amount of reading can prepare a graduate student for the experience of listening to the frustration of parents who have tried to get good medical or psychological care for a developmentally disabled child or adult. Many of the readers of this chapter will rarely or perhaps never come across an individual with an intellectual or developmental disability in their professional lives. Those of you who do will be rewarded many times over for listening to them as you would to any other person.

ACKNOWLEDGEMENT

Thank you Dr. Susan M. Heimlich for your reactions to the chapter draft and sensible editing suggestions. Thanks, too, for your friendship and collegiality over the past 25 years.

REFERENCES

Allen, J. D. (2003). *Gay, lesbian, bisexual and transgender people with developmental disabilities: Stories of the Rainbow Support Group.* Binghamton, NY: The Haworth Press.

American Association on Intellectual and Developmental Disabilities [AAIDD]. (2009a). *Selected highlights: Definition of intellectual disability.* Retrieved December 28, 2009, from http://www.aaidd.org/content_100.cfm?navID=21

American Association on Intellectual and Developmental Disabilities [AAIDD]. (2009b). *Selected highlights: Autism.* Retrieved December 28, 2009, from http://www.aaidd.org/content_2159.cfm

American Psychiatric Association [APA]. (2000). *Diagnostic and statistical manual of mental disorders* (4th ed.) text revision. Washington, DC: American Psychiatric Association.

Baxter, H., & Kerr, M. (2002). Barriers to health care services and the role of the physician. In V. P. Prasher & M. P. Janicki (Eds.), *Physical health of adults with intellectual disabilities.* Oxford, UK: Blackwell Publishing.

Beange, H. (2002). Epidemiological studies. In V. P. Prasher & M. P. Janicki (Eds.), *Physical health of adults with intellectual disabilities.* Oxford, UK: Blackwell Publishing.

Bouras, N. (Ed.). (1994). *Mental health in mental retardation: Recent advances and practices.* Cambridge: Cambridge University Press.

Braddock, D., Hemp, R. E., & Rizzolo, M. C. (2008). *The state of the states in developmental disabilities* (7th ed.). Boulder, CO: University of Colorado department of psychiatry and Coleman institute.

California Department of Developmental Services [DDS]. (2007). *Selected highlights: Autism Report.* Retrieved December 28, 2009, from http://www.dds.ca.gov/AutismReport_2007.pdf

Castellani, P. J. (2005). *From snakes pits to cash cows: Politics and public institutions in New York*. Albany: State University of New York Press.

Cornell University. (2009). *Selected highlights: Employment and disability institute at industrial and labor relations*. Retrieved September 10, 2009, from http://www.ilr.cornell.edu/edi/pcp/

Crocker, A. C., Cohen, H. J., & Kastner, T. A. (Eds.). (1992). *HIV infection and developmental disabilities: A resource for service providers*. Baltimore, MD: Paul H. Brookes.

Davidson, P. W., & O'Hara, J. (2007). Clinical services for people with intellectual disabilities and psychiatric or severe behavior disorders. In N. Bouras & G. Holt (Eds.), *Psychiatric and behavioral disorders in intellectual and developmental disabilities*. Cambridge: Cambridge University Press.

Garwick, G. B., & Swanson, C. K. (1992). Treatment of sex abusers with developmental disabilities and HIV infection. In A. C. Crocker, H. J. Cohen & T. A. Kastner (Eds.), *HIV infection and developmental disabilities: A resource for service providers*. Baltimore, MD: Paul H. Brookes.

Greenspan, S. I., & Wieder, S. (1997). Developmental patterns and outcomes in infants and children with disorders in relating and communicating: a chart review of 200 cases of children with autistic spectrum diagnoses. *Journal of Developmental and Learning Disorders, 1*(1), 1–38. Retrieved October 11, 2010 from http://autism.bibliomaker.ch/BM_DIRECTORY/B/BM000000320/5947/GRE1.PDF

Health and Human Services [HHS]. (1980). *Mental retardation and the law: A report on the status of current court cases*. Office of Human Development, President's Commission on Mental Retardation, Washington, DC.

Herr, S. S., Gostin, L. O., & Koh, H. H. (Eds.). (2003). *The human rights of persons with intellectual disabilities*. Oxford: Oxford University Press.

Hodapp, R. M., Burack, J. A., & Zigler, E. (Eds.). (1990). *Issues in the developmental approach to mental retardation*. Cambridge: Cambridge University Press.

Lathe, R. (2006). *Autism, brain and environment*. London: Jessica Kingsley Publishers.

Lennox, N. (2002). Health promotion and disease prevention. In V. P. Prasher & M. P. Janicki (Eds.), *Physical health of adults with intellectual disabilities*. London: Blackwell Publishing.

Levy, B. L., & Sidel, V. (Eds.). (2006). *Social injustice and public health*. Oxford: Oxford University Press

Mandlawitz, M. R. (2005). Educating children with autism: Current legal issues. In F. R. Volkmar, R. Paul, A. Klin, & D. Cohen (Eds.), *Handbook of autism and pervasive developmental disorders: Assessment, interventions, and policy* (3rd ed., Vol. 2). New York, NY: John Wiley & Sons.

Marcus, L. M., Kunce, L. J., & Schopler, E. (2005). Working with families. In F. R. Volkmar, R. Paul, A. Klin, & D. Cohen (Eds.), *Handbook of autism and pervasive developmental disorders: Assessment, interventions, and policy* (3rd ed., Vol. 2). New York, NY: John Wiley & Sons.

McGee, G. G., & Morrier, M. (2005). Preparation of autism specialists. In F. R. Volkmar, R. Paul, A. Klin, & D. Cohen (Eds.), *Handbook of autism and pervasive developmental disorders : Assessment, interventions, and policy* (3rd ed., Vol. 2). New York, NY: John Wiley & Sons.

McGuire, D., & Chicoine, B. (2006). *Mental wellness in adults with Down syndrome: A guide to emotional and behavioral strengths and challenges.* Bethesda, MD: Woodbine House.

Mount, B. (2000). *Person-centered planning: Finding directions for change using personal futures planning.* Amenia, NY: Capacity Works.

O'Brien, J. (1989). *What's worth working for? Leadership for better quality human services.* Responsive Systems Associates, Lithonia, Georgia. Retrieved September 13, 2009, from http://thechp.syr.edu//whatsw.pdf

Office of Mental Retardation and Developmental Disabilities [OMRDD]. (2005). Selected highlights: New York State-CARES Initiative. Retrieved September 10, 2009, from http://www.omr.state.ny.us/nyscares/hpnycares.jsp

Pawlyn, J., & Carnaby, S. (Eds.). (2009). *Profound intellectual and multiple disabilities: Nursing complex needs.* Chichester: Wiley-Blackwell.

Rosenthan, E., & Sundram, C. J. (2003). Recognizing existing rights and crafting new ones: Tools for drafting human rights instruments for people with mental disabilities. In V. P. Prasher & M. P. Janicki (Eds.), *Physical health of adults with intellectual disabilities.* London: Blackwell Publishing.

Schopler, E. (2005). Cross-cultural program priorities and reclassification of outcome research methods. In F. R. Volkmar, R. Paul, A. Klin, & D. Cohen (Eds.), *Handbook of autism and pervasive developmental disorders: Assessment, interventions, and policy* (3rd ed., Vol. 2). New York, NY: John Wiley & Sons.

Schreibman, L. (2005). *The science and fiction of autism.* Cambridge: Harvard University Press.

Shannon, J. B. (Ed.). (2000). *Mental retardation sourcebook.* Health Reference Series. Detroit: Omnigraphics, Inc.

Sullivan, R. C. (2005). Community-integrated residential services for adults with autism: A working model (Based on a Mother's Odyssey). In F. R. Volkmar, R. Paul, A. Klin, & D. Cohen (Eds.), *Handbook of autism and pervasive developmental disorders: Assessment, interventions, and policy* (3rd ed., Vol. 2). New York, NY: John Wiley & Sons.

Sundram, C. J., Platt, I. L., & Cashen, J. A. (1991). *A report by the New York State Commission on Quality of Care (CQC) for the mentally disabled.*

The Arc of the United States. (2009). *Selected highlights.* Retrieved September 10, 2009, from https://www.thearc.org.

The New York Times Editorial. June 2, 2009. *Communities, innovation and Washington.*

Thorn, S. H., Pittman, A., Myers, R. E., & Slaughter, C. (2009). Increasing community integration and inclusion for people with intellectual disabilities. *Research in Developmental Disabilities, 30*(5), 891–901.

Volkmar, F. R. (2005). International perspectives. In F. R. Volkmar, R. Paul, A. Klin, & D. Cohen (Eds.), *Handbook of autism and pervasive developmental disorders: Assessment, interventions and policy.* (3rd ed., Vol.2). New York, NY: John Wiley & Sons.

CHAPTER FIFTEEN

Disabled Women and Domestic Violence

Notes from the Field

Paul Feuerstein

INTRODUCTION

The number one issue of women with disabilities in the United States is domestic abuse. It is not a new issue. My agency, Barrier Free Living (BFL), an agency in New York City serving people with disabilities, commissioned a study of the public's perceptions of people with disabilities. While "access," "jobs," and "health care" were common issues identified, no one thought of domestic violence.

Surveys of women with disabilities tell a different story. A recent survey showed domestic abuse to be the number one concern of women with disabilities (www.unitedspinal.org, 2009). People with disabilities not only have higher rates of abuse, but also stay in abusive relationships twice as long: 11.3 years versus 7.1 years in situations of physical abuse, 8.3 years versus 4.1 years in situations of sexual abuse (Baylor College of Medicine).

This chapter will address the factors that lead to domestic violence being hidden among disabled women, and the role of the caseworker in helping to bring to light the abuse so that the client may begin the process of recovery. Using the paradigm of the Duluth Power and Control Wheel (www.theduluthmodel.org), the chapter discusses how the vulnerability of a disabled person intersects with an abuser's need to control. It describes modalities that go beyond the complex process of healing to aid a disabled abused person build a firm foundation upon which to create an independent life.

A large percentage of the people we work with are disabled prior to becoming victims of domestic violence. We have found a strong correlation between domestic violence and early childhood abuse. The rate of abuse of children with disabilities is significantly higher than for their able-bodied counterparts. Studies show that one in three children with an identified disability that qualified them for special education services are victims of some type of maltreatment (i.e., either neglect, physical abuse, or sexual abuse), whereas 1 in 10 nondisabled children experience abuse. Children with *any type of disability are* 3.44 times more likely to be a victim of some type of abuse compared to children without disabilities (Sullivan & Knutson, 2000). One study found that children with developmental disabilities were at twice the risk of physical and sexual abuse compared to children without disabilities (Crosse, Elyse, & Ratnofsky, 1993).

ABUSE OF PEOPLE WITH DISABILITIES: THE SHAMEFUL SECRET

We live in a culture that discounts the value of people with disabilities. Within our culture, there are institutional environments that set the tone for abusive behavior. Foster care, group homes, and institutions have an increased risk of victimization when compared with natural families. Abusers often have a caregiver role, which gives them power and control over their victims, and frequently a stronger relationship with police and regulatory authorities than the victims themselves.

In other cases, domestic violence can be the cause of an individual's disability. An emergency room study of head assaults found that while stranger assaults tended to focus on the jaw, intimate violence assaults tended to focus on the upper part of the head (Arosarena et al., 2009). These are areas of the head that lead to vision or hearing loss or traumatic brain injury. A resident of Freedom House (BFL's shelter) became disabled when her abuser threw her out of a second story window.

Frequently, disabled victims are not identified because of a "don't ask, don't tell" culture within disability agencies. Prior to 1986, my agency fit into the same profile. I had been working with people with disabilities since 1979. In 1986, as I was interviewing a deaf woman for a job as a counselor in our program, she reported that she had 13 years experience working with disabled victims of domestic violence. I was interested, but dismissed the thought of working with this population because I believed that we did not have victims in our own agency. I hired her and she began to teach us the questions to ask about abuse. We found that we had plenty of victims amidst us.

Consequently, one of the first recommendations I make to people working with people with disabilities is to include questions about abuse in the intake process. At that early stage, an individual may not be open about a history of abuse, but a message has been sent that the subject is open for discussion. I worked with a young woman who was referred for therapy by her vocational counselor. She denied abuse in the intake process, but after three months of therapy, she revealed that she had been sexually abused by her father from the age of 12. She blamed her father for her massive stroke at the age of 18 that left her in a wheelchair with aphasia and significant other cognitive deficits.

Once the issue of domestic violence is identified, it is critical that a multifaceted evaluation is undertaken. There is often a complex relationship between trauma issues, concrete needs, and the individual's capacity for independent living. More often than not, the abuser is also the victim's caregiver. Women with disabilities are often easy targets for individuals in need of power and control. We have found a close interrelationship between childhood abuse and adult domestic violence.

Leigh Ann Davis of the ARC of the United States reports that "People with severe intellectual disabilities may not understand what is happening or have a way to communicate the assault to a trusted person. Others with a less severe disability may realize they are being assaulted, but don't know that it's illegal and that they have a right to say no. Due to threats to their well-being or that of their loved ones by the abuser, they may never tell anyone about the abuse, especially if committed by an authority figure that they learn not to question" (Davis, 2009).

DYNAMICS OF ABUSE

As a result of childhood experiences, many individuals will not identify what is happening to them as abusive. To explain the dynamics, we have taken the Duluth Model of Power and Control to a new level which adds additional dynamics due to disability. See Figure 15.1.

High levels of dependence fit into the cycle of Power and Control. Control of Supplemental Security Income (SSI) checks, for example, often begins with the family of origin. In some cases, we have worked with victims that did not know that they had a source of income. In other cases, disabled young adults have referred to the first day of the month as "my mother's bonus day." Restricting access to transportation is another common theme. In an early phase of our program, we placed a support team in a domestic violence shelter in order to provide access for deaf women and their children. Not a single adult who came into that program knew how to travel on a city bus by herself.

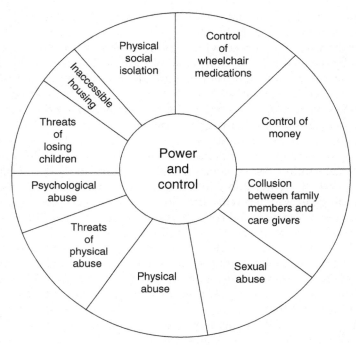

FIGURE 15.1
Power and Control Wheel for People with Disabilities

Withholding wheelchairs and medications is a variation on the same theme. Individuals live in fear of angering their caregiver because they know their punishment would be the withholding of medications, a wheelchair, a text telephone (TTY), or assistance with personal needs. One wheelchair-user who came into our shelter lived in a four-story walk-up apartment. She had been dependent on her husband to help her get in and out of bed, buy food, and prepare her meals. When she got a court order of protection to get him out of the house, members of her church helped her survive for a few months, but they were not able to sustain the effort.

Restricting access to friends and means of communication is a critical aspect of power and control because information is empowerment. A common theme of deaf women in our program has been withholding or limiting the use of a telecommunication device for the deaf (TDD) by their abusers. In moments of rage, the adaptive equipment has been destroyed. Because of the isolation, it is often difficult for a victim with disabilities to get the help they need.

One particularly telling threat used by abusers is the loss of children if the victim ever reveals the abuse to authorities. All too often the threat is real. If police find an abusive situation in which children have been witnesses to the abuse of a mother with a disability, they will often have the children put in foster care for "failure to protect." If the mother is deaf or has a communications issue, she will often be charged with "educational neglect." A thread of our work is helping mothers with disabilities get their children returned.

THE ROLE OF THE CRIMINAL JUSTICE SYSTEM

If police come across a situation of domestic violence that involves an individual with impaired communication, they will often interview the abuser to find out what has happened. The potential for the victim getting the help needed is compromised. Part of our agency's work is educating police about the issue and about appropriate interventions to be sure they get the whole story.

One of BFL's most effective partnerships is with the district attorney's office in Brooklyn, NY. Joe Hines, the current Brooklyn DA, has been an advocate for battered women since he was old enough to stop his father beating his mother. He developed a team approach using collaborations between his assistant district attorneys (ADAs) and his social work department. In 2000, BFL began a program with the Brooklyn DA's office called "Barrier Free Justice." The partnership combined social workers in the district attorney's office, civil attorneys from South Brooklyn Legal Services and BFL. It ensures that every victim with a disability coming through the district attorney's offices is interviewed by a social worker in the DA's office. BFL staff is collocated in the DA's office to engage victims as they begin the process of pressing charges.

The retelling of the story, often multiple times, is a retraumatizing experience. Compounding this, the adversarial nature of the court system is also difficult to navigate for individuals who have been trained to please. A social worker on our team will often take a disabled person to Court to provide emotional support. She may act as an advocate as well to prepare the victim for testimony, ask for a smaller court room or one that does not permit spectators. They may also ensure that the abuser is not allowed to contact with the victim/survivor during court process. Our workers will collaborate with civil lawyers to address custody issues, visitation, and, for many, divorce. As they help a victim through that process, the beginning of a trusting relationship develops. Trust is one of the core issues we address in the beginning and middle phases of our work.

ESTABLISHING TRUST

BFL has found that helping individuals with their concrete needs is one of the most effective ways to establish trust. Trust is a core issue for us, because many of our clients have been betrayed by everyone claiming to love them, and there is little reason for individuals to trust us given the traumas they have endured. Judith Herman, in her book *Trauma and Recovery,* asserts that "traumatic events overwhelm the ordinary systems of care that give people a sense of control, connection and meaning" (Herman, 1997).

Trust begins with engaging victims about their most basic needs. It is difficult, if not impossible, to get victims to address long-term issues if basic needs have not yet been addressed. Acquiring safe, accessible housing and financial independence are among the first priorities that must be addressed, which is not to say that other important work cannot be done until those issues are settled. Generally, the women[1] we serve are willing to begin to address other issues when they see movement on their concrete needs.

Our case managers do a thorough evaluation of concrete needs as a woman enters our program. Housing and financial issues are intractably linked. It is rare that a landlord will rent a tenant an apartment without a credit check, but economic abuse often leaves the victim mired in debt. An abuser will open credit in the name of the victim or run up a great deal of joint debt and fail to pay. This leaves our victims with a poor credit rating and makes starting over all the more difficult. In our exploration of the issue, there are no quick fixes to rehabilitate an individual's credit rating. The only solution we have found is to pay off the debt, but that is usually beyond the means of the people we serve.

There have been situations in which a staff has been able to negotiate with a single creditor. For example, our nonresidential team worked with Ms. A, a woman with schizoaffective disorder who is in recovery from substance abuse. When Ms. A began attending the program, she had worked for the Metropolitan Transit Authority for nearly 25 years. Her abuser demanded that she give him large sums of money for food, car insurance, and anything else he desired. If she did not give him the money, he would

---

[1]Our program works with men as well. Ninety-five percent of the victims we work with are women; so I will refer to the people we serve in the feminine.

threaten her, sometimes physically striking her. As a result, Ms. A was in rental arrears of nearly $12,000 and could barely afford to feed herself, even though she earned a salary of around $60,000 per year. During the course of intensive counseling and support, Ms. A developed a safety plan. She contacted her two sons in North Carolina, who invited her to come live with them and escape the abuse. Her social worker connected her with Adult Protective Services who assisted her in going to court to have her rental arrears waived. With our support, Ms. A made it safely to Metropolitan Transit Authority (MTA) retirement. She got a plane ticket to North Carolina, and has joined her sons. Ms. A reports that she is safe and healthy and has not seen or heard from her abuser since leaving New York. She continues to have contact with her social worker via telephone.

BEHAVIORAL HEALTH MODALITIES

Our social workers evaluate individuals for the emotional impact to trauma and the need for mental health intervention. Judith Herman introduces the concept of "Complex Post Traumatic Stress Disorder," a cluster of symptoms that occur when a victim has a long history of abuse or has survived extreme situations (Herman, 1997). The symptoms include: Alteration of Affect Regulation (including preoccupation with suicide, self-injury, explosive, or inhibited anger which may alternate, alternating compulsive, or inhibited sexuality); Alteration of Consciousness including amnesia or hypermnesia of trauma, dissociative episodes, reliving traumatic experience); Alteration of Self-Perception (including helplessness, paralysis, shame, guilt, or stigma); Alteration in Perception of Perpetrator (including preoccupation with the relationship, attributing total power to the abuser, acceptance of the belief systems of the perpetrator); Alteration in relation to others (including isolation, withdrawal, disruption of intimate relationships, persistent distrust); and Alterations in systems of meaning (including loss of sustaining faith, a sense of hopelessness, and despair).

Part of BFL's role is psychoeducational, that is, helping women realize that they are not alone. This is a major source of relief for many of the women with whom we work, who often believe that their personal situation is unique. When they meet others who are experiencing isolation, stigma, depression and anxiety, and the sense of powerlessness over their own lives, they come to the realization that they are not alone. Part of the work happens in a one-to-one relationship.

An important part of our intervention involves group work. When women hear each other's stories, they can identify common themes and begin to create a circle of mutual support. New members of the group benefit from hearing the stories of women who have left their abusers and have begun to put their lives together. The senior members of the group benefit, because they see that their experiences are a source of hope for group members who are not as far along in their healing journey. When we first started our program, a Center for Self-Help existed as part of the City University of New York. Frank Riesman studied the effects of "helper therapy." He found that helpers often benefited more from the helping relationship than the person being helped (Riessman, 1965). In fact, in our initial years of research with newly disabled people, we saw a qualitative difference between program participants who just came to be recipients of services and those who were involved in helping others.

My favorite illustration was a young man named Raymond who was a victim of crime. His little brother, who belonged to a Chinatown gang, was beaten up by rival gang members. Raymond went to the head of the rival gang and confronted him about what had been done to his brother. Raymond was shot in the back the next day, severing his spine. He refused to believe that he would never walk again. Hoping to effect a cure, his family sent him back to China to be healed by Chinese physicians. He returned to the United States in his wheelchair, having been told that the American doctors had done such a bad job that the Chinese doctors could not fix him. Raymond had been studying to be a draftsman, which was still a possible vocational goal, but he refused to go back to school until he could walk. Raymond's English was very good. When we had another Chinese young man come into our program with no English skills, we convinced Raymond to be his tutor. Once he took on the task, the difference was dramatic. Raymond became active in group. When we lost our federal funding, Raymond was involved in organizing a protest in front of Federal Plaza. The last we heard from him, Raymond had gotten a job with a home care agency as the person who fielded emergency calls at night.

We have gotten some of our survivors involved with the Voices of Women Empowerment Project. Survivors are trained to be advocates and public speakers to push for more services for victims of domestic violence. One of our survivors is a member of Safe Horizon's Domestic Violence Hotline Advisory Board as well as the fatality review committee for the Mayor's Office to Combat Domestic Violence. Besides her own empowerment, she has been a role model for many women in our program.

Beyond psychoeducation, there is the need for intense verbal therapy. Our social workers work to create a safe place in which women can tell their stories. People suffering with posttraumatic stress disorder (PTSD) have a constant conflict about approaching stories of abuse. Women vacillate between avoidance and being overwhelmed with the reliving of the experience of abuse. Encouraging them to tell their story helps them to put it in perspective. A colleague of mine uses the analogy of a scab over an infected wound: Healing does not begin until the scab is opened and the wound is cleaned out. It is the analogy she uses to describe the process of delving into the story to begin a journey of healing.

I often use the analogy of social worker as midwife. Our staff is assisting, encouraging, coaching, and supporting women in the process of rebirth. The real labor is being done by the women themselves, and we can only play a supporting role in the process. The real heroes are the women. Given the challenging nature of our work, I believe that is an important distinction. If a women moves from victim to survivor, it is on the basis of her hard work, and we can only take partial credit. However, if a woman cannot break out of her victim role, it is beyond our ability to transform her, and we must not beat ourselves up if a person does not succeed.

ESCAPING ABUSE

From day one of intervention, safety planning is a critical component of our program. In our nonresidential program, many women are still living with their abusers, and it is helpful to develop a safety plan for these individuals. An escape kit is developed which includes a copy of the Medicaid card, entitlement papers, birth certificates, as well as a supply of medications and materials for personal care needs. We encourage that this be entrusted to a close friend or neighbor to facilitate a quick getaway if the situation becomes violent. When a woman comes into our shelter, we assess her readiness to take the steps to become anonymous in her new community. We work on developing her skills to assess the safety of relationships, places, and situations and to work out a plan of action if she should run into her abuser or someone he knows.

Interdependence

While that process proceeds, parallel processes are needed to develop an interdependent lifestyle.[2] For a majority of women in our program, their abuser is also their caregiver. Many have not had the experience of living

---

[2]Unless we are survivalists, none of us live independently. We depend on family, friends, super markets or dry cleaners down the block or our coworkers. The difference between this and dependence is the extent to which we depend upon very few resources to help in our activities of daily living and the extent to which the help is mutual versus unidirectional.

alone. When BFL began its domestic violence program, we were able to fund a support team for deaf victims of domestic violence located in a general domestic violence shelter. The women we served were in their late 20s to late 30s and had multiple children. None of them knew how to travel on a city bus by herself. We had to teach them how to pay the fare, how to read a schedule and a bus map to determine which bus route would get them to their destination. Staffs accompanied them on their first trips until they felt confident enough to do it on their own. One of our guiding values is "when people build the skills and the mind set to become interdependent, they are less likely to accept abuse."

Occupational Therapy's Evaluation Tools

It was shortly after we gained experiences in these areas that we decided that we needed to add another aspect to our program. We found that Occupational Therapy (OT) needed to be an important component of our program. Many people think of OT as a discipline that enables job readiness. While that is part of what occupational therapists do, there are many other aspects of their work that have to do with interdependence. We have graduate-level OT interns that do a thorough evaluation of every adult who comes into our domestic violence programs. They use a battery of tools. The Allen Cognitive Level tool is a simple craft project that determines the way the subject learns new skills. The Koleman Evaluation of Living Skills creates a numerical score for a variety of activities of daily living (ADL). This acts as a baseline for our work in capacity building. The Abused Women's Self-Efficacy Scale measures a subject's comfort with talking about domestic violence and taking action for their own safety. The Beck Depression Inventory creates a baseline on the subject's affect. On the basis of the test battery, history taking, and the observation of the occupational therapist, a plan is developed to address areas of daily living in need of intervention. Some women have fairly good ADL skills. Others have next to none.

Habilitation

While "rehabilitation" is often a term used with newly disabled individuals, it refers to the relearning of activities to compensate for the limitations of a disability. We often find the need for *habilitation*—including people who are learning about ADLs for the first time. We have had women in our program who never knew that they had a source of income, Supplemental

Security Income (SSI). We have others who knew they had income, but it was taken over by an abuser. Teaching budgeting and money management skills is one of the building blocks of our program. Each of our residential programs has a training kitchen. Our OTs work with residents on planning meals, shopping for food, and preparing meals. As part of our self-help orientation, our domestic violence shelter has a cooking group that is held before every weekly community meeting to prepare dishes to share with their fellow residents and staff.

Another major ADL skill that we need to address is time management. When women come into shelter, there are a lot of tasks to be accomplished. It is often the first time in their lives that they have had to manage their children by themselves. Mothers, grandmothers, aunts, and other relatives have often played a role in child rearing in the past. Now women are in the equivalent of a witness protection program. Grandma cannot come over and watch the kids for a few hours, because she must never know where the family is located. Time management often requires our occupational therapists to become like case managers. Frequently, they have to work on follow-up activities to be sure that a resident makes a doctor's appointment. It may require cuing and other reinforcement to help the person remember the appointment. A resident may need problem-solving help to plan how to get to that appointment in a timely way. There may be a need for follow-up after the appointment to make sure the resident fills a prescription, follows through on getting an orthopedic device, or sets up ongoing physical therapy. It may require going through a similar process with residents more than once before they can pick up the skills needed to do it themselves.

Safety in the Outside World

Even after a woman leaves shelter and starts a new life, planning for safety can require limited contact with relatives and friends who might inadvertently disclose to the abuser where the victim and her children are living. Helping women manage their time as they balance their own needs with those of their children is an important skill set. If a woman does not succeed in finding time for herself, the temptation to find a solution through another relationship can loom larger. Entering a relationship out of need can lead to the replication of the dynamics from which she has just escaped.

If a woman or a child with a disability has regular connections with particular health-care providers, it can be a way an abuser can track down a victim. Often health-care providers are located in an unsafe neighborhood which can expose an individual to contact with the abuser or people who know him. Freedom House has a nurse on staff to help with the coordination of health-care issues. Our nurse does an evaluation of health-care needs and works to find appropriate providers in safe neighborhoods. In some cases, a disability or medical condition makes changing a provider problematic. We had a child at Freedom House with a rare form of cancer which was only being treated at Memorial-Sloan Kettering Hospital or a hospital in Baltimore, MD. Our nurse was able to make arrangements with the child's doctor and support staff to change the child's appointments to a time only known by the doctor and one support staff and to have the child enter the hospital through an alternate door.

Stress Management

Juggling all of these issues mandates a focus on stress management. Our OT interns introduce stress management exercises in our community meetings and hold groups and individual sessions that focus on learning stress management skills. Our residents verbalize what they find most stressful, discussing the positive and negative aspects of stress and participating in breathing and other stress reduction exercises, often with a guided visualization. We have added a yoga group and started a drumming circle as other creative ways to address stress.

Positive Parenting Intervention

For better or worse, we learn how to be parents from our own parents. At its most dysfunctional, we treated a grandmother, a mother, and her children for the trauma of maternal sexual abuse. We hoped to break the pattern by the third generation.

Positive parenting begins with an orientation to childhood development. Many mothers have not developed realistic, age-appropriate expectations for their children. Our parenting groups led by social workers address positive discipline techniques, developing negotiating skills with children, establishing boundaries, and managing daily frustrations. We help mothers build strong parent–child relationships through the creation and maintenance of family traditions, such as daily exercises like bath time rituals and bedtime stories. It may involve a mother in planning a special event. We take our mothers and children to the zoo, the park, and to other special events. Oftentimes, our workers are leading by example, in a nonjudgmental way. They make sure that the children have something to eat and drink and have the supplies needed to keep them clean and dry. On our first trip to the zoo, many mothers showed up without food, drink, or diapers and expected their children to have a good time. By the next trip, mothers brought the essentials.

We have learned that the real family secret in domestic violence is that abused women do not feel that they are very good mothers, a message they receive from their abusers, who reinforce the message every time they run into challenging situations with their children. Helping women see that motherhood is more art than science, and that it requires flexibility and creativity that will be different for each child is a critical part of our program. Women are taught to understand that every challenging situation is unique and that parenting in general and single-parenting in particular is challenging and demanding. Hearing each other's stories and providing support to each other is a powerful way for women to build up their own skills and confidence in their role as mother. When we see women adopting positive parenting, we can see an increase in their children's self esteem as well as their own.

CONCLUSION

Working with victims with disabilities is the most challenging work that any of us have attempted. The strength of multidisciplinary collaboration has been a critical component of our success. Different disciplines approach issues with different questions. Different aspects of a family's story are revealed to different workers. Important information often comes from nontraditional sources like resident aides or maintenance workers. We train our paraprofessionals to be our eyes and ears, but not to attempt to be "junior therapists." We train all of our staff in basic crisis intervention techniques using the Crisis Prevention Institute's curriculum (http://www.crisisprevention.com/). More information on this subject is available on our website http://bflnyc.org/BREAKINGBARRIERSDV.asp and by subscribing to our monthly newsletter, "Breaking Barriers in Domestic Violence" at http://bflnyc.org.

REFERENCES

Arosarena, O. A., Fritsch, T. A., Hsueh, Y., Aynehchi, B., & Haug, R. (2009). Maxillofacial injuries and violence against women. *Archives of Facial Plastic Surgery, 11*(1), 48–52.

Baylor College of Medicine Study. http://www.bcm.edu/crowd/index.cfm?pmid=1507.

Berkley Planning Associates (1995–1996). Study Crisis Prevention Institute (CPI): Nonviolent Crisis Intervention Training. (n.d.). *Crisis Prevention Institute (CPI): Nonviolent crisis intervention training.* Retrieved April 15, 2010, from http://crisisprevention.com

Crosse, S., Elyse, K., & Ratnofsky, A. (1993). *A report on the maltreatment of children with disabilities.* Washington, DC: National Center on Child Abuse and Neglect, U.S. Department of Health and Human Services.

Davis, L. A. (2009). *Fact sheet people with intellectual disabilities and sexual violence,* www.thearc.org

Herman, J. L. (1992). *Trauma and recovery.* Boulder, New York, NY: Basic Books Inc.

Riessman, F. (1965). *Social Work, 10*(2), 27–32.

Sullivan, P., & Knutson, J. (2000). Maltreatment and disabilities: A population-based epidemiological study. *Child Abuse & Neglect, 24*(10), 1257–1273.

United Spinal Association. Retrieved May 31, 2010, from http://www.unitedspinal.org/2009/03/12/no-excuse-for-abuse-and-neglect

CHAPTER SIXTEEN

Jail Diversion Models for People with Mental Illness

Charles Amrhein and Virginia Barber-Rioja

INTRODUCTION

In 2005, the Sheriff of Los Angeles County told a reporter, "I run the biggest mental hospital in the country" (Lopez, 2005). The Los Angeles County Jail has become to be known as the largest provider of psychiatric services in the United States. Rikers Island, the jail that serves the five boroughs of New York City, follows close behind along with the Cook County Jail of Chicago. In fact, the top ten largest providers of psychiatric services are not primarily hospitals or clinics, but are all incarceration settings (Torrey, Kennard, Eslinger, Lamb, & Pavle, 2010).

This relative overincarceration of people with mental illness compared to those without mental illness has complex roots and a total solution will require complex initiatives on behalf of many different systems. Still, the criminal justice system itself has grown to see the high levels of incarceration of people with mental illness as a problem. This view is shared by policy makers from across the political spectrum, with conservative and liberal officials working toward shared goals in projects designed to help this problem. This chapter will throw light on the forces that have led to this current state and the efforts toward a remedy from within the criminal justice system.

Jails, as opposed to the longer-term setting of prisons, are the incarceration settings that are used for new arrestees held in pretrial detention and those who have been sentenced to shorter-term periods of incarceration. Prisons admit offenders after the conviction and sentencing phases of court processing have concluded and the offender is transferred from a jail to prison. Jails have extensive turnover as they process new arrestees, many of whom are released on bail conditions pending court proceedings, and the group of defendants who are given sentences as a result of low-level misdemeanor offenses or other shorter-term jail incarcerations. In a recent study by Steadman, Osher, Robbins, Case, and Samuels (2009), they found that of 20,000 adults who were arrested and admitted to five different jail settings, approximately 14.5% of men admitted to the jails and a dramatic 31% of the women, were people with a mental illness. Together this group was 16.9% of the total jail admissions. The researchers use these rates to speculate about the number of people with mental illness who are arrested annually. In 2007, they reported that 13 million people were admitted to US jails. Of those, this research suggests that 2 million people with mental illness were arrested and admitted to jails over the course of the year.

As a mental health advocate, Laurie Flynn, who was Executive Director of the National Alliance for the Mentally Ill, notably said in an interview for the *New York Times*, "Part of mental illness in America now is that you are going to get arrested," (Butterfield, NYTimes.com, accessed June 4, 2010).

This chapter will review the nature of the problem and various program models that divert individuals with mental illness from the criminal justice system into treatment. In a broad sense, "jail diversion is the avoidance or radical reduction in jail time achieved by linkage to community-based services" (CMHS National Gains Center, 2007, p. 9). Steadman's jail diversion logic model includes two types of interventions: identification and enrollment of the target group at any point of contact with the criminal justice system, and then linkage to comprehensive and appropriate community-based services. The goal of these interventions is to improve mental health/individual outcomes, and public safety outcomes. The opportunities for diversion occur along a continuum as the person penetrates deeper into the court and incarceration systems, from the point of arrest, to pretrial detention in jail, to prison, and back to the community for community-based supervision provided by probation and parole (Munetz & Griffin, 2006). Diversion can occur at many points along the criminal justice process, whether first police contact or arrest, arraignment, later court appearances, or after conviction. Therefore, we will also provide an overview of how an arrestee moves through the criminal justice system, from the point of arrest through serving time, and the diversion opportunities that occur at each step along the process.

DEINSTITUTIONALIZATION

The story of *deinstitutionalization*, a policy shift by the states to move people with debilitating mental illness from institutions to care in the community, is one that has been told many times. Often blamed for the increase in people with mental illness in jails and prisons, this policy direction was adopted by the states and supported by the federal government. Born out of an excess of hope placed in new antipsychotic medications that were introduced in the 1950s, deinstitutionalization was expected to be a shift towards treatment in the community. However that would have been a project that would require more comprehensive resources and investment than what eventually came to pass. The medication was provided, but the intense service provision and psychotherapeutic efforts that remain necessary to maintain stable functioning in the community were not delivered. Instead, the community mental health systems across the states have withered under many pressures. Early in his first term, President George W. Bush appointed a commission to investigate the state of psychiatric treatment in the United States, chaired by Michael Hogan. Hogan offered another famous comment that has reverberated even further than Laurie Flynn's words to the *New York Times* about the inevitability of arrest for people with mental illness. Hogan wrote in his formal letter to the president summarizing the report's findings that "America's mental health service delivery system is in shambles" (Hogan, 2002).

SENTENCING POLICY AND INCREASING LENGTH OF INCARCERATION

A headline on the front page of The *New York Times* read "ASYLUMS BEHIND BARS: Prisons Replace Hospitals for the Nation's Mentally Ill" (Butterfield, 1998, p. A1). This problem has many sources. Many writers have attributed this current state to the deinstitutionalization movement, a policy that most states began in the 1960s (Lamb, Watson, Luchins, & Weinberger, 2005), but it is only one factor among many. Another factor has been the increasing rates of incarceration in general. In 2002, the U.S. prison population had swollen to 1.9 million (Bureau of Justice Statistics, 2010). Just 8 years later, that number rose around 20%, to 2.4 million. The headlines announcing the number of people incarcerated in 2008 also included those on parole or under probation supervision, for a total of 7.3 million people, or 1 in every 31 adults (Liptak, 2008).

The heavy use of incarceration and criminal sanctions began to increase in the 1980s with the drug war and mandatory sentencing. Laws were passed requiring judges to follow mandatory sentencing guidelines, in effect reducing the discretion of judges to consider extenuating or mitigating circumstances in determining the length of a sentence. Another factor that increased the number of people in prison was that the length of sentences for many crimes was increased. Throughout this expansion of incarceration that has continued to the present time, many people with mental illness have been swept up into the ever widening net of imprisonment. This expansion is not limited to incarceration, and in fact criminal supervision has also increased. In 1980, there were 1.3 million Americans under the supervision of a parole or probation officer. By 2008, that number had increased to 5 million people (Bureau of Justice Statistics, 2010).

Compounding the issue of community supervision, parolees and probationers with mental illness are more likely to violate their supervision conditions and be sent back to jail (Skeem & Eno Louden, 2006). Once incarcerated, the person with mental illness stays in jail longer. In 1998, detainees at Rikers Island in New York City spent an average of 42 days in jail, but those with a mental illness stayed an average of 215 days (Butterfield, 1998). Inmates with mental illness are less likely to earn early release and the quality of the treatment of their illness makes the time they serve more challenging. As one advocate has put it, "if you have a mental illness in jail, you will do longer time, and harder time" (Sultan, 2010).

BAIL REFORM AND THE BEGINNING OF PRETRIAL SERVICES

It is often a surprise to our contemporary sensibility that the current approach to bail and pretrial release is relatively new. While the United States Constitution prohibits what it calls "excessive bail," the accepted understanding of this prohibition began to evolve in the 1950s (Lotze, Clark, Henry, & Juzkiewicz, 1999). In 1960, the U.S. Supreme Court in *Bandy v. United States*, held that

> The fundamental tradition in the country is that one charged with a crime is not, in ordinary circumstances, imprisoned until after a judgment of guilt ... The traditional right to freedom during trial ... has to be squared with the possibility that the defendant may flee or hide himself .... It is assumed that the threat of forfeiture of one's goods will be an effective deterrent to the temptation to break the conditions of one's release ... But this theory is based on the assumption that a defendant has property ... Can an indigent

be denied freedom, where a wealthy man would not, because he does not happen to have enough property to pledge for his freedom?
—Bandy v. United States, 1960

The court held that a defendant without property who is thus denied bail is therefore denied "equal protection under the law" which is guaranteed by the constitution's equal protection clause. Further, the presumption of innocence adds another complicating layer to the detention of people charged with a crime who, legally, remain innocent until the court finds to the contrary.

This trend in criminal legal thinking was joined with policy influence from a grassroots community project developed in 1961 in New York City. At that time Louis Schweitzer founded the Vera Institute of Justice and began the Manhattan Bail Project (Lotze et al., 1999; Thomas, 1976). This project interviewed arrestees, assessed their community ties, and made recommendations to be considered at the bail hearing. They showed that a substantial number of people jailed as pretrial detainees were offered relatively low bails but were too poor to arrange for the bail. They also produced evidence that showed that people with strong community ties were likely to appear on following court dates if released while awaiting trial. During the third year of operation, the recommendations that had begun conservatively were recommending that 65% of interviewed arrestees be released on recognizance, and they found that less than 1% of this group failed to appear (Lotze et al., 1999).

Schweitzer's findings and model began to grow in influence and 5 years later Congress passed the Bail Reform Act of 1966, enhancing the opportunities for defendants in the federal court system to be released on recognizance. This law also provided for conditional pretrial release, contingent upon the supervision of released defendants who had to follow certain conditions.

Another Supreme Court case from 1962 began to exert its influence as the decade proceeded. In *Robinson v. California*, the Supreme Court held that the mere fact of being addicted was not enough to warrant imprisonment. The law in California made the addiction itself a crime, even if the person was to have "never used or possessed any narcotics within the State and has not been guilty of any antisocial behavior there" (*Robinson v. California*, 1962, p. 660). The court said that addiction was a disease: "narcotic addiction is an illness. Indeed, it is apparently an illness which may be contracted innocently or involuntarily" (*Robinson v. California*, 1962, p. 667). Further, the court said by way of analogy, "Even one day in prison would be a cruel and unusual punishment for the 'crime' of having a common cold" (*Robinson v. California*, 1962, p. 667). Reframing the issue of addiction as an illness had deep implications for policy responses to the problem, calling into question the limits of law enforcement influence on addiction and pointing toward treatment responses as a more logical solution to the addiction itself.

Within this climate came a logical extension of the bail reform movement, enhanced conditions for release that integrated vocational activities with other social or clinical services. Cases were identified in which there were underlying problems that contributed to the criminal behavior and social services were arranged to address those problems, with the assumption that as the root problem was alleviated, so too would criminal behavior lessen. Prosecutors began to experiment with allowing charges to be reduced or dismissed if certain conditions were met, such as employment or other activities like treatment or vocational training. Pretrial diversion became the term that referred to cases where defendants were offered the opportunity to have their charges dismissed in exchange for successful participation in services that offered social benefits. The promise of dismissal of charges began to be used as a motivator to drive adherence to services or the treatment plan. In 1967, the President's Crime Commission recommended that pretrial diversion be expanded and two federal agencies were funded to start projects at sites across the country (Nolan, 2001). The Department of Labor's Manpower Administration was funded with a focus on developing employment in pretrial diversion, and the Department of Justice's Law Enforcement Assistance Administration was also funded. Soon jurisdictions across the country developed pretrial services as a normal part of their local criminal justice system.

By 1985, the American Bar Association recommended "that every jurisdiction establish a pretrial services agency or similar facility, empowered to provide supervision for released defendants" (American Bar Association, 1985). Pretrial services exist today to provide multiple services (Lotze et al., 1999). They first assess family ties, employment, and other factors that go into determining the level of flight risk for a defendant so that judges can make informed decisions about the need for bail. They also support pretrial diversion and referrals to treatment and social services and monitor participation for the courts in exchange for dismissal of charges upon successful completion (Clark, 2004).

The work of pretrial diversion, made possible by the bail reform movement, mostly occurs outside of the courthouse by an agency independent of the court. These programs revolutionized the opportunities for courts to influence and collaborate with social service providers. Pretrial diversion agencies have become expert in a variety of social service needs, from substance abuse and mental health treatment, to vocational training and youth services. A vast number of social service providers have, in turn, grown to meet the needs of pretrial diversion clients. Another critical change was the development of trust by judges and prosecutors who have come to rely on pretrial services as an effective way of addressing public safety while also remedying large-scale social problems and needs. The group that was primarily targeted for pretrial diversion included first-time offenders charged with nonviolent misdemeanors. With the heavy support offered by the federal government through the Department of Labor and Law Enforcement Assistance, pretrial diversion became an option for many with substance abuse disorders.

THERAPEUTIC JURISPRUDENCE AND THE PROBLEM-SOLVING JUSTICE MOVEMENT

The growth of jail diversion has arisen within a context of multiple factors: deinstitutionalization, increased sentences, increased prison populations, the drug war, and for the last 20 years the problem-solving court movement. The contemporary problem-solving court movement began in 1989, when Dade County, Florida began its first specialized drug court (Berman & Feinblatt, 2001; Huddleston, Marlowe, & Casebolt, 2008). This model had a judge trained in understanding the treatment process and who closely monitored the progress of participants who were sentenced to treatment instead of incarceration, but with the added element of close judicial supervision that relied on graduated sanctions designed to change behavior in addition to rewards for successful achievements. While pretrial diversion services worked offsite from the courthouse, the drug court brought the diversion agency straight into the courtroom, with the judge working in a manner that has been referred to as "therapeutic" judging. In many jurisdictions, agencies providing case management through pretrial services became the provider of case management services for the drug court (Clark, 2004).

The reported success of the drug court model resulted in a wave of jurisdictions developing similar courts as an additional criminal justice response designed to reduce the reliance on incarceration. Drug courts have grown to over 2000 in number (Huddleston et al., 2008). As these courts grew in influence, the potential of the model began to be explored with changing other types of behavior that often resulted in criminal recidivism. The application of problem-solving justice has grown as a model where the use of the court's authority to influence behavior change for the better has been used with domestic violence, prostitution, chronic low-level misdemeanors in community courts, and mental health problems among other models. The state of New York funded an institute, the Center for Court Innovation, whose mission is to develop and study such problem-solving courts (Berman & Feinblatt, 2001). Over a similar time period, a legal theory arose that has been called therapeutic jurisprudence, which has not only the fair administration of justice as a goal, but in addition seeks to achieve a social benefit and minimize the damage that can result from court proceedings (Wexler, 1992). It has been defined as "the study of the extent to which substantive rules, legal procedures, and the roles of lawyers and judges produce therapeutic or anti-therapeutic consequences for individuals involved in the legal process" (Hora, Schma, & Rosenthal, 1999). The drug court model informed by therapeutic jurisprudence theory has resulted in a general problem-solving court model with many potential applications. The model has several common elements: immediate intervention, a nonadversarial process where the court parties collaborate as a team to support the change process or treatment, an involved, hands-on judge with advanced knowledge about the treatment process, and treatment resources or social service supports with clearly defined rules and goals (Berman & Feinblatt, 2001). The models typically require case management or clinical staff who do the work of connecting the defendant to services and liaison with the service providers.

THE CRIMINAL JUSTICE PATHWAY AND THE SPECTRUM OF DIVERSION OPPORTUNITIES

Involvement in the criminal justice system means progressively moving deeper into a complicated and layered system. The first level of contact is with an arresting officer. When an officer makes an arrest, the person is typically taken for booking where the details of arrest are recorded and the person is moved to jail or a detention setting. The next step is the formal arraignment by a court. This is where the person is formally told of the charges he or she is facing. The defendant is expected to enter a plea and often, this is where the conditions of pretrial release are addressed. The judge may order continued detention pending future court appearances, set conditions for bail, or order the person released on his or her own recognizance, "ROR'ed." The next stage is to return to court for a preliminary hearing or await action by a grand jury. The judge or the grand jury may decide to continue with the case or conclude that there is not enough evidence to warrant prosecution. During this phase, usually the defense attorney and prosecutor consider negotiating a plea.

Most cases in the United States, around 90%, reach negotiated dispositions as plea bargains or plea arrangements (Alschuler, 1979). These plea arrangements may be worked out over the course of several adjournments where the court parties update the court on the direction they are pursuing to resolve the case. If the defendant enters a plea of guilty, or if the person is tried and found guilty, then the case is typically adjourned for sentencing. During this time, the offender, who now stands convicted, may be allowed to remain in the community pending the sentencing phase or not. This is particularly relevant for many jail diversion models where the offender pleads guilty and then is allowed to return to the community while the sentencing is deferred.

Munetz and Griffin (2006) have conceptualized the pathway of criminal justice involvement, and the various opportunities for diversion along this pathway, with their sequential intercept model. This model helps map out the various points along the criminal justice process where diversion may occur. They "envision a series of 'points of interception'" (2006, p. 544) where interventions to prevent the person from "penetrating deeper into the criminal justice system." The first intercept point is the prevention of law enforcement contact through effective and comprehensive clinical services. The next point is the use of specially trained law enforcement teams who use arrest as a last resort and who aim to divert individuals with mental illness to emergency treatment systems. If the officers make an arrest, then diversion may still be possible at the post-booking phase.

Post-booking diversion programs can occur at several points. Pretrial service programs can engage the participant at the point of arraignment and before conviction. Some pretrial programs connect the defendant to services while the court proceedings continue simultaneously. Others provide diversion that takes the person away from the prosecution process entirely while they participate in treatment. Such models may require a plea of guilty while the sentence is deferred or they may defer prosecution itself without requiring a plea of guilty while the person enters treatment. If the participant completes the expected then the charges may be dismissed or reduced. These models work most often with low-level, nonviolent misdemeanor offenders, however there has been expansion of programs to cover the diversion of people with felony charges and some programs that consider candidates with a history of violent behavior.

PREBOOKING DIVERSION

Crisis Intervention Teams: Diversion Before an Arrest

Many police calls result in encounters with people with untreated mental illness and on occasion tragedy has resulted. Iman Morales was standing naked on a ledge of a Brooklyn building when police were called (Hauser, 2008). He thrust at an officer with an eight-foot-long fluorescent light and a police lieutenant ordered the officer to use a taser gun. Following use of the taser device, Morales fell off the ledge and suffered a fatal head injury. The tragic nature of this accident was obvious, and eight days later the lieutenant who ordered the use of the taser committed suicide (Gendar, Boyle, & McShane, nydailynews.com, accessed October 11, 2010). Survey data have often found that police officers do not feel adequately trained in managing crises related to people with mental illness (Dupont & Cochrane, 2002).

The goal of prebooking diversion is to divert the offender at initial contact with the criminal justice system (Steadman, Morris, & Dennis, 1995). Police officers play a very important role at this point of the process. Responding to situations involving mentally ill individuals has become a main role of law enforcement agencies. Deinstitutionalization of the 1960s and 1970s, stricter civil commitment criteria, cutbacks in mental health funding and a decrease in society's tolerance of mentally ill people living in the community are all factors that have increased the likelihood of police encounters with people with mental illness. When police officers encounter people with psychiatric symptoms, they are instructed by mental health codes to initiate a psychiatric emergency apprehension whenever the person is either a danger to self or others or is unable to provide for basic physical needs so as to protect him/herself from serious harm (Teplin, 2000). However, although the law legitimizes the police officers power to intervene, they can use their discretion when deciding whether the person who exhibits symptoms of mental illness needs to be arrested (Lattimore et al., 2003; Templin, 2000). In essence, officers have three choices: they can resolve the matter informally, transport the emotionally disturbed person to a psychiatric hospital, or arrest the person (Teplin, 2000). Any intervention that does not lead to the arrest of the mentally ill when charges could have been filed is considered prebooking diversion as it avoids the individual's involvement with the criminal justice system.

The American Bar Association's Criminal Justice Mental Health Standards state that when a mentally ill individual is under police custody exclusively as a result of noncriminal behavior or minor criminal behavior, the police officer should transport the individual to an appropriate facility for evaluation or negotiate a voluntary disposition (American Bar Association, 1985, p. 40). This rapid intervention requires that police officers be adequately trained in mental health issues and/or appropriate collaborations between law enforcement and human service agencies and mental health systems. For example, collaboration between social workers and police officers was already identified by Treger in 1975 as a vehicle to divert mentally ill individuals away from the criminal justice system and into the public mental health system. Social workers can assist law enforcement agencies to quickly identify symptoms of psychiatric illness in individuals under police custody so that individuals can be immediately linked to service providers at the time of the crisis when they are in real need of mental health services.

In 1998, a national survey of all major police departments was conducted to investigate the types of partnerships between law enforcement and mental health systems that have been implemented to improve prebooking diversion (Deane, Steadman, Borum, Veysey, & Morrisey, 1998). Results showed that only 45% of police departments had some type of specialized response to individuals with mental illness in crisis, while 88% provided some training for officers on mental health issues. Of the police departments with some specialized response program, most conformed to one of three models:

- *Police-based specialized police response (3.4% of police departments):* This model consists of sworn officers who receive specialized mental health training and serve as the first-line police response to crisis involving individuals with mental illness and act as liaison to the formal mental health system.
- *Police-based specialized mental health response (11.5% of police departments):* Mental health professionals are employed by the police department in this model to provide on-site and telephone consultation to police officers in the field.
- *Mental health-based specialized mental health response (30% of police departments):* In this model, partnerships between police and mental health crisis teams exist. Therefore, mobile crisis teams respond when requested by police. Mobile crisis units are independent from the police department and are part of the local community mental health services.

An example of a police-based specialized police response model, and probably the most prominent and widely recognized type of prebooking diversion is the Memphis Crisis Intervention Team (CIT) Model. Partly as a result of an incident involving the police shooting of a mentally ill person, this model was developed in 1988 by Dr. Randolph Dupont from the University of Tennessee, and Major Sam Cochran from the Memphis Police Department (Compton, Bahora, Watson, & Oliva, 2008). The Bureau of Justice Assistance estimates that there are currently more than 400 existing CIT programs operating nationally (Bureau of Justice Assistance, 2010).

The CIT model diverts individuals with severe and persistent mental illness when the charges are minor in nature and do not involve the victimization of others. They improve the interactions between police officers and persons with mental illness, reduce injuries of officers and individual in crisis, and link mentally ill individuals to appropriate treatment in the community. What makes this model different from others is that it provides officers within the patrol division with specialized expertise to allow for crisis interventions to occur in real time. Designated CIT officers answer traditional police calls, but can quickly take the lead on calls identified as behavioral crises by 911 dispatch protocol or fellow officers (Dupont & Cochran, 2002).

The two main components of the CIT model are selection and training. Special emphasis is placed on experienced officers who volunteer for the team. Officers volunteer for different reasons such as personal experience with individuals with mental illness, recognition of the limitations of traditional law enforcement interventions, or a history of special crisis intervention skills. The selection procedure includes an extensive interviewing process and evaluations for supervisors. In addition, history of the citizen's complaints or positive feedback plays an important role in the selection process (Dupont & Cochran, 2002).

Officers undergo a 40-hour comprehensive training that emphasizes mental health-related topics, crisis resolution skills and de-escalation training, as well as access to community-based services. The training format consists of didactics and workshops, on-site visitation and exposure to mental health facilities and interaction with mentally ill individuals, and role playing through scenario based de-escalation skill training.

This model of police response to mental health emergencies has been described as the "most visible pre-booking jail diversion program in the U.S." (Steadman, Deane, Borum, & Morrissey, 2000), and in 1999, the White House Conference on Mental Health considered it a best practice model. A comprehensive review of extant research on CIT programs (Compton, Bahora, Watson, & Oliva, 2008) revealed that the CIT model may be an effective model of prebooking diversion by connecting individuals with mental illness who come into contact with law enforcement with appropriate psychiatric services in the community. Research suggests that the training component of the CIT model has a positive impact on officers' beliefs and knowledge regarding mental health issues, and CIT-trained officers reported feeling better prepared in handling crisis situations involving individuals with mental illness (Compton, Bahora, Watson, & Oliva, 2008).

Postbooking Diversion

With the 1960s, came the rapid growth of pretrial diversion and treatment in lieu of incarceration became a widespread practice among courts. Postbooking diversion programs divert people with mental illness from the criminal justice system after they have been arrested and formal charges have been filed. These programs have grown rapidly from approximately 54 jail diversion programs in existence in 1992 (Steadman, Morris, & Dennis, 1995) to over 300 of these programs operating nationally today (Steadman & Naples, 2005), making this type of diversion the most prevalent in the United States. Out of 500 jail diversion programs in the country in 2007, 65% are classified as postbooking (CMHS National Gains Center, 2007).

Postbooking programs can be either jail-based or court-based. Steadman et al. (1999) identified some key elements of postbooking programs at either the arraignment court or the jail:

1. Diversion programs screen individuals in contact with the criminal justice system for the presence of mental illness.
2. They employ mental health professionals to evaluate the defendants for treatment in the community.
3. Once a defendant has been found appropriate, diversion programs negotiate with prosecutors, defense attorneys, community-based treatment providers, with the goal of developing community-based treatment disposition in lieu of prosecution or as a condition of a reduction in charges.
4. Finally, diversion programs link individuals to treatment programs in the community.

Court-based diversion programs can take place at any time prior to sentencing. These programs can be decentralized, diverting individuals from multiple court parts with multiple judges, or centralized, diverting individuals through special jurisdiction courts such as mental health courts. In general, the goal of the diversion program does not end with diverting the individual, but it also includes monitoring and supervising the individual involved in treatment in the community, and reporting back to the court with updates on treatment compliance, although this varies among jurisdictions.

Mental Health Courts

As part of the larger movement of therapeutic jurisprudence and directly flowing from the success of drug courts, mental health courts were developed as a type of post-booking diversion program where all defendants are handled on a single court docket (Steadman, Davidson, & Brown, 2001). The first widely recognized MHC that spun out of the drug court tradition was developed in 1997 in Broward County, Florida. In the year 2000, President Clinton signed Senate Bill 865 into law (Public Law 106-515, America's Law Enforcement and Mental Health Project) to provide states with grants to establish up to 100 demonstration MHCs (Watson, Hanrahan, Luchins, & Lurigio, 2001). Since the establishment of the first MHC, there has been a rapid increase in the number of these types of courts. Today, there are at least 100 MHCs in the country (National GAINS Center, 2004) in 34 different states (Redlich, Steadman, Monahan, Robbins, & Petrila, 2006).

Steadman et al. (2001) proposed four characteristics shared by all MHCs: all mentally ill defendants are handled on a single court docket, there is a collaborative team which includes a clinical specialist who recommends and makes linkages to treatment, availability of appropriate clinical placement is assured prior to the judge making a ruling regarding diversion, and the court engages in specialized monitoring for participants with possible sanctions for noncompliance. Although most MHCs report that participants are not forced to take medication, defendants are often excluded from participation unless they comply with prescribed medication. Moreover, medication noncompliance just as failing to participate in psychosocial programming, is often considered a violation of the conditions of their release resulting in subsequent sanctions such as reprimands from the judge, increased supervision time, and remand to jail. Jail as a sanction is usually considered as a last resort when all other clinical efforts and lesser sanctions have failed. Additional requirements usually include regular court review hearings, meetings with case managers or counselors, and increased urine toxicology screenings. While avoiding jail and prison may be reinforcing for positive behavior, participants receive additional incentives for successfully complying with the negotiated treatment plan. Frequently charges are either dropped or reduced, or the initial conviction is vacated (Redlich, Steadman, Monahan, Petrila, & Griffin, 2005). Finally, participation in all MHCs is voluntary (Redlich, 2005).

Despite these common elements, unlike the drug treatment model, there is no common model for MHCs and they differ in a number of ways such as whether a guilty plea is necessary prior to entry to the program and whether punishment should be used for noncompliance with treatment (Petrila, 2003). Mental Health Courts also vary in the required inclusion criteria (Redlich et al., 2005) with some MHCs requiring that participants meet the criteria for serious and persistent mental illness, whereas others are less strict and require only "demonstrable mental health problems" (p. 607) and not necessarily an Axis I psychiatric diagnosis. A second generation of MHCs has been described after comparing eight long-existing courts with seven courts that had not been previously described in the psycholegal literature (Redlich et al., 2005). Four dimensions are used to describe the second generation of MHCs. First, newer courts are more open to accept felony charges. Of the eight first-generation courts, only two accepted felonies whereas all of the second generation accepted felonies. In addition, courts in the second generation were more open to accept violent offenses looking at the totality of circumstances. For instance, some MHCs would accept defendants charged with more serious offenses that include an element of violence, if it is determined that symptoms of mental illness played a substantial role in the offense (a challenging assessment question likely answered through various guidelines unique to the jurisdiction), and that the level of risk for future violence is found to be manageable without jeopardizing public safety. Second, newer MHCs are more likely to use post-plea adjudication models. Six of the second generation of MHCs only enrolled participants after they had entered a plea. As a result, MHCs' participants are being referred later on the criminal justice process. First-generation courts tend to refer defendants within the first 48 hours after their arrest, while the time from referral to enrollment ranged from 0 to 129 days in the second-generation courts. Third, the second-generation courts are more likely to use jail as a sanction. Possibly as a consequence of accepting more felonies, second-generation courts were more willing to remand participants to jail as a result of noncompliance. However, many of the courts studied by Redlich et al. (2005) found that although jail was effective to regain compliance in some participants, it had a detrimental effect on others. Finally, as opposed to first-generation courts that use a combination of mental health court workers, community mental health providers, and probation officers to supervise participants, second-generation courts are more likely to utilize staff linked to the MHC. First-generation courts are more likely to only use community mental health providers for supervision, while six of the second-generation courts used both treatment providers and personnel linked to the MHC to monitor participants' progress.

The fact that judges hearing cases in MHCs have been specially trained in mental health issues and that all parties involved work as a team that distinguishes MHCs from traditional criminal courts and traditional jail diversion programs that do not rely upon a problem-solving court model. An article published in 2009 (Schwartz, 2008) in U.S. News and World Report about the Allegheny County Mental Health Court describes the unique efforts to create a "therapeutic" atmosphere that some mental health courts pursue:

> Judge John Zottola's courtroom often feels more like a kindergarten award ceremony than part of the criminal justice system. Every Thursday on the fifth floor of a Romanesque-style courthouse, defendants shuffle to a podium to receive compliments, encouragement, and applause, whether it's for sticking to their treatment, wearing a nice outfit, or staying clean and sober. Even defendants who've slipped up on probation are unlikely to be thrown back in jail. Instead, most face a stern but kind warning, along with orders for more rigorous treatment or reporting schedules. 'Don't make me look bad,' Zottola tells them (Schwartz, 2008).

It is precisely this adoption of nontraditional roles by lawyers and judges that has been criticized by some law scholars and advocacy groups. With the goal of rehabilitating individuals with psychiatric disabilities, judges typically work as part of an interdisciplinary team that includes the defense attorney, court social workers, and community treatment programs (Stefan & Winick, 2005). This represents an important change in the role of the judge where he or she is viewed as the "coach not arbiter" (Petrila, 2003, p. 10). The role of the defense attorneys assumes an additional dimension within a collaborative framework where he or she plays a role that supports a therapeutic outcome in addition to thinking in terms of the defendant's best interest, and where the defender attempts to collaborate with the court team rather than maintaining a strictly adversarial stance (Breeding, 2006; Petrila, 2003).

Some advocacy groups and law scholars have claimed that these enhanced roles for judges and defense attorneys complicates the issue of client representation. They assert that judges and attorneys should focus strictly on the participants' rights and due process rather than to represent a more clinical view of what is the client's best interests. This view maintains that interdisciplinary teams and a goal of helping meet a need that is in the client's best interest leads to paternalism and diffuses the defender's obligation to zealousy defend the client's legal rights (Breeding, 2006; Erickson, Campbell, & Lamberti, 2006; Stefan & Winick, 2005). Seltzer (2005) has argued that there may be situations where attorneys believe that rejecting a MHC option and staying in a conventional court is indeed in the defendant's best interest, but that the pressure of speeding the release of a mentally ill defendant may conflict with the attorney's ability to make a thorough investigation of the prosecutor's case, thus jeopardizing representation of the defendant.

Pretrial Diversion and the TASC Model

Pretrial diversion originated in the 1960s when treatment in lieu of incarceration was tried by several states (New York, Connecticut, and Illinois) (Bellassai, 2010). The year 1967 brought out the Report of the President's Commission on Law Enforcement and Administration of Justice which made recommendations for pretrial diversion. This led to the development of programs that targeted first-time offenders charged with nonviolent misdemeanors (Nolan, 2001). In these programs each participant had to be unemployed or underemployed, and job development, training, and employment were primary goals of the intervention. Upon successful completion, the original charges would be dismissed. Throughout the first half of the 1970s, there was an explosion of diversion programming across the United States. Supported by both the Department of Labor and the Department of Justice through its Law Enforcement Assistance Administration (LEAA), pretrial diversion became an option for many with substance abuse disorders. The Treatment Alternatives to Street Crime (TASC) model of pretrial diversion gained the backing of the federal government, and President Nixon notably spoke at a National TASC conference in 1973 (Bellassai, 2010).

TASC programs around the country are court-based, post-adjudication case management models that offer the following services: screening, assessment, linkage to community-based treatment, case management, and judicial supervision. After referring the defendant to community-based treatment, TASC monitors treatment progress and compliance. If the individual is not compliant with the conditions of his/her release, TASC is responsible to submit to the courts a violation of conditions notification, which may result with the individual being returned to criminal justice processing.

Under the Drug Abuse Office and Treatment Act of 1972, the TASC model originated as a federal initiative in response to the increased number of substance-involved offenders revolving through the criminal justice system. The first TASC programs were implemented in Wilmington, Delaware, and Philadelphia, Pennsylvania and were initially funded through the LEAA and the National Institute of Mental Health (NIMH). In 1982, LEAA was discontinued, but there was a resurgence of interest in the TASC programs through the Bureau of Justice Assistance (BJA), which took up the work of the LEAA. Currently, many TASC programs have expanded their state and federal funding through private donations or grants.

Today there are over 150 individual TASC programs around the country in 32 states. TASC programs initially focused on pretrial diversion of first-time offenders with substance abuse disorders. However, the TASC model progressively expanded to divert repeat offenders charged with both violent and nonviolent crimes, and to serve a variety of populations including individuals with mental illness and co-occurring diagnoses. Some programs continue to use the original name; others have changed the name to reflect their role in their own communities while generally retaining the TASC acronym. In New York State, TASC stands for Treatment Alternatives for Safer Communities. All programs share the same goal of providing a treatment intervention to stop the cycle of arrest, incarceration and release. The National Institute of Justice (NIJ) labeled TASC a "best practice" model in 1986.

New York City TASC Mental Health Diversion Programs

In New York City, the Education and Assistance Corporation (EAC) adopted the national TASC model to divert defendants with substance abuse disorders. However, in the mid-1990s, EAC added a mental health division to divert individuals with mental illness and co-occurring disorders. In 1999, pilot programs were developed in Brooklyn to provide diversion, linkage to community-based treatment, case management, and monitoring for seriously and persistently mentally ill (SPMI) adolescents and adults including individuals released from local correctional facilities and detention centers and individuals reentering the community from state prisons.

The success of these programs gave rise to a full-fledged comprehensive mental health diversion program in the Bronx in 2001, with the establishment of the Bronx Mental Health Court. All of these projects requires extensive collaboration between multiple systems that focused on the criminal justice system and the treatment world. The New York State Division of Probation and Correctional Alternatives (DPCA) (recently renamed the Office of Probation and Correctional Alternatives), having provided some of the original funding for the Bronx Program, found it worthy of replication and provided funds to start a similar model in Queens in 2007.

The NYC TASC Mental Health Diversion Programs provide post-booking, court-based diversion at any time after arraignment to defendants charged with violent and nonviolent misdemeanors and felonies. Diversion is both centralized (Bronx TASC staffs the Bronx Mental Health Court and Queens TASC evaluates and case manages most of defendants out of the Queens Mental Health Court) and decentralized (by obtaining referrals from any court outside of the special jurisdiction courts). All NYC TASC Mental Health diversion programs use a deferred sentence model for the adjudication and diversion of defendants, which gives the courts the ability to require and monitor the treatment services that meet the clinical needs of the client. After a defendant has been found clinically eligible by the mental health team and after all parties have consented, he or she is required to enter a plea of guilty generally to the most serious charge at which point the sentence gets deferred until successful completion of the treatment plan designed by the TASC program. Typically, defendants charged with felonies are monitored for a period of 12–24 months, and defendants charged with misdemeanors are monitored for a period of six to nine months. After successful completion, charges are either dropped or reduced, or the initial conviction is vacated. However, if defendants violate the conditions of their release by not complying with treatment, engaging in violence or being rearrested, they are at risk for receiving the alternative sentence, which is established at the time of the guilty plea.

Both the Bronx TASC Mental Health Court Program and Queens TASC Mental Health Diversion Program place special emphasis on the assessment process employing clinical forensic psychologists and forensic psychiatrists to conduct these evaluations. The screening and evaluation process, based in core clinical and forensic principles of professional examination, review of collateral sources of information, and violence risk assessment and management, ensures that clients receive accurate and comprehensive diagnoses and placement in the most clinically appropriate community-based services.

Because of the emphasis on maintaining independent clinical-forensic assessment resources within the programs, these particular models do not reject cases based simply on the basis of violence involved in the offense or in the person's criminal history. Whether charged with a violent offense, or whether the presence of violence becomes known through collateral sources, such individuals receive a comprehensive risk assessment examination using clinical judgment in combination with structured risk assessment tools. The goal however is to enhance treatment planning in order to determine if there are suitable clinical resources that can fairly be expected to reduce such a risk. Finally, the employment of specialized mental health clinicians at the screening and assessment phase also ensures that defendants make rational and voluntary decisions regarding their treatment alternatives. Although clinicians do not provide legal counsel, a thorough explanation of the voluntariness of participating in diversion through TASC, as well as the plea requirement and conditions of release, increases the chances that defendants make informed decisions addressing some of the concerns raised by advocates and mental health law scholars previously mentioned.

The clinical focus does not end after the assessment process, but carries for the length of the diversion process. These programs have come to recognize both the client and the treatment provider as the targets for communication and coordination. The role of the mental health team goes beyond the more traditional compliance monitoring by providing ongoing support, crisis intervention, clinical reassessment as needed, and consultation for the treatment providers with respect to individual client needs and general clinical issues.

Boundary Spanners: The Critical Ingredient in All Diversion Models

A common element of the different types of diversion programs described in this chapter is the constant interaction among different systems, such as the court, correctional and mental health systems. After visiting at least 43 jail diversion programs, Steadman (1992) argued that a key element for the effective functioning of these programs is the presence of "boundary spanners" or workers in positions that mediate or manage the interactions between different systems with distinct and some times conflicting goals. In the context of diversion programs, these systems include mental health, correctional and judicial staff. These boundary spanning positions can be held by different employees with different job titles within their organization (Steadman, 1992).

In mental health diversion programs, whether mental health courts or not, workers must operate within multiple contexts and be able to bridge these different domains, learning how these different systems work, their unique terms and common practices, and then be able to go between these systems, effectively engaging them, in order to serve their clients. The work crosses disciplines and training backgrounds and a skill-set is necessary that is rarely taught in professional training programs. When a referral is made to the Bronx Mental Health Court a case manager must go to court and interact with the attorneys of the client, then do a comprehensive screening of the client, a task that requires extensive efforts with the corrections department. If during this screening there are obvious untreated symptoms, then the worker must contact Rikers Island psychiatry services to arrange treatment before discharge. With supervision and follow-up assessment by the clinical director or other clinician, specific target symptoms can be followed in tandem with the jail psychiatry providers, observing the course of symptoms and tracking the effectiveness of medications or other interventions and obtaining necessary information for discharge planning. The same case manager or clinical director will need to go to court and communicate the results of the evaluation to the judge, defense attorney, and the prosecutor's office. Finally, if the defendant has been found eligible and the defendant and all court parties are in agreement with a diversion disposition, the workers must then support the discharge from jail, engage available treatment providers, including medical and housing providers, and arrange linkages. This work crosses these different systems that often may not work well together, and this boundary spanning function reaches across many levels, including helping the community providers understand how they may be effective with a population they might hesitate to accept.

Because the expectations of the different systems are some times in conflict, boundary spanner positions tend to be challenging and high-demand roles. However the function of these roles, as Steadman has outlined in depth (1992) are critical to the success of most any diversion program.

CONCLUSION: THE LAST STEPS IN THE CRIMINAL JUSTICE PROCESS

When someone with mental illness is discharged from jail or prison, the support that is provided to adequately link the person to community treatment resources is often minimal. The Department of Corrections of the City of New York was confronted with a lawsuit demanded a standard for discharging people with mental illness from jail that is similar to the standards for discharging patients from a psychiatric hospital unit. The New York state courts held in *Brad H. v. Giuliani* (Barr, 2003) that the jail assumes an obligation to provide levels of discharge support at levels similar to a hospital. Proper discharge planning is an essential element of any psychiatric treatment plan. Without it the person may "fall through the cracks" and fail to engage in follow-up treatment that will maintain his or her mental health and well-being. Given the assumption that poor engagement with treatment is a contributing factor to the increasing population of people with mental illness in the criminal justice system (Torrey et al., 2010), then failure to help transition inmates back to the community with adequate treatment resources will likely lead to a revolving door effect, where the person eventually returns to the criminal justice system.

Similarly, probation and parole systems are recognizing that they provide an important function in maintaining the stable functioning of this population by collaborating with the mental health system. It is estimated that there are over 4 million people in the United States under some sort of community supervision like probation or parole (Bureau of Justice Statistics, 2010). In fact, recent data show that probationers and parolees with mental illness are twice as likely as those without mental illness to fail on supervision (Skeem & Eno Louden, 2006). Probation and parole departments have been developing special tracks often called dedicated caseloads, where officers are given special training in working with people with mental illness and a smaller caseload in order to focus on linking with treatment services and use more of their time to serve this higher-need population. In some models, the probation or parole officer works out of a mental health clinic, and in other models, a social worker is placed in a probation or parole office. Probation and parole officers are being trained in techniques such as motivational interviewing, an effective skill for helping maintain someone in treatment. Skeem and Petrila (2004) have referred to specialized caseload work such as this as problem-solving supervision. Skeem's work (2007) has even taken the concept of the therapeutic alliance from research of psychotherapy and analogized it to a construct of a working alliance between a figure who represents a mandating agency, like a probation officer or a case manager from a mental health court and a probationer or client. This line of research is investigating if the element of the quality of the personal relationship between legally mandated treatment clients and the person who represents the mandating agency in order to determine if the higher the quality of the relationship the better the clinical and public safety outcomes.

Prison and jail reentry programs similarly seek to ensure that inmates who return to the community are provided with the services they require in order to reduce the risk of rearrest and decompensation. These programs will often provide medication for an interim period before seeing a new mental health treatment provider, along with beginning the process of activating necessary benefits and ensuring appropriate referrals are made.

Successful drug and mental health courts were developed as a type of post-booking diversion away from any stage of the criminal justice process. In the end, successful diversion away from any stage of the criminal justice process and engagement in clinically-appropriate and effective treatment requires ensuring linkage to adequate services that meet the clinical needs of the defendant or offender. Still, as Munetz and Griffin (2006) have put it, the "ultimate intercept" for moving people away from the criminal justice system is "an accessible, comprehensive, effective mental health treatment system" that prevents the criminalization of people with mental illness in the first place (p. 545).

REFERENCES

Alschuler, A. W. (1979). Plea bargaining and its history. *Columbia Law Review, 79*(1), 1–43.

American Bar Association. (1985). *Criminal justice standards* (Chapter 10). Washington, DC: Author.

Bandy v. United States, 81 S. Ct. 197 (1960)

Barr, H. (2003). Transinstitutionalization in the courts: *Brad H. v. City of New York*, and the fight for discharge planning for people with psychiatric disabilities leaving Rikers island. *Crime & Delinquency, 49*(1), 97–123.

Bellassai, J. P. (2010). A short history of the pretrial diversion of adult defendants from traditional criminal justice processing. Accessed on May 23, 2010, at www.napsa.org/publications/diversionhistory.pdf Washington, DC: Pretrial Services Resource Center.

Berman, G., & Feinblatt, J. (2001). *Problem solving courts: A brief primer.* New York: Center for Court Innovation.

Breeding, J. (2006). The case of Sohrab Hassan: Assault on Liberty in the Texas mental health courts. *Journal of Humanistic Psychology, 46,* 243–254.

Bureau of Justice Statistics. (2010). Correctional populations, key facts at a glance. Retrieved from http://bjs.ojp.usdoj.gov/content/glance/tables/corr2tab.cfm

Bureau of Justice Assistance. (2010). Law enforcement/mental health partnership program. Retrieved from http://www.ojp.usdoj.gov/BJA/grant/LE_MHPartnership.pdf.)

Butterfield, F. (1998). Asylums behind bars: A special report. Prisons Replace Hospitals for the Nation's Mentally Ill. *The New York Times.* Published March 5, 1998. Retrieved from http://nytimes.com

Clark, J. (2004). *Non-specialty first appearance court models for diverting persons with mental illness: Alternatives to mental health courts.* Delmar, NY: Technical assistance and policy analysis center for jail diversion.

CMHS National GAINS Center. (2007). *Practical advice on jail diversion: Ten years of learning on jail diversion from the CMHS National Gains Center.* Delmar, NY: Author.

Compton, M. T., Bahora, M., Watson, A., & Oliva, J. (2008). A comprehensive review of extant research on crisis intervention team (CIT) programs. *Journal of the American Academy of Psychiatry and the Law, 36,* 47–55.

Dupont, R., & Cochran, S. (2002). Police and mental health linked programs: Promising Practices—The CIT Model. In G. Landsberg, M. Rack, & L. Berg (Eds.), Serving mentally ill offenders: challenges and opportunities for mental health professionals. New York: Springer Publishing.

Erickson, S. K., Campbell, A., & Lamberti, S. (2006). Variations in mental health courts: Challenges, opportunities, and a call for caution. *Community Mental Health Journal, 42*(4), 335–344.

Gendar, A., Boyle, C., & McShane, L. (2008). NYPD Lt. Michael Pigott, who ordered fatal tasering of naked man, left suicide note: It's my fault. Daily News. Published October 2, 2008, Accessed October 11, 2010 at nydailynews.com

Hanrahan, P. (2000). Mental health court: Promises and limitations. *Journal of the American Academy of Psychiatry and the Law, 28*(4), 476–482.

Hauser, C. (2008). Police lieutenant in taser case commits suicide. *The New York Times.* Accessed on June 28, 2010 at http://cityroom.blogs.nytimes.com/2008/10/02/police-lt-in-deadly-taser-case-commits-suicide/?scp=1-b&sq=iman+morales&st=nyt

Hogan, M. (2002). October 29, 2002, accessed at http://mentalhealth.samhsa.gov/publications/allpubs/nmh02-0144/default.asp on June 4, 2010.

Hora, P., Schma, W., & Rosenthal, J. T. A. (1999). Therapeutic jurisprudence and the drug court movement: Revolutionizing the criminal justice system's response to drug abuse and crime in America. *Notre Dame Law Review, 74*(2), 439–555.

Huddleston, C. W., Marlowe, D. B., & Casebolt, R. (2008). *Painting the current picture: A national report card on drug courts and other problem-solving court programs in the United States, 2, 1.* Alexandria, VA: National Drug Court Institute.

Lamb, R., Watson, A., Luchins, D., & Weinberger, L. E. (2005). The shift of psychiatric inpatient care from hospitals to jails and prisons. *Journal of the American Academy of Psychiatry and the Law, 33*(4), 529–534.

Lattimore, P. K., Broner, N., Sherman, R., Frisman, L., & Shafer, M. (2003). A comparison of prebooking and postbooking diversion programs for mentally ill substance-using individuals with justice involvement. *Journal of Contemporary Criminal Justice, 19*(1), 30–64.

Liptak, A. (2008). U.S. prison population dwarfs that of other nations. *The New York Times,* April 23, 2008. Accessed on June 4, 2010 at nytimes.com.

Lopez, S. (2005). Mentally ill in the jail? It's a crime. *Los Angeles Times.* December 11, 2005.

Lotze, E., Clark, J., Henry, D. A., & Juzkiewicz, J. (1999). *The pretrial services reference book.* Washington, DC: Pretrial Services Resource Center.

Munetz, M., & Griffin, P. (2006). Use of the sequential intercept model as an approach to decriminalization of people with serious mental illness. *Psychiatric Services, 57,* 544–549.

Nolan, J. L. (2001). *Reinventing justice; the American drug court movement.* Princeton: Princeton University Press.

Petrila, J. (2003). An introduction to special jurisdiction courts. *International Journal of Law and Psychiatry, 26*, 3–12.

Redlich, A. D. (2005). Voluntary, but knowing and intelligent. Comprehension in mental health courts. *Psychology, Public Policy, and Law, 11*(4), 605–619.

Redlich, A. D., Steadman, H. J., Monahhan, J., Petrila, J., & Griffin, P. A. (2005). The second generation of mental health courts. *Psychology, Public Policy, and Law, 11*(4), 527–538.

Redlich, A. D., Steadman, H. J., Monahan, J., Robbins, P. C., & Petrila, J. (2006). Patterns of practice in mental health courts: A national survey. *Law and Human Behavior, 30*, 347–362.

Robinson v. California, 370 U.S. page 660 (1962).

Schwartz, E. (2008). Mental health courts: How special courts can serve justice and help mentally ill offenders. US News and World Report. February 7, 2008. Accessed June 15, 2010 at http://politics.usnews.com/news/national/articles/2008/02/07/mental-health-courts.html

Seltzer, T. (2005). Mental health courts. A misguided attempt to address the criminal justice system's unfair treatment of people with mental illnesses. *Psychology, Public Policy, and Law, 11*(4), 570–586.

Skeem, J., & Petrila, J. (2004). Problem-solving supervision: Specialty probation for individuals with mental illness. *Court Review, 40*, 8–15.

Skeem, R. J., & Eno Louden, J. (2006). Toward evidence-based practice for probationers and parolees mandated to mental health treatment. *Psychiatric Services, 57*, 333–342.

Steadman, H. (1992). Boundary spanners: A key component for the effective interactions of the justice and mental health systems. *Law and Human Behavior, 16*(1), 75–87.

Steadman, H. J., Cocozza, J. J., & Veysey, B. M. (1999a). Comparing outcomes for diverted and nondiverted jail detainees with mental illness. *Law and Human Behavior, 23*(6), 615–627.

Steadman, H. J., Davidson, S., & Brown, C. (2001). Mental health courts: Their promise and unanswered questions. *Psychiatric Services, 52*(4), 457–458.

Steadman, H. J., Deane, M. W., Morrissey, J. P., Westcott, M. L., Salasin, S., & Shaoiro, S. (1999). A SAMHSA research initiative assessing the effectiveness of jail diversion programs for mentally ill persons. *Psychiatric Services, 50*, 1620–1623.

Steadman, J. H., Morris, S. M., & Dennis, D. L. (1995). The diversion of mentally ill persons from jails to community-based services: A profile of programs. *American Journal of Public Health, 85*(12), 1630–1635.

Steadman, H. J., & Naples, M. (2005). Assessing the effectiveness of jail diversion programs for persons with serious mental illness and co-occurring substance use disorders. *Behavioral Sciences and the Law, 26*, 163–170.

Steadman, H. J., Osher, F., Robbins, P., Case, B., & Samuels, S. (2009). Prevalence of serious mental illness among jail inmates. *Psychiatric Services, 60*, 761–765.

Stefan, S., & Winick, B. J. (2005). Foreword. A dialogue on mental health courts. *Psychology, Public Policy, and Law, 11*(4), 507–526.

Sultan, B. (2010). Personal communication.

Teplin, L. A. (2000). *Keeping the peace: Policediscretion and mentally ill persons.* National Institute of Justice Journal 244. Washington, DC: National Institute of Justice. Available at www.ncjrs.gov/pdffiles1/jr000244c.pdf

Thomas, W. (1976). *Bail reform in America.* Berkeley: University of California Press.

Torrey, E. F., Kennard, A., Eslinger, D., Lamb, R., & Pavle, J. (2010). More mentally ill persons are in jails and prisons than hospitals: A survey of the states. Treatment Advocacy Center and National Sheriff's Association. Accessed on May 30, 2010 at National Institute of Corrections Library, http://nicic.gov/Library/024454

Watson, A., Hanrahan, P., Luchins, D., & Lurigio, A. (2001). Mental health courts and the complex issue of mentally ill offenders. *Psychiatric Services, 52*(4), 477–481.

Wexler, D. B. (1992). Putting mental health into mental health law. Therapeutic jurisprudence. *Law and Human Behavior, 16*(1), 27–38.

CHAPTER SEVENTEEN

Program Evaluation with Vulnerable Populations

Nancy A. Hepler, Frank Guida, Maria Messina, and
Mohamed Kanu

INTRODUCTION

Evaluation is a process to determine merit, worth, or value of a program or practice, product, personnel, policy, or proposal. Evaluation is distinguished from research by the immediate utility of its findings and conclusions; consideration of variables such as costs, ethics, and legal and political dimensions; and the use of "transdisciplines," that is reliable and valid tools from many fields of inquiry, rather than using one scientific method for all studies (Scriven, 1991; Stodolsky, 1974).

This chapter will describe evaluation procedures for programs that feature vulnerable populations and include evaluation considerations; client demographics; informed consent/confidentiality; participatory evaluation with vulnerable populations; evaluation methods appropriate for the population; evaluation design; data collection; adherence to evidence-based practices; fidelity to the intervention model; and dissemination of findings.

EVALUATION CONSIDERATIONS FOR VULNERABLE POPULATIONS

As with every search for new knowledge, evaluation standards require the evaluator to start with what is already known. The evaluator should establish a theory-driven (Chen, 1990) or evidence-based design supported by thorough and insightful review of current literature. The literature base should include prior research findings and identify gaps the proposed method is designed to address. If a sufficient literature base has not yet been developed, then the evaluator should develop preliminary designs that test the receptiveness of the population being studied; the appropriateness, reliability and validity, and sensitivity of proposed methods, and preliminary findings that support the proposed design.

At all times, the evaluator must be aware of and conform to the ethics, guidelines, laws, and regulations that protect the civil rights, privacy, anonymity, confidentiality, and health and well-being of each participant in any study, such as the CFR45 Part 46, CFR 42 Part 2, the Family Right to Privacy Act (FERPA), 2008, the Health Insurance Portability and Accountability Act (HIPAA), 1996; among others.

Evaluators should strive to give an authentic voice to participants of evaluation studies, particularly those coming from minority, emerging or historically disenfranchised or underserved, underrepresented populations (Substance Abuse and Mental Health Services Administration, 2009). Members of the study population should be integrally involved in the design, implementation, and reporting of the study to increase validity, reliability, cultural appropriateness, and relevance. The genuine involvement of members of the study population also expedites the dissemination of findings within the population. Involving members of the target population include representation on a Program Advisory Board, Quality Assurance (QA) committee; consumer/patient satisfaction surveys; and interviews and focus groups.

CLIENT DEMOGRAPHICS

The first responsibility of the evaluator is to provide the demographics of the intended client or patient base. Specific demographic variables could include gender (males, females, transgender), race, education, number of children, sexual orientation, criminal justice history, age, employment, income, residence (i.e., shelter, street, someone else's apartment, etc.), mental health status, current or past substance abuse (including primary drug of abuse), physical history (including HIV/Hep C status, smoking cigarettes), etc. As an example, it is important to program funding sources, such as federal agencies, to determine if an evidence-based practice is effective in a particular target population. Often, not all ethnic populations have been included in the demographics of the original studies that established the effectiveness of evidence-based practices, and so a funding source may offer funding to study a particular population. For instance, a Substance Abuse and Mental Health Services Administration (SAMHSA) grant program may target minority women, coming out of prison or jail, between the ages of 21–65, who have a co-occurring disorder, and who are at risk for or are HIV positive. In applying for the funding, it is important to assure the potential program funders that the population enrolled in the program is the actual population envisioned by the funders to receive the services the grant provides.

INFORMED CONSENT/CLIENT CONFIDENTIALITY AND PROTECTION

It is also the responsibility of all staff involved in an evaluation study to know all ethics, laws, regulations, and guidelines to protect the study population including all pertinent international, national, state, local, and professional standards. In the United States, for example, each staff member involved in research or evaluation using human subjects must complete the National Institutes of Health (NIH) web-based training course. Upon completion of the course, the staff member receives a certification of completion with a certification number. If an Internal Review Board (IRB) approval is needed for the study, each staff member must submit the certificate as part of the IRB application. The training is provided by NIH on its website (National Institutes of Health, 2008).

The purpose of this section is to give a brief overview of human subject protection. This section will include the following:

- A brief history of human subjects protection
- Additional protections for vulnerable populations
- Conditions under which IRB approval is required
- Issues with participant protection.

A Brief History of Human Subjects Protection

Hippocrates is credited with the most well-known oath taken by doctors to protect the well-being of their patients in the course of medical treatment. Evaluation participants are protected by the same international laws and regulations that protect human subjects of medical research. Federal and State laws and regulations interpret international and national law or provide additional protections. Agencies and institutions who serve as guardians of individuals, such as corrections institutes, hospitals and other treatment facilities, and state educational agencies (SEA) and local educational agencies (LEA) may provide additional protections and safeguards. Additional guidelines have been codified to protect vulnerable populations among them CFR 42, Part 2; the Family Educational Rights and Privacy Act (2008); and the HIPAA (1996).

Professional organizations, such as the American Medical Association, the American Psychological Association, the American Evaluation Association, and the American Educational Research Association have additional professional standards which must be met for studies to be published in their peer-reviewed journals. In the event that there is any conflict among regulations, the most restrictive of regulations must be met.

The World Medical Association Declaration of Helsinki (1964; amended 1975, 1983, 1989, 1996, 2000, and 2004) put forth Ethical Principles for Medical Research Involving Human Subjects which assert that the individual's rights and well-being must be put ahead of science in medical experiments. It also requires that researchers, including evaluators, be aware of the ethical, legal, and regulatory requirements including: assessment of the risks and benefits of the study and clear demonstration that the benefits outweigh the risks; plan for informed, voluntary consent; and protection of the participant from risk of coercion. Additional provisions are included for studies that are combined with medical care: the risks, effectiveness, and burdens must be tested against usual care methods; every patient must be assured of care whether or not she/he agrees to participate in the study; the staff must inform the participant which procedures are part of the study; all findings both positive and negative must be published.

The Belmont Report-Ethical Principles and Guidelines for the Protection of Human Subjects (1979) established the three fundamental principles of research with human subjects: respect for persons, beneficence, and justice. The Belmont Report provides the foundation for Title 45 Code of Federal Regulations, Part 46, Protection of Human Subjects (45 CFR Part 46).

Additional Protections for Vulnerable Populations

The Declaration of Helsinki acknowledges that some populations are vulnerable and need special protections and specifies economically and medically disadvantaged populations, those who cannot consent for themselves (e.g., adults under conservership, children), those who may be giving consent under duress (e.g., adjudicated or incarcerated individuals, employees), those who will not benefit personally from the research (e.g., members of a control group), and those for whom research or evaluation is combined with care. Also included are people who are legally incompetent, physically or mentally incapable of giving consent, and legal minors for whom legal guardians must give consent. CFR 42, Part 2 (2002) provides additional protections for the confidentiality of the medical records of people participating in alcohol and/or drug treatment programs. In addition to establishing rights to education, the Family Educational Rights and Privacy Act (2008) defines under what conditions parents must provide consent to collect data from their children, conditions under which active or passive consent are required, and restrictions on the data that can be collected. The HIPAA (1996) privacy rule protects the privacy of individually identifiable health information.

Conditions Under Which Institutional Review Board Approval is Required

Most program evaluations do NOT require approval from an IRB because the data collected are publicly available, the subject is identified only by an ID number, randomization of subjects to groups does not occur, nor are subjects assigned to a group (control) that does not receive the services promised. IRB approval is required whenever the research or evaluation includes identifiable human material or identifiable data. Unidentifiable group data such as sociodemographics, group statistical reports such as school suspensions and expulsions or uniform crime reports, and survey data that do not collect individually identifiable data may be used without the approval of an IRB. If, however, the sociodemographic, crime, school, treatment, or other data are collected and stored in such a way that an individual can be identified and linked to the data, then the evaluation would require the prior approval of an IRB. This is as true of use of secondary databases (data that have been previously collected by the evaluator or others that are used for a different study) as it is for primary data (data that are collected by the evaluator conducting the current study).

If an evaluator believes the study is exempt, then an application can be made to the IRB using a form that requests and explains the reasons for the exemption. Investigators cannot make their own determinations about exemptions. At times, the funding source (e.g., federal funding sources such as SAMHSA) will consult an IRB on behalf of applicants. The IRB will determine whether or not approval is needed or the evaluation activities are exempt.

Issues for Participant Protection

Funding for evaluation studies, such as those to improve mental health or educational achievement or decrease substance abuse, often target vulnerable populations. While insurance including Medicaid pay for some services, the important evidence-based services such as Assertive Community Treatment (ACT) Teams, Integrated Dual Disorder Treatment (IDDT) which have demonstrated effectiveness are only funded by discretionary federal grants or private foundations. Since participation in evaluation studies is attractive to vulnerable individuals, any study must be designed to protect the people who participate.

Equitable Selection

Selection into a study must be equitable and forbid the exclusion of women and minorities in study populations. If women or minorities are excluded, the evaluator has to provide a written justification. For example, if the evaluation studies' focus is alcohol consumption in fraternity pledges, then women are not included in the study because only males pledge fraternities. The evaluator is required to explain and justify the exclusion of women in the study.

Assuring Informed Voluntary Consent

Informed consent provides the opportunity to the participant to assess whether or not she/he wants to participate in the study. The description of the study should be clear and complete and include the study's procedures, risks and benefits, and rights and responsibilities of the participant. Guidelines require disclosure of relevant information, verification that the participant comprehended the information and a voluntary signed agreement free of coercion and undue influence (National Institutes of Health, 2006).

Evaluators are required to provide additional vigilance against coercion in vulnerable populations which include cognitively impaired subjects, children, pregnant women, people who are incarcerated, and people who are economically or educationally disadvantaged. The only person who can consent to participation is the participant or a legally authorized representation (e.g., a parent or a guardian) (National Institutes of Health, 2006). Releases of information are also governed by HIPAA (1996) and Family Educational Rights and Privacy Act (FERPA) (2008).

In the situation where another responsible party consents for the participant, the evaluator is required to get an informed assent from the participant. For example, if a parent signs consent for a minor adolescent to participate in a study, the researcher is also required to obtain an informed assent from the adolescent. The evaluator is required to know and comply with all consent procedures (National Institutes of Health, 2006).

Reducing Risk and Assuring Balance of Cost and Benefit to Participants

Evaluation staffs are required to identify and minimize risks to participants, to adequately provide for safety of participants and to provide for procedures in the event that a participant experiences harm. Evaluation staffs are also required to balance the risk to the participant with a benefit to the participant and to convey the risks and the benefits clearly to the participant as part of the consent procedures. At no time can treatment be withheld if a person refuses to participate in an evaluation study. In that case, the person would receive usual care from the program or be referred to appropriate care within the agency or to another provider in the community.

PARTICIPATORY EVALUATION WITH VULNERABLE POPULATIONS

The evaluation staff should involve members of the community and target population in every phase of the evaluation process from development of the application through the program implementation, evaluation, and dissemination. This will help ensure that the program is culturally appropriate and sensitive to the needs of the target population (SAMHSA, 2009). Involvement of members of the target population from the beginning through the planning, development, intervention, QA, report writing, and dissemination is required by many funding sources. Examples include the United States Department of Health and Human Services Health Resources Services Administration (HRSA, undated), and SAMSHA (2009). Member involvement strengthens planning, development, implementation, evaluation, and dissemination in many ways. Members of a population can interpret the population's culture; represent the evaluators and program to the population; facilitate introductions and entry to the population; ensure cultural competency of instruments, procedures, and methods; provide insights into findings; and help disseminate findings back into the community (Hepler & Renfro, 1999).

Finally, the members of the community know whether they have an authentic voice; their cooperation is contingent upon their perceptions of whether the evaluators are doing something to them or with them. As an example, people who live in public housing have seen many researchers come and go and know that the researchers will only be there for the short time they are funded so "we will wait you out" (Wingfield, 1999).

Persons who are vulnerable, minority, and/or have been historically disenfranchised need protections and support in being meaningfully involved. Licensing standards, regulations, and funding sources require that participants be involved in governance in a meaningful way. To provide for meaningful participation, evaluators should provide opportunities to members of the target population that are accessible, appropriate, comfortable, safe, and demonstrate that the input from the representatives is being used. Meeting these requirements will vary depending on the population. Care must be taken so that the representative feels comfortable sharing input. As an example, a sole consumer on an advisory board is not as likely to actively participate as consumers who have other peers to support the participant point of view. As a result, some regulations require 51% representation of consumers. Others require a separate Consumer Advisory Board whose recommendations carry weight in the decision-making process. As with any set of advisors, participants on advisory boards should receive training about the evaluation; its goals and objectives and procedures; and how to participate including rights, roles, and responsibilities of advisors. Participants should also receive reports of how input has been incorporated into the evaluation and program implementation.

EVALUATION METHODS APPROPRIATE FOR THE POPULATION

Few studies have been published for many of the vulnerable populations discussed in this book. Often, standard evaluation procedures and methods that have proven effective in studying members of the general population are not appropriate, reliable, or valid for members from some minority populations. To be valid, evaluation methods need to be appropriate for the culture of the population. Many rigorous scientific methods assume prior knowledge about the study population that may not be available in an emerging population. This section will discuss issues related to establishing a body of scientific literature about a new population and the need to look for convergent validity among methods whenever studying a new population for which there is little established scientific literature. Issues that will be addressed in this section include the following:

- Methods that capture emerging knowledge including capturing observations of key informants such as staff, administrations and members

of the population, their family members, advocates, and clinical case studies.
- Matching methods to the evaluation questions and population to include ethnographic, qualitative, and quantitative methods.

Methods That Capture Emerging Knowledge

Observational and Interview Techniques

In order to sense the pulse of what's happening "on the ground" with a given intervention or program, the evaluator may conduct participant observation, focus groups, or key informant interviews which may capture new or unexpected developments within the group or matter under study. Participant observation provides data from first-hand, potentially serendipitous, observations of people in their "natural settings" whether a day program for persons with mental illness, an adolescent therapeutic community for drug treatment, or a shooting gallery for injection drug users. Focus groups are a form of qualitative research in which a facilitator asks a group of people about their attitudes toward a product, service, concept, or idea. Each focus group discussion will produce data and insights that would be less accessible without interaction found in a group setting — listening to others' verbalize experiences stimulates memories, ideas, and experiences in participants (Morgan, 1997). Using open-ended questions avoids delimiting or providing cues for a topic and allows an informant room to move in new and unanticipated directions. For example, the Diabetes Co-Morbidity Initiative (DCI) developed a workbook to teach severely mentally ill (SMI) consumers how to manage their diabetes. In order to see if the workbook was effective or could be improved, the evaluator conducted focus groups with consumers at participating programs and received feedback about its strengths or weaknesses. Since there were fewer line staffs or consumer advocates in the DCI, key informant interviews were efficient means for gaining insights in support of or in addition to those of consumers. A key informant is an individual who is articulate and representative of the group under study and provides key insights and interpretations. Feedback about the effectiveness or level of difficulty in the workbook was shared with the developers who then integrated relevant points to increase the material's effectiveness. This process of including consumers in the development of a program creates a sense of ownership and pride and almost guarantees their participation.

Case Study Methodology

Case study methodology, also known as single-subject design, is the intensive study of a single individual, organization, business application, or community by using in-depth longitudinal methods in the real-life context for a single event: a case. Case studies are common in medicine, law, and business and are also used by social science and educational researchers and evaluators. Case studies are useful as a first study when influencing variables are unknown, for example, in the evaluation of business innovations (Brinkerhoff, 2003). Case study methodology follows the same design steps as any other study design and uses some similar methods, both qualitative and quantitative, such as interviews and surveys; the focus on a single case is the primary difference (Brinkerhoff, 2003; Stake, 1995). A major difference, however, is that a case is not selected randomly, as in experimental design, but rather for its known richness of information. The findings from case studies cannot be generalized to the general population as can experimental studies. Rather, their value comes from the richness of the data collection and their power to study a case in great depth and to identify and eliminate variables and hypotheses.

As an example, case studies were conducted on all school districts in the United States with student entry (first grade) average test scores lower than the 10th percentile, but high graduation rates with high-school test scores at or above the national average. Researchers used a standardized valid, reliable protocol from an earlier case study to collect data, conduct interviews, and record observations to elicit successful strategies that contributed to the phenomenal success of the school districts over the course of a student's tenure in the system (Hepler et al., 1987). The results of the studies were used for both policy decisions, specifically that students who enter school in the lowest percentile can learn and school districts should be funded to serve them, and for program design.

Needs Assessment

One of the more common forms of evaluation studies, especially for populations where little is known, is needs assessment. Needs assessments are conducted for the purposes of planning prior to securing resources for community and program development. Standards of practice and funding agency regulations require that members of study populations be genuinely involved in the assessment of their needs and service gaps (e.g., Substance Abuse and Mental Health Services Administration, 2009).

Two frequently used methods for assessing community needs are the nominal group process and the Delphi technique.

The nominal group process is a "structured meeting that attempts to provide an orderly procedure for obtaining qualitative information from target groups who are most closely associated with a problem area" (Fink, Kosecoff, Chassin, & Brook, 1984, p. 980). It involves the recruiting of participants or stakeholders who take part in a discussion with the intent to rank competing priorities.

The Delphi technique, on the other hand, involves pooling expert participants through mail or self-administered questionnaire to elicit expert opinion necessary to reach a consensus on an issue (McDermott & Sarvela, 1999).

Often, needs assessments are conducted in an expedient way to accomplish a specific goal and thus are targeted with a narrow focus. As an example, archeologists (Robinson, 2009) are finding evidence that an African-American neighborhood in Indianapolis that was cleared for urban renewal in the 1960s was not blighted as initially assessed. Recovered artifacts suggest middle-class wealth rather than items that would be found in a blighted community. At the time of the urban renewal, community members, including a state legislator who resided in the community, were not involved in the discussion and were not heard when they issued formal protests of the destruction of their community.

The example above illustrates that needs assessments should include a wide view of the community being assessed and its members. Often, needs assessments are conducted using local statistics such as sociodemographics, key informant surveys of service providers, and/or survey methods such as random mail or digit dialing telephone surveys. Such needs assessment methods, however, do not often fully assess the needs of populations with low occurring numbers in the general population and may miss capturing the perceptions of its members. Needs assessments that collect data from captive populations such as consumer or patient surveys may be more successful in eliciting needs from the target population. However, these surveys exclude members of the population who are not yet engaged in services that may be disenfranchised or otherwise different and thus are biased in favor of the members who have access to services.

Needs assessment methodology requires a comparison, for example: (1) gaps analysis, which is the comparison of an ideal standard to actual community perceptions of crime and neighborhood disorganization; (2) comparison of one population or community to another to demonstrate health disparities; or (3) a comparison of one time period to another to demonstrate the declining resources in a community. Therefore, accurate assessment should use standardized protocol with established validity and reliability with the target population or similar target populations. If the methods have not been used with the target population, they should be reviewed by members of the population for appropriateness; pretesting of the methodology is also advised.

Matching Methods to the Evaluation Questions and Population

Reliability refers to consistency; that is, "whether the process of the study is consistent, reasonably stable over time and across researchers and methods" (Miles & Huberman, 1994, p. 1). Internal consistency raises questions about the truth value, whether or not the findings make sense, are credible, and authentic (Miles & Huberman, 1994).

Validity refers to the extent to which a measure or method truly measures what it purports to measure and how well it does so (Scriven, 1991). There are many kinds of validity. *Face validity* concerns whether a measure appears to measure what it claims to measure. *Construct validity* concerns the presence of a theoretical construct in the measure or method. *Content validity* determines whether a measure adequately samples the content it proposes to measure. *Criterion-related validity* concerns the predictive ability of the measure. *Convergent/Discriminant validity* is the correlation of a measure or method to other measures or methods for the same and different constructs. *Internal validity* requires findings with internal coherence (Eisner, 1991), and concepts that are systematically related (Strauss & Corbin, 1990).

Evaluation often includes both quantitative and qualitative methods. Quantitative methods collect and analyze numerical data, such as the number of sexual partners within a specified time period, or scores on the Beck Depression Inventory; while qualitative methods collect and analyze raw, in-depth data that consist of words or pictures (Bernard, 1994); for example, the complex social and personal meanings men having sex with men (MSM) attach to "bare backing" (anal sex without a condom). Combined, the two methods can present a sophisticated description of the behavior under evaluation. One type of qualitative methodology, ethnography, is the systematic and holistic study of human behavior in a particular context or community as perceived by the members of that community through intensive fieldwork. Most commonly, ethnographic research generates qualitative data which are "a source of well-grounded, rich descriptions and explanations of processes in identifiable, local contexts" (Miles & Huberman, 1994, p. 278). The use of his methodology allows chronological order to be preserved, actions and their consequences observed in real time, and differences between the ideal or formal rules and actual behavior captured, which elucidate the underlying cultural organizing principles of social action documented (Barret, 1991). Quantitative data can more easily access a larger number of participants and gauge, for example, the incidence and prevalence rates, or significant reduction in PTSD symptoms from a baseline to a follow-up time period.

Evaluation methods must be appropriately geared toward the new population under study. For example, where literacy or cognitive functioning is in question, a qualitative approach to collecting client data with open-ended questions would be more suitable because the evaluator could work with the client to find common language to get the point across. However, if the objective is to determine the frequency of a specific behavior, for example, how many times per month the clients check their glucose levels, a quantitative approach would be appropriate.

EVALUATION DESIGN: BALANCING SCIENCE AND THE NEEDS OF THE PARTICIPANTS AND OTHER STAKEHOLDERS

The root word in evaluation is value; evaluation is a process of determining the value of something, for example, a new policy, process, program, or practice. Evaluations require the same scientific rigor as research regardless of the methodology being used. A comprehensive evaluation may include a quasi-experimental design (measuring outcomes for one group receiving program interventions over multiple time periods), and a report which includes a review of the literature, theoretical framework, purpose, methodology, findings/results, discussion, and conclusions.

Constructing Evaluation Logic Models to fit the Intervention and Population

The evaluation design should be expressed in a program logic model, which should demonstrate the relationship of the identified needs, resources, goals, objectives, and outcomes. Program logic models are required by many funding sources including governmental agencies such as the World Bank, Ontario Canada Ministry of Health, U.S. Centers for

Disease Control (CDC), HRSA, and SAMHSA as well as nongovernmental agencies such as the United Way. Logic models can be found on the Centers for Disease Control Evaluation Working Group website (CDC, 2009).

Meeting Reporting Needs of Stakeholders (QA/CQI, Compliance, Outcomes)

As part of the QA/continuous quality improvement process, the evaluator can inform clinical practice by attending case conferences and informing clinical staff regarding clients' progress in treatment based on clients' baseline and follow-up scores on local instruments. For example, in the evaluation of a SAMHSA-grant-funded program, the evaluator attends the program's case conference every Tuesday with results of a depression scale and Post Traumatic Stress Disorder (PTSD) inventory, and is able to confirm psychiatric diagnoses at intake and report depression and PTSD symptom reduction (or increase) at 6-month follow-up. In this manner, the staff feels that the evaluator is an integral part of the process. At times the evaluator can seem to be the eyes and ears of the entire program. At another SAMHSA-funded program, the evaluator, because of extensive program staff turnover, has become the *de facto* symbol of the program and the government program officer (GPO) has taken to calling the evaluator directly when he has a question, comment, or complaint. Albeit an extreme case, it illustrates the QA/CQI role of the evaluator, who not only performs *t*-tests with dependent samples or analyses of repeated measures, or calculates clients' session attendance logs, but is an integral part of the treatment process, so that the program stays on track in meeting its goals and objectives.

Process Evaluation

Process evaluation is primarily concerned with documenting the process of implementation. Process evaluation is an important part of any comprehensive evaluation. At minimum, process evaluation should include an accurate description of the interventions and outcomes produced by the program. This is important for evaluators to be able to link the process to outcomes or to explain different outcomes in similar studies. Process evaluations should use sound methodological practices such as dose logs which record the number of units of service a client receives, participant observation to capture how the intervention is implemented "on the ground," and attendance at case conference to assess, from a different vantage point, how treatment is affecting clients.

Outcome Evaluation

Outcome evaluation methods measure the posttreatment effects. Ideally, outcome evaluations should use experimental designs. Unfortunately, cost, ethical and other constraints often make experimental designs difficult or impossible. In those cases where an experimental control group design is not possible, a quasi-experimental design should be used. Expected outcomes from an evaluation would include behavioral changes (e.g., changes in management of diabetes like diet, exercise, weight loss, medical visits) and the consequences of the changes in behavior (e.g., decreases in HbA1C, lipid and urine profile, and hospitalizations due to complications of diabetes).

Data Collection

Selecting Instruments

Evaluators should use reliable and valid instruments for data collection that are consistent with the goals and objectives of the program. In reviewing the published reliability and validity information, evaluators should ascertain the populations for which reliability and validity have been established and choose instruments which have been found valid and reliable for the target population. Cultural appropriateness should also be established. Cultural competency refers to the ability, knowledge, and skills to work, communicate, and interact effectively with individuals from different cultural, educational backgrounds/communities, age groups, or gender orientations. Awareness of one's own worldview and biases as well as knowledge of other cultures or communities (Martin & Vaughn, 2007) better enables a service provider, evaluator, or researcher to develop competency and work well in a cross-cultural setting. Ideally, staffing should reflect individuals who are familiar with or are from the same backgrounds as the population to be served (SAMHSA, 2009). Linguistic and multicultural competences are crucial to work with a target population whose primary language is not English. Materials, brochures, or visual aids as well as the evaluation methods and instruments should be suitable and consistent for the age/gender/ethnicity of the target population.

ADHERENCE TO EVIDENCE-BASED PRACTICES

Adherence is the extent to which an evidence-based practice has been fully implemented. Most funders require that the intervention used to improve mental health, or decrease PTSD symptoms or increase reading achievement is an evidence-based practice, by which the practice has been tested in a randomized, control-group clinical trial and found to be significantly effective in improving the outcomes it was designed to target. For example, Seeking Safety, a specialized group therapy intervention for treating PTSD and substance abuse is a present focused therapy addressing three domains (cognitive, behavioral, interpersonal) in 25 treatment topics. The group therapy can be implemented once a week for 25 weeks, or twice, even three times per week for a shorter interval; however, all 25 topics should be covered for full effect. Seeking Safety (Najavits, 2002) is manualized with an adherence section. To demonstrate adherence to any given topic, say topic #6-asking for help, the evaluator should be present during the group therapy session featuring this topic, and will take note of the length of session, number of group members, and the extent (via rating scales) to which the group facilitator implemented the topic according to the topic curriculum in the Seeking Safety manual. This process would be followed for all other topics, and the average of all the 25 topic rating scales would signify the level of adherence to the intervention in the program.

FIDELITY TO THE INTERVENTION MODEL

Fidelity refers to the degree to which a program's logic model or complete array of specific interventions is faithfully reproduced in practice. As an example, the Institute for Community Learning (ICL) health-care providers, a psychiatrist, psychologists, and case managers, for the SMI with diabetes, developed a program to teach SMI persons at residential or day programs how to manage their diabetes. The program consisted of behavioral, medical, and educational interventions modeled around the treatment of diabetes. In the pilot study, line and supervisory staffs were purposefully trained how to teach SMI persons to utilize the program to maintain wellness. ICL developed an instrument to measure fidelity by identifying the essential elements of the diabetes training model and then sent their Clinical Coordinator to observe and implement the fidelity measure while diabetes trainings were in session. The evaluators analyzed the data and fidelity levels of high, medium, or low, were calculated. A score of low fidelity indicated the need for a booster training session to help staff get on track. High fidelity meant that the program was being implemented as intended.

DISSEMINATION OF FINDINGS

Although always last but certainly not least, the evaluator's written and often oral report of findings is perhaps the most important of evaluation activities. Almost all funders require some type of evaluation report, often quarterly, sometimes semiannually, and even monthly. Ther results of qualitative and quantitative process and outcomes should be reported in clear, lucid, and easily understandable tones. Sophisticated data analyses results such as multivariate analyses of repeated measures can and should be presented in laymen's terms. Whenever possible the reports should contain actual comments by the consumers targeted by the program, often in the form of consumer satisfaction surveys. Copious tables and charts help the funders to better understand and digest results. Excerpts from the reports should go into agency newsletters and marketing materials. If outcome results are particularly positive and robust, reports should become manuscripts and submitted to refereed journals in the field so that other evaluators and clinicians may replicate best practices.

REFERENCES

Barret, R. A. (1991). *Culture and conduct: An excursion into anthropology* (2nd ed.). Belmont, CA: Wadsworth.

Bernard, H. R. (1994). *Research methods in cultural anthropology.* Newbury Park, CA: Sage Publications.

Brinkerhoff, R. (2003). *The success case method.* San Francisco, CA: Berrett-Koehler Publishers, Inc.

Centers for Disease Control (CDC). (2009). CDC evaluation working group resources. Retrieved from http://www.cdc.gov/eval/resources.htm#logic%20 model. Accessed July 30, 2009.

Chen, H. (1990). *Theory-driven evaluations.* Newbury Park, CA: Sage Publications.

Code of Federal Regulations Title 45 Public Welfare Department of Health and Human Services Part 46 Protection of Human Subjects (CFR 45 Part 46). Revised June 23, 2005. http://www.hhs.gov/ohrp/humansubjects/guidance/45cfr46.htm. Accessed July 30, 2009.

Eisner, E. W. (1991). *The enlightened eye: Qualitative inquiry and the enhancement of educational practice.* New York, NY: Macmillan.

Family Education Rights and Privacy Act (FERPA). (2008). 20 U.S.C. 1232g: 34 CFR Part 99. December 9, 2008.

Fink, A., Kosecoff, J., Chassin, M., & Brook, R. H. (1984). Consensus methods: Characteristics and guidelines for use. *American Journal of Public Health, 74*, 980.

Hepler, N., Stringfield, S., Seltzer, D., Fortna, R., Stonehill, R., Yoder, N., et al. (1987). *Effective compensatory education programs for extremely disadvantaged students.* Portland, OR: Northwest Regional Educational Laboratory.

Hepler, N. A., & Renfro, J. A. (1999). Show me the money: Grant writing workshop presented for the U.S. Substance Abuse and Mental Health Services Administration (SAMHSA) in various cities across the nation.

Martin, M., & Vaughn, B. (2007). *Strategic diversity & inclusion management magazine* (pp. 31–36). San Francisco, CA: DTUI Publications Division.

McDermott, R. J., & Sarvela, P. D. (1999). *Health education evaluation and measurement: A practitioner's perspective.* New York, NY. The McGraw-Hill Companies, Inc.

Miles, M. B., & Huberman, M. A. (1994). *Qualitative data analysis: An expanded sourcebook* (2nd ed.). Thousand Oaks, CA: Sage.

Morgan, D. L. (1997). *Focus groups as qualitative research* (2nd ed.). Thousand Oaks, CA: Sage.

Najavits, L. M. (2002). *Seeking safety: A manual for PTSD and substance use treatment.* New York, NY: Guilford Press.

National Institutes of Health (NIH). (2006). *Guidelines for writing informed consent documents.* Office of Human Subjects Research Information: Sheet 6.

National Institutes of Health (NIH). (2008). *Protecting human research participants.* NIH Office of Extramural Research. Retrieved from http://phrp.nihtraining. com/users/login.php Cited July 30, 2009.

Robinson, D. (2009). Urban dig rewrites lost neighborhood history. Broadcast on National Public Radio July 23, 2009. Retrieved from http://www.npr.org/templates/story/story.php?storyId=106799382&ft=1&f=1008 Also available at http://www.newsmatters.org/urban-dig-rewriting-lost-neighborhoods-history/

Scriven, M. (1991). *Evaluation Thesaurus.* Newbury Park, NY: Sage.

Stake, R. (1995). *The art of case study research.* Thousand Oaks, CA: Sage.

Stodolsky, S (1974). *Open education: A challenge to evaluators.* Report #29. ERIC Clearinghouse on tests, measurement and evaluation. Princeton, NJ.

Strauss, A. L., & Corbin, J (1990). *Basics of qualitative research: Grounded theory procedures and techniques.* Newbury Park, CA: Sage.

Substance Abuse and Mental Health Services Administration (SAMHSA). (2009). *Guidelines for assessing cultural competence.* Retrieved from http://www. samhsa.gov/Grants/guide_culture.aspx. Accessed July 31, 2009.

The Health Insurance Portability and Accountability Act (HIPAA). (1996). *Health resources and services administration (HRSA).* Health Center Program Stature: Section 330 of the Public Health Service Act (42 CFR Part 51c; 42 CFR Parts 56 and 45 CFR Part 74).

The National Commission for the Protection of Human Subjects of Biomedical and Behavioral Research. (1979). *The Belmont report: Ethical principles and guidelines for the protection of human subjects of research.* April 18, 1979. Retrieved from http://ohsr.od.nih.gov/guidelines/belmont.html

Wingfield, S. (1999). The need for a long-term commitment of services in public housing. A presentation to the contractors meeting for building safer public housing communities through locally initiated research partnerships jointly sponsored by the National Institute of Justice and Housing and Urban Development.

World Federation of Doctors Who Respect Human Life. (1964). *The Medical Code of Ethics, Declaration of Helsinki, 1948*. Retrieved from http://www.euthanasia.com/belgium.html#code

CHAPTER EIGHTEEN

Mental Health Meets New Media

A Powerful New Portal for Increased Access to Mental Health Services

Jill Wolski Ordoñez and Michael Cheng

INTRODUCTION

The emergence of new media as a major communication tool in the 21st century represents a new opportunity for the mental health system, an opportunity that up to this point has been largely untapped. New media includes communications and media venues over the web including chat, email, video, social networking, message boards, and texting, all of which may be accessed wherever there is an Internet connection, including stationary or laptop computers, and hand-held mobile devices. Since new media communication opportunities follow people wherever we are, it only makes sense that the mental health service system should adapt to the reality of a wired culture and capitalize on these new venues to provide positive support.

New media is also inherently a good fit for the mental health field, because at its essence new media relies on interactivity. Comments on blogs, You-tube or Facebook postings, or conversations via chat or messaging boards, are just a few examples of the interactivity of new media. The mental health field relies primarily on positive, helping relationships to support consumers in distress and these helping relationships, if brought to new media venues, could have a resoundingly positive impact on people in distress, people who increasingly are found online, engaging in new media.

More than anything, adapting mental health services to new media offers increased access to services. Potential mental health consumers who may have opted out of the mental health service system in the past

375

will have a whole new way of opting into services. And these "services" can look completely different from traditional mental health service provision. Where face-to-face counseling was provided in the past, chat, email, or video Camcorder exchanges between consumer and therapist can be offered. Where hotline crisis intervention services were offered to those thinking about suicide in the past, texting, chat, and messaging boards can now be offered for quick access in a time of greatest suicidal crisis. Where phone-based or agency-based information and referral services were offered in the past, consumers will be able to find information and referral on mental health issues quickly—via online, easy-to-use resource databases, and information libraries, all of which can engage consumers via user comments, feedback, and linkages to topic-based message boards. So many interactive and creative services may be offered online, the limits to these services may be only encumbered by our own abilities to imagine the type of services we want to provide.

It has been said that the internet has provided a democratizing effect by placing more people on equal playing fields to access information. It is also well-known that the mental health field has long struggled with the forces of stigma, shame, and lack of awareness and knowledge that have prevented people from accessing the services they need. Finally the internet platform and accompanying new media will provide the ultimate democratizing force in the field of mental health by providing multiple and easily accessible venues for mental health support and treatment online. These new venues will not be necessarily tied to insurance and will be accessed whenever the consumer needs the support via whatever portable or stationary technological device, the consumer has at hand.

This chapter will examine two particular niche in the mental health field, crisis intervention, and information and referral services, two areas where mental health consumers have traditionally made a first step into the mental health system, and two areas that are especially adaptable to the online, new media environment. Traditionally, non-for-profit mental health agencies have provided these services, and because the non-for-profit sector is generally able to adapt to new models of service provision faster than establishment agencies connected to government, it is no surprise that they have also been the frontrunners in adapting mental health provision, online.

CrisisChat.org and e.MentalHealth.ca are examples of how crisis intervention and information and referral mental health services can adapt to the online, new media environment. Not only do these projects propose new technological platforms to provide these services, but they also are the frontrunners in providing training and standards to guide online service provision. These projects are described in detail in the upcoming chapter, as well as shown as examples for how online services can easily have national and international implications.

MENTAL HEALTH UNMET NEEDS

Unmet mental health needs to place a huge burden on our society. In any given year, it is estimated that 20% of individuals are affected by mental disorders (Regier et al., 1993).

According to the National Co-Morbidity Study, 57% of Americans will be diagnosed with a psychiatric disability over the course of their lifetimes. Among these disorders, anxiety disorders and substance abuse problems are most common. Within a given year, it is estimated that close to three in ten adults will have a psychiatric disability (NIMH). In younger populations, it is estimated that one in every five children and adolescents are affected by psychiatric disabilities.

While psychiatric disabilities are relatively common, about half of all people with psychiatric disabilities never receive treatment (Grant & Potenza, 2006). In the adolescent years, about 70% of adolescents never access treatment. At the same time, young people delay treatment for their mental health concerns; they are also more likely to have one. Many mental health difficulties, including suicidal behavior, depression, anxiety, and drug and alcohol use increase markedly in mid-to-late adolescence and young adulthood. Often, the delay between the onset of symptoms and the provision of effective treatments is 5–15 years. In this intervening time, mental health issues can become more persistent and occur in more serious forms by the time the adolescent becomes an adult (Swanson, Rosie, & Philipa, 2007).

THE INTERNET AND THE OPPORTUNITY FOR MENTAL HEALTH

Americans of all ages are engaging in "new media" more than ever and trends suggest that this engagement will continue to grow. Interventions using new media such as email, chat, messaging boards, social networking, and internet information platforms offer new solutions to the traditional barriers to accessing the mental health system.

In the last decade, Americans of all ages have adapted to a new communication landscape, one in which the internet prevails. According to a Pew Internet Research poll 93% of adolescents between the ages of 12–17 are online and 83% of young adults between the ages of 18–32 are online. In fact, internet usage has been increasing in all age groups, most dramatically in age groups 45+ (Jones & Fox, 2009).

Mobile technology has also revolutionized the ways we communicate, and never more so than with teenagers and text messaging. While in 2005, 51% of teens used texting to communicate, in 2009, a full 72% of teens used text messaging. One in three teenagers send more than 100 text messages per day, or 3000 text messages a month (Lenhart, Ling, Campbell & Purcell, 2010). Upward trends in texting are also found in all age groups, even in older adults as research suggests 35% of adults aged 55–64 using texting in 2009. In fact, the average U.S. mobile phone subscriber now sends and receives more text messages than voice calls (Lenhart, 2010).

Lastly, not only is society adapting these new media communications as broadband access continues to grow, but access to any services online will also grow. Seventy-seven percent of the American public between the ages of 12–54 had access to broadband technology in 2008 versus 49% in 2005 (Jones & Fox, 2009).

CASE STUDY BEFORE ONLINE ADAPTATION OF MENTAL HEALTH SERVICES

It is the year 2000. The Internet is still a young phenomenon, most people still use Windows 98, and Myspace, Facebook, Twitter do not yet exist.

Meet Robert, your average twenty-something college student who enjoys hanging out with his friends and who enjoys sports. But Robert has a secret . . . He is incredibly shy. So shy, that he can't raise his hand in class, out of fear of being embarrassed. In fact, he would rather skip class and receive a failing grade on a presentation, rather than have to speak in front of a class. He is so shy in fact, that he has never gone to a school dance, nor has he ever asked a girl out . . . Even with friends, family or his family doctor, there is no way that he'd tell them about his troubles . . .

Lately however, Robert discovers that alcohol seems to help his anxiety and shyness. It seems to really help him relax, and for a few weeks, he feels much more confident and even asks out a co-ed in his class. But what starts off as an occasional drink at social events quickly grows into daily drinking before classes. He suspects there might be something wrong, but doesn't know what to do about it.

By the final term of the school year, his grades have fallen to the point where he is failing most of his classes. And due to his antics while drunk, he has managed to lose all but one or two friends. Robert eventually drops out of school, telling himself that college "just wasn't for me".

What's wrong with Robert? Was he simply 'unmotivated' to get help? Or was there something else that could have been done to help him?

It is highly likely that Robert today will have access to broadband internet access. The barriers to access that Robert faced in first scenario, may be mitigated by the following present-day online tools:

Robert was unaware that he had a problem: free, online screening questionnaires for a variety of mental health problems can be found online, as information about mental health conditions can be offered online.

Robert didn't know where to go for help: online community resource directories make it easy for the general public and professionals alike to find information.

Robert didn't feel comfortable accessing "help" because of stigma and shame: The anonymity of using online support services helps to reduce embarrassment, making it easier and less threatening to make that first step in asking for help. An online emotional support chat line or a messaging board with posts specific to alcohol are examples of these types of services.

MOVING FACE-TO-FACE MENTAL HEALTH SERVICE PROVISION TO NEW MEDIA MODALITIES

The mental health field has historically strongly favored face-to-face approaches, for obvious reasons. Face-to-face therapy and support has been found to be highly effective. But, with the advent of new media technologies, it is incumbent to think beyond this traditional box and begin to investigate the effectiveness of new media modalities.

Not only is access improved with online outreach and intervention, but research in online mental health provision has also uncovered the following advantages over face-to-face, traditional approaches:

- Ambiguity of the Receiver — since the "helper" cannot be seen or heard, the "client" is less likely to experience the type of transference that may interfere with helpful communication (Gilat & Shahar, 2007).
- Lack of Distracting Environmental Factors — the client and helper are left to more clearly focus on the helping relationship (Gilat & Shahar, 2007).
- The "Online Disinhibition Effect" — the phenomenon documented soundly by mental health practitioners online which explains the tendency for high disclosure and the low inhibition of emotional expression in an online environment (Gilat & Shahar, 2007; Suler, 2004).

While there will always be a place for traditional face-to-face mental health service provision, online services can make it even easier for many people to make the first step into services as well as provide an alternative level of help that may seem more comfortable for some because of the above-mentioned factors.

In recent years, online mental health service provision, on a fee-for-service basis, has proliferated on the internet. Now, anyone who has internet access and the money to pay for it (online therapy is generally not paid for by insurance companies), can access an online therapist of their choice. The International Society for Mental Health Online (www.ismho. com) has grown into a thriving community for online therapists where information is shared on best practices, upcoming conferences, and links to the significant body of research compiled by these pioneers in online mental health service provision.

While online therapy seems to be a logical first step into the new communications landscape for the mental health field, online therapy does not truly capture the potential of new media and also is limited to those who can pay for it. CrisisChat.org and eMentalHealth.ca are additional examples that show how traditional mental health services can be adapted to new media to expand mental health service provision beyond what we would have thought was possible, beyond traditional therapist–client relationships and beyond fee-for-service contracts.

AN ONLINE ENTRY POINT TO MENTAL HEALTH SERVICES

CrisisChat.org and eMentalHealth.ca have taken existing mental health service systems and successfully transitioned them online. CrisisChat.org was built from the existing network of crisis call centers in the United States and Canada. eMentalHealth.ca was built from the resource directories that community mental health providers have traditionally maintained for their communities.

Taking the Crisis Hotline Online

Since the first telephone crisis line started in the United States in 1967, they have proliferated across the United States and the rest of the world. Crisis hotlines are credited with saving the lives of thousands of people, by being readily accessible in the moment of greatest need, at the moment when a person may be most despairing, closest to taking their life.

Crisis centers are often the initial link in the human service chain. Many other health and social service organizations turn to hotlines not only to handle their after-hours calls, but as the first step for clients entering their programs. Often, whether or not a person gets help can be determined by that first call to a hotline.

Despite their ability to help people in need, crisis centers can only do this if a person calls. Many crisis centers report that younger generations are not calling crisis lines in percentages proportionate to their population or their documented level of distress, as teenagers are likely to attempt suicide at rates higher than older age groups. Also, many people have shifted their preferred communication methods from the telephone to electronic means such as email, texting, discussion boards, and social networking and are simply not served by the traditional telephone helpline anymore.

Online crisis service provision can be an effective solution as it poses as a solution to reach people whom would otherwise not call a traditional telephone hotline, let alone access mental health services. Just as hotlines have been a conduit for helping many people into the formal mental health treatment system, as it is an easier, relatively nonthreatening first step, online crisis provision is likewise a stepping stone for a whole host of other people in distress who see even calling a hotline as a difficult first step.

Online crisis intervention services can also reach hard-to-reach populations. These may be populations that are traditionally difficult to engage in traditional mental health care, such as teenagers, the homebound, people with social anxieties and phobias, and people of all ages who view asking for help with stigma and shame. These populations may find that accessing online services is an easier first step.

But shouldn't the new media generation simply learn how to use "old media," like telephones? Interestingly enough, there was a time when crisis intervention and information and referral services (I&R) were provided only face to face. But, it was the development of the telephone which allowed this to shift toward telephone-based service. Similarly, just as there was a shift from face-to-face service delivery to telephone-based service delivery in the 1950s, if trends follow the same path there will a parallel shift to new media, never replacing the old method of service provision, but merely adding a new dimension and point of access, congruent with modern communication venues.

Pioneers in Online Emotional Support

Online crisis services first began with the Samaritans UK in 1994 through email. Since this time, various entrepreneurial crisis centers, both large and small, across the globe have begun offering some sort of online direct service, including, but not limited to: SAHAR, Israel; The Low Down, New

Zealand; The National Veterans Chat Line, USA; Lifeline, Rochester, NY, USA; The Crystal Cathedral, California, USA; The Rape and Incest Support Network (RAINN), USA; The Trevor Project, USA; Boys Town, USA; Kids Crisis Link, Vancouver, Canada; The Support Network, Edmonton, Canada.

These centers have largely been pioneers in the new practice of providing crisis services online, moving forward with the service despite skeptics who have questioned the effectiveness of providing services online. In fact, these centers have found that the services are very effective. In the experience of SAHAR, based in Israel, for example, not only are hundreds of people given support each day, but successful rescue has also been sent to many people on the verge of attempting suicide. The basic premise that the internet can be successfully exploited to provide suicide prevention services has been demonstrated by the success of these centers (Barak, 2007). These online crisis centers also report widely that the people who reach out are able to express themselves very openly in online venues. Research in online mental health provision has documented the online disinhibition effect, previously mentioned, which describes the tendency of people to open up more and say more about themselves online than in a phone or face-to-face (f2f) interaction. The outpouring of emotional and situational details by users of online support services may in fact point to increased effectiveness of online support services over phone or f2f interactions. Continued research may more clearly document the differences in effectiveness between different modes of communication.

In addition, these pioneering centers have reported that volume of service is steady, and in some cases outstripped the ability of the center to keep up with online demand. The Samaritans UK, for example, began offering text-based crisis service in 2004 and by 2007 stopped advertising it because of the outstanding demand for the service. The Low Down, NZ, in another case example, began chat services in 2008 and after 12 months of service had to double staff size to keep up with demand. SAHAR, Israel, has also chosen not to market its service on social networking sites because increased marketing on such a popular platforms may increase service demand beyond the current ability to provide service.

Advantages of a Full Service Web Platform

One of the distinct advantages to offering mental health crisis services online is that multiple levels of service can be offered via a website platform. These levels can be both passive service provision (search for information, reading of blog, and messaging boards) and interactive (posting, texting, chatting, contributing to messaging boards, and submitting art, poems, or video to an online community, etc.). Service can also be provided directly (via chat, email, or text with a counselor) or indirectly (messaging boards, information, blogs, etc.). The ability to offer differing levels of service may be what encourages someone to accept help for the first time. The following are examples of websites that offer support and intervention in varying methods online.

Examples of innovative sites targeted toward youth include:

- Reachout.com is an initiative of the Inspire USA Foundation and launched in March 2010. The idea for such a website was brought to the USA from Australia as the result of a similarly successful site in that country. Reachout.com has been largely promoted by the Substance Abuse and Mental Health Services Administration (SAMHSA). The site offers information on mental health concerns to youth in a non-judgmental and safe atmosphere. Information is offered on topics such as family issues, relationship problems, depression, and more. It features major sections titled, "Hear From Others Who Have Been There and Made It," "Help Yourself," "Help a Friend," and "Help Others." Through these tabs, both information and interactive discussion boards can be accessed. Inspirational stories of young people who have been through tough times but have recovered abound on the site, via text and video stories. Video from the SAMHSA supported "WeCanHelpUs" national campaign also is embedded in the website, creating another venue for positive, inspiring messaging, encouraging young people to access help.
- MindYourMind.ca, offers similar positive messaging and information services online for youth, and is based in Canada. From its home page, the main tabs are "Reach Out," "Get Help," and "Give Help." The site also contains inspiring stories of youth struggling with mental health issues as well as a place to view artwork created by youth expressing painful emotions and mental health struggles. Youth are also asked to submit artwork and stories, becoming creators of the site.

Both sites offer significant content that speak to youth. There are other sites throughout the world that offer similar positive messaging and inspiring stories and a platform for youth, many of them with excellent graphics and design that really speak to youth. Most of these platforms do not, as of yet, combine an option for direct contact with a counselor.

SAHAR and the Low Down are good examples of "full service" mental health platforms, offering both the types of information and interactivity offered in the above platforms as well as the option to directly connect with a counselor for support.

- SAHAR (www.sahar.org.il), the online crisis service in Israel, has also been offering multiple levels of service since its inception in 2001, in Hebrew. SAHAR offers synchronous (instant messaging) and asynchronous (discussion boards) options for communication as well as information for people in need. It may be less threatening for a person in distress to access information the first time they access the site, but they may come back later for a chat/email session. This makes online crisis services more dynamic and flexible, able to reach a diverse range of people, some who may not be ready to directly reach out, but still can benefit from the positive messages, educational materials, and resources posted on a website.
- The Low Down: (www.thelowdown.co.nz) is an initiative of the Ministry of Health in New Zealand. It offers a very friendly website interface where talking actors and actresses actually welcome visitors to the site if you click on them. The actors then continue to lead visitors throughout the site, introducing them to site options where visitors can learn about depression or about what to do if you or someone else you know is depressed or in imminent danger. Another tab leads to an area where visitors can choose to register for chat or view/write on a messaging board. Short video clips of the online counselors giving personal introductions and a welcome to the service are available to view so that visitors may feel more comfortable talking with a counselor. Lastly, a large section of the site is devoted to testimonial videos of other young people, many of whom are celebrities, talking about their own struggles with depression and success in overcoming it. The entire site has a wonderfully welcoming and fun feel to it that successfully defeats feelings of stigma or shame in accessing services.

CRISISCHAT.ORG: BUILDING A FULL-SERVICE MENTAL HEALTH PLATFORM

As with SAHAR and Low Down, CrisisChat.org is a full-service online crisis site that will offer service via direct, indirect, passive, and active options. People accessing the site will be able to pick and choose among these interventions based on their own comfort level as well as need, perhaps visiting the site the first time for information and the second time to talk to a chat specialist.

CrisisChat.org is a project of CONTACT USA, a national crisis center accreditation organization which provides standards and technical support for crisis centers across the United States. CONTACT USA has firmly established buy-in and interest in the project from crisis call centers throughout its existing network and within the overlapping crisis center networks of the National Suicide Prevention Lifeline and the American Association of Suicidology. CONTACT USA has provided seed funding for the project and is currently seeking national foundation funding to launch a national office that would assist call centers around the county with the technical expertise in how to transition center operations from hotline-based service to hotline and online-based services.

The CrisisChat.org project will link crisis call centers throughout the United States onto one universal platform and provide technical assistance to help them, "take the crisis hotline, online." CrisisChat.org is a practice demonstration project. It establishes the first ever national website platform which all crisis hotline centers can join to provide easy, consistent access to crisis intervention and emotional support services to any American with internet access via computer or mobile device. The project will also establish the first ever codified guidance to crisis centers on how to provide online services. New service provision standards, guidelines for operations, materials on how to train staff and volunteers, and advice on how to handle questions regarding liabilities and intervention procedures, have been produced by CONTACT USA. Additionally, CONTACT USA will provide centers with consults, materials, and statistics that may assist local centers in securing funding for the new online service provision.

The initial pilot of the project began in the Summer of 2010, with two primary crisis center partners: United Way 2-1-1/CONTACT Lifeline in Albany, NY, a program of Family and Children's Service of the Capital Region, and Austin Travis County Integral Care in Austin, TX. Centers in Arkansas, Louisiana, and Delaware are also poised to join the portal to provide service to their areas of the county. Additional centers throughout the United States will be added onto this portal until there is a crisis center that services every part of the county, to anyone in need of service as long as they access the services from a computer from an IP address within the United States.

The CrisisChat.org platform will start out by offering chat service, a mental health library, and mental health screening tools. In the future, the site plans to offer multiple, direct, and interactive service options, including, but not limited to: individual chat, email, texting, and support on social networking sites, and mental health screening tools.

CrisisChat.org will offer indirect and passive methods of accessing help that may complement the direct service options mentioned above or be used as a first step to seeking service. These include a mental health library and local resource database, which will be powered by eMental-Health.ca and will be explained at length in the following section.

EMENTALHEALTH.CA: KNOWLEDGE IS EMPOWERMENT

The website eMentalHealth.ca (eMH) was created in 2005, and makes it easy for consumers and professionals to find out anything and everything about mental health. eMH was initially launched in Ottawa as a pilot project. Following a successful launch, eMH was quickly approached by partners in other communities, interested in having eMH for their local areas. The database includes national mental health organizations, as well as provincial resources for every province in Canada. The crucial and unique aspect of eMH is its partnerships with local communities to populate local mental health-specific databases. Currently, eMental-Health.ca covers a growing number of regions in Ontario and British Columbia, with expansions planned elsewhere.

eMentalHealth is an initiative of the Provincial Centre of Excellence for Child and Youth Mental Health, which in turn is funded by the Ministry of Child and Youth Services, of the government of Ontario, Canada. eMentalHealth.ca has received favorable feedback in the Canadian mental health community and government, including praise in the Parliament of Canada (Jaffer, 2006), and accolades in a Health Canada report which recommended eMentalHealth as a "Canadian best practice [to] be funded to expand this portal service across Canada" (Leitch, 1997).

The main components of eMentalHealth.ca are:

- Local mental health resource directories which contain information about mental health services in a local community. A visually pleasing clickable directory of resources is easily searchable by simply clicking on headings. Although Information and Referral (I & R) services such as 2-1-1 exist to provide general mental health resource information, eMH provides more specialized MH resource information (such as names of individual providers and their specialties).
- A "Mental Health Library" contains a series of articles about mental health topics which have been written and reviewed by professionals and

mental health consumers alike. Knowledge is power, as the old saying goes. However, knowledge can also bring empowerment. Studies have shown that people who have good "mental health literacy" are more knowledgeable about their health and their mental health will have superior outcomes compared to those who are not (Jorm et al., 1997).

■ Easy-to-use screening tools for common mental health disorders, that use validated screening questionnaires. If a person is wondering if he or a client has post-traumatic stress disorder (PTSD), they can simply fill out the backend screening questionnaire and if enough items are positive, then the scored questionnaire can be printed out and taken with the patient to see a health professional.

■ A calendar of local mental health-themed events.

■ Mental health news, a selection of main news items relating to mental health.

■ A google style search box, which makes it easy to search by keyword for all the content on the site. A smart parser allows the user to type in synonyms, but which will still map to the correct target term.

While the mental health information pages, screening, and other tools are consistent regardless of geography, the dynamic portion of eMH is the local, mental health-specific resource database. The databases are built off of existing paper or electronic resource directories that already exist in communities throughout Canada (and soon as well in the United States). eMentalHealth.ca's local "community partner," could be a mental health clinic, a mental health advocacy group, a crisis center or an existing 2-1-1 service. The community partner agrees to be the agency that is responsible for populating and updating the resource database for its community. This method uses the power of internet technologies to improve upon what they always have done, providing mental health resource information to the community.

Information for the resource database is migrated from existing directories into the new online, dynamic directory. Once in the eMentalHealth.ca directory, the information is available to the public. Not only is the service name, description, and contact information included in the profile, but a Google map also shows alongside the profile for the ease of use. Additionally, if the information is incorrect or needs updating, a simple online form (that can be filled out by anyone) is available to submit to an administrator of the community partner for the verification of source and validity. In this way, the community is empowered to make corrections and additions to the resource database and it truly becomes a dynamic, user-created platform, similar to Wikipedia or other online platforms that harness the power of collective wisdom.

The database is also easily accessible from one universal national portal (eMentalHealth.ca or eMentalHealth.us), similar to CrisisChat.org's national portal. A user from any area of either country simply clicks on a map of the country to indicate the locality in which they would like to search for information. Clicking on a local city from a list brings the online mental health consumer to a local page.

Database Maintenance

The idea of a database of mental health services and resources is not new, but in practice, it is generally an expensive, laborious, and resource-intensive process to set up and maintain a database. What is the secret?

- Low-cost, custom-built database using open-source technology (i.e., MySQL/PHP). Compared to proprietary database software, it is an ideal solution for nonprofit organizations, as any community can use the system without having to pay commercial licensing fees.
- The database is accessed online via a web browser, without needing any software to be installed on a computer. Thus, as long as the local administrator has internet access, the database can be managed from anywhere.
- Distributed content management. Since local community partners know their resources the best, it is they who manage their local database. In most cases, these are local partners who already had their own list or database of mental health services. eMentalHealth.ca. thus, represents an easier way for them to keep their resources up to date online, as well as giving them the opportunity to make their resources available for the community. This further benefits the agency by enhancing their presence in the community. Rarely is there any one single community partner that knows all resources; many communities have multiple partners who administer the database, thus distributing the workload. Because front line service providers at these agencies regularly use eMentalHealth.ca, there is further added incentive to ensure the information is up to date.

eMentalHealth.ca as an Evidence-Based Health Informatics Intervention

Although the idea of making information available online appears intuitive, is there evidence that this is a helpful practice? Consumer health informatics is a field that, "analyzes consumers' needs for information and studies and implements methods of making information accessible to consumers" (Eysenbach, 2000). Evidence in the field of health literacy shows that health outcomes are superior when people have good "health literacy," which is knowledge about health and wellness, and how to take care of one's medical health.

Though there is a shortage of research in the specific area of mental health informatics, the consensus nonetheless is that consumers are very satisfied with easy access to health information, and there are no studies that demonstrate any evidence of harm (Gibbons et al., 2009). Furthermore, medical health information on eMentalHealth.ca. is written by a multidisciplinary team of health professionals (including consumer input) in accordance with recognized health literacy guidelines such as using plain language.

CASE STUDY AFTER THE ADAPTATION OF ONLINE MENTAL HEALTH SERVICES

Let's meet Robert again, but this time, let's imagine him in an alternate universe. Robert is your average twenty-something college student, but this time, it is the year 2012 rather than year 2000. Twitter and Google are used as verbs, even middle school students have Facebook, and your great grandmother Betty knows what email is.

Robert has troubles with severe anxiety, and has discovered that alcohol appears to help.

Website: Thanks to a Facebook friend, he learns about an alcohol/ mental health website tagged by a friend on her Facebook page. He gets onto the site and finds that there is an information sheet on "substance abuse." He finds it interesting to learn that binge drinking on the weekend is considered a substance abuse problem.

Self-assessment test: He clicks on the, "Wondering if you might have an alcohol problem?" link and takes a quick, validated screening questionnaire for alcohol use problems. In a matter of seconds, he learns that "You may have problems with alcohol use," and the page gives a listing of local mental health and addictions services. "See a counselor? No way!" but he is intrigued enough to keep surfing around the site, comfortable in the anonymity and privacy of his room.

Discussion board: He sees the discussion boards on the site, and reads one specifically on college drinking. He reads questions and comments from other college students who are facing or have faced similar challenges. He is surprised to find that one posting is from a younger man, in his late 20's who is offering support to a young woman who is struggling with a drinking problem. The man talks about how he hid his drinking problem for years in college, under the veil of his collegial successes, including high grades and high performance as a scholarship athlete. This man reminds Robert of himself! He is shocked but also inspired to do things differently.

Chat now: Robert notices a prominent "chat now" button on the site and decides, "hey, what the heck, let's just give this a try ... After all, no one will know its me!" He clicks on the chat button and after providing some basic info, he ends up chatting with a chat specialist named, "Nikki" from the crisis center that serves his area. He starts out by simply asking the chat specialist what she thinks he should do. When she kindly tells him that she cannot give direct advice but then asks him what he is concerned about, Robert begins to open up. Feeling safe in the anonymity of the chat, he tells Nikki about his longstanding problems with anxiety, worsened by the pressures of college. He tells her about his discovery that alcohol appeared to help in the beginning, but that now it has gotten out of control to the point where he may have to drop out of school. He tells about his fear of disappointing his parents, who have worked hard all their lives just in order to send him to school. The chat specialist validates his concerns.

Robert is a 20 year old male, more common that you'd imagine. He is not someone who would ever call a hotline that he believes is for people who are really messed up. He is also not someone who would call his college health center to schedule a counseling appointment.

But, over the course of a month, Robert found himself back on the website, chatting with a chat specialist at all hours of the night. More than once, at 2 a.m., he found himself despondent, regretful, alone and drunk in his dorm room and also found himself accessing the site again and chatting with a specialist. Through these interactions, Robert felt safe because the chat specialist couldn't see him and didn't even know his real name. Robert logged in for chat anonymously each time and when asked what his name was by the chat specialist, gave the pseudonym of "Tom." While on chat, the specialists with whom Robert interacted offered him compassion and acceptance at a time when he was desperately disappointed in himself and felt ashamed and alone in his struggle with depression and increasing substance abuse. The chat specialists encouraged Robert to access formal help and offered him referrals to mental health and substance abuse counselors several times.

Breakthrough: Although hesitant in the beginning, thanks to the trust built up through his chat sessions, Robert finally agrees to see a counselor on campus. Even so, he continues to rely on the chat service sporadically, in addition to seeing his live counselor.

In this way, through a simple link on Facebook, Robert, a college student who was completely uneducated regarding his own struggles with mental health and substance abuse, not only learned about his own issues and was able to maintain his sense of privacy and dignity in doing so, was also able to establish a non-threatening connection with chat specialists who assisted him (to his surprise) in his darkest hours. While Robert would have been one of the least likely candidates to accept help at the college counseling center, he came to understand that he needed help and also came to realize that accepting help felt good and it was worth it to make an effort to start seeing a counselor.

And how is Robert doing now? Thanks to his counselor, Robert finds a healthier way to manage his anxiety and stress, without needing alcohol. He manages to stay in school, graduates with honors, and goes on to contribute to society in a meaningful way. The simple presence of a Facebook tag and a "CHAT NOW" button on a website helped to bring Robert to this healthier place.

CONCLUSION

Robert's final outcome is assisted by not only the presence of a simple chat button, but also by an initial connection via a place he often visits, Facebook. In addition, the range of options for him to engage, from information on drinking to messaging boards to live chat, all help him engage in a "service" that he does not see as a "service." While he is intuitively following his own lead, first from information then to a screening tool, and next to a messaging board and chat, he is deciding how he will receive help at every turn, and doing it in a way that feels comfortable to him. While he may not see this as a service, as it does not look or feel like one in the traditional sense, truly the sum of all the ways he engaged in his search for help can be seen as the "intervention" or "treatment" provided.

The power of mental health services provided in new media formats can be great and far reaching, moving beyond many traditional barriers to accessing care. All online service options are helpful individually but the sum of the parts can equal a powerful whole. With online mental health service options, the opportunity to meet the historically unmet mental health needs of society suddenly becomes closer to possible.

When the mental health establishment begins to expand the notion of "mental health treatment" to a combination of online "interventions," including but not limited to, crisis chat service, the sharing of poems and art on emotional turmoil, the exchange of experiences on a message board or a moderated group chat room, and the perusal of information on disorders online, the mental health field will truly understand and witness the power of harnessing new media. When the mental health establishment recognizes that meeting the consumer where they are at means providing services that can be accessed via computers and hand-held mobile devices, the consumers will be best served. When these shifts in consciousness occur, and funding priorities follow suit, these new approaches will be invested in by both the private and public sectors and will prove to have far-reaching positive impacts on the mental health wellness of our society.

REFERENCES

Eysenbach, G. (2000). Consumer health informatics. *British Medical Journal, 320,* 1713–1716.

Gibbons, M. C., Wilson, F., Samal, L., Dickersin, K., Lehmann, H., Aboumatar, H., Finkelstein, J., Shelton, E., Ritu, S., & Bass, E. (2009). *Impact of consumer health informatics applications.* Evidence Report/Technology Assessment No. 188. (Prepared by Johns Hopkins University Evidence-based Practice Center under contract No. HHSA 290-2007-10061-I). AHRQ Publication no. 09(10)-E019. Rockville, MD. Agency for Healthcare Research and Quality, October 2009.

Gilat, I., & Shahar, G. (2007). Emotional first aid for a suicide crisis: Comparison between telephonic hotline and internet. *Psychiatry, 70*(1), 12–18.

Grant, J. E., & Potenza, M. N (2006). In J. Sydney, & S. Fox (Eds.), *Textbook of men's mental health.* APA Publishing (January 28, 2009).

Jaffer, M. (October 10, 2006). Speech to the Senate, Parliament of Canada, Ottawa, ON, Canada. Retrieved May 10, 2010, from http://www.parl.gc.ca/39/1/parlbus/chambus/senate/deb-E/033db_2006-10-03-e.htm?Language=E&Parl=39&Ses=1

Jones, S., & Fox, S. (January 28, 2009). Generations Online in 2009. The Pew Research Center's Internet & American Life Project. Retrieved from www.pewinternet.org, October 14, 2010.

Jorm, A. F., Korten, A. E., Jacomb, P. A., Christensen, H., Rodgers, B., & Pollitt, P. (1997). Mental health literacy: A survey of the public's ability to recognise mental disorders and their beliefs about the effectiveness of treatment. *Medical Journal of Australia, 166*(4), 182–186.

Leitch, K. (1997). *Reaching for the top: A report by the Advisor on healthy child & youth.* Ottawa: Health Canada.

Lenhart, A., Ling, R., Campbell, S., & Purcell, K. (April 20, 2010). Teens, cell phones and texting: Text messaging becomes centerpiece communication. Pew Internet and American Life Project. Retrieved from http://www.pewinternet.org/Reports/2010/Teens-and-Mobile-Phones.aspx

Lenhart, A. (September 2, 2010). Cell phone and American Adults. Pew Internet and American Life Project. Retrieved from http://www.pewinternet.org/Reports/2010/Cell-Phones-and-American-Adults.aspx

National Co-Morbidity Study. Retrieved from http://www.hcp.med.harvard.edu/ncs/ftpdir/table_ncsr_LTprevgenderxage.pdf

Nielson Mobile (September 2008). Retrieved from http://www.bizreport.com/2008/09/nielsen_ mobile_texting_vs_talking.html

Regier, D. A., Narrow, W. E., Rae, D. S., Manderscheid, R. W., Locke, B. Z., & Goodwin, F. K. (1993). The *de facto* US mental and addictive disorders service system. Epidemiologic Catchment Area prospective 1-year prevalence rates of disorders and services. *Archives of General Psychiatry, 50,* 85–94.

SAMHSA's National Mental Health Information Center Retrieved from http://mentalhealth.samhsa.gov/publications/allpubs/CA-0006/default.asp

Suler, J. (2004). *The psychology of cyberspace.* Book published online www.usr.edu/~suler/psycyber/disinhibit.html

Swanson, R., & Collin, P. (2007). Engaging, understanding and including young people in the provision of mental health services. *International Journal of Adolescent Medical Health, 19*(3), 325–332.

CHAPTER NINETEEN

Health Literacy and Human Services Delivery

Sandra A. Smith

Health literacy matters. While definitions abound, health literacy is recognized as the currency that enables adults to obtain the benefits of the health-care system, to take care of themselves and others, and to exert some control over their health and its determinants.

The U.S. Institute of Medicine has described the nation's vision for a health literate society in which people have the skills to use information to improve health behaviors and participate in health care; and health systems provide clear information along with support to facilitate health promoting practices (Nielsen-Bohlman, Panzer, & Kindig, 2004; Healthy People, 2020; U.S. Department of Health, 2009). The national public health objectives for the decade supports this vision and sets the challenge to "improve the health literacy of the population." This objective represents a significant evolution in health literacy research and practice. The original objective set in 2000 was to "improve the health literacy of persons with low literacy skills" (U.S. Department of Health and Human Services, 2009, HC/HIT-1). The update integrates research showing that achieving health literacy presents a complex challenge, not only to patients with reading difficulty, but also to all who seek health and all who provide health and human services.

This chapter explores the meaning, measure, and practice of health literacy, with particular attention to its implications for vulnerable populations and those who serve them. The intention is to assist the reader in navigating through differing conceptual models of health literacy, their attendant research approaches, and intended outcomes of intervention. This chapter first examines the clinical approach that dominates health literacy research and practice in the United States and focuses on patients in the health-care system. The chapter then describes a broader emerging health promotion approach to health literacy that may be more relevant for vulnerable populations with limited access and participation in the health-care system and for social services providers working in community settings. It should be emphasized that these different approaches are not mutually exclusive, but, rather, complementary. Both are important and necessary to achieve the vision of a health literate society. A multidimensional approach to addressing health literacy through social service programs will improve program design and service.

THE MEANING OF HEALTH LITERACY

The multiple disciplines involved in health literacy research and practice have not achieved a standard lexicon. In research articles, government reports, news media, and industry white papers, terms related to literacy and health literacy have been used imprecisely and interchangeably. This is not surprising since the terms "health" and "literacy" are understood differently within and across disciplines, and their meanings change with time and place to reflect society and culture. To clarify the subsequent discussion, consider the evolving meanings of *functional literacy* and *functional health literacy*.

Functional Literacy

Traditionally, the term "functional literacy" refers to basic cognitive skills taught in school, the three Rs, "Reading, 'riting, and 'rithmetic." These fundamental literacy skills are functional in that they enable a person to acquire knowledge about any subject, and so, it is presumed, to function in any social context. In this limited view, literacy is viewed narrowly as the ability to read and write. It is considered a fixed individual trait unrelated to context, social support, or resources. While literacy scholars have since defined additional categories or advanced levels of literacy and the term "functional literacy" has taken on deeper meaning and purpose for the Information Age, the term typically describes the fundamental literacy skill set—the traditional three Rs.

Multiple Functional Literacies

The National Literacy Act of 1991 marked a significant evolution in the meaning of "literacy" for U.S. adults. The legislation recognized that the three Rs which enabled people to function adequately during a simpler time are insufficient to participate in the information economy, particularly in health and social services, with their complex, highly technical, and rapidly changing knowledge base, logic, language, and culture.

> Literacy means ... ability to read, write, and speak in English, and compute and solve problems at levels of proficiency necessary to *function on the job and in society, to achieve one's goals, and develop one's knowledge and potential.* [emphasis added] (National Literacy Act of 1991, Public Law 102-73)

This understanding of adult literacy in the Information Age reflects literacy scholars' broader, more practical, sociocultural view in which literacy is shaped within social practices and relies on critical reflection to make meaning from information and apply it in context. From this perspective, literacy always is used for some practical purpose (function), and involves social interaction. Over time, with need, opportunity, and resources, a person may develop *multiple functional literacies* at different levels of proficiency (Culligan, 2005). For example, an individual may attain proficient computer literacy as an office worker and moderate financial literacy to manage the family budget, while demonstrating low functional health literacy for using the health-care system and maintaining personal, family, and community health.

Traditionally, functional literacy has meant being able to read and write and use numbers. In the Information Age, being functionally literate means putting into practice, in real-life situations, a wide range of cognitive and noncognitive skills, including communications, problem solving, interpersonal, and lifelong-learning skills in order to participate in society and exert control over one's life.

THE CLINICAL APPROACH: LOW HEALTH LITERACY AS A CLINICAL RISK

Clinical research interest in health literacy grew out of National Literacy Act of 1991, which funded the National Adult Literacy Survey (NALS) to assess the literacy skills of U.S. adults. Health literacy studies initially appeared in the medical literature shortly after the NALS results, published in 1993, showed widespread low functional literacy among U.S. adults. NALS did not intend to set standards for adequate adult literacy and was not designed to comment on what skills adults need to function in general or in any particular context. Rather, NALs was designed to estimate the literacy skills demonstrated by adults at the time. Still, in the first decade of health literacy research, standards were inferred and it was widely reported that "half the adult population lacks the literacy skills necessary to utilize the healthcare system." This interpretation of NALS results as standards of adult literacy by the media and experts in many fields generated significant controversy, is not substantiated by the evidence, but nonetheless still prevails (National Academy of Sciences and National Research Council, 2005).

Most health literacy studies have been conducted since 1993 in academic medical centers in the biomedical research model. Reports focus on *low* health literacy as a risk to patients and health-care systems. Low health literacy is viewed as limited ability to comprehend medical and health-care information transmitted from experts to patients and is attributed to inadequate basic literacy skills. Thus, low health literacy has been treated as a cognitive deficit in patients, which clinicians need to identify and manage. This line of research has associated low reading skill in a clinical setting with medication errors, unnecessary testing and treatment, poor outcomes, high health-care costs, and inequities in access and outcomes.

The 2003 National Assessment of Adult Literacy (NAAL) showed little change in literacy levels in the decade since the 1992 NALS. This follow-up survey included questions related to health and health care that were used to estimate the level of health literacy in adults. Results showed 88% of the population with "less than proficient" health literacy skills, suggesting only about 12% of adults could comprehend most printed information about health and health care. This finding confirmed nearly 300 studies showing that the complexity and specialized vocabulary of most medical and health care information exceeds the literacy skills of intended readers.

CLINICAL MEASURES OF HEALTH LITERACY DRIVE RESEARCH

The perceived need to identify patients with low literacy skills continues to drive research; the majority of studies have pursued clinically feasible tests to identify patients with limited literacy skills, particularly inability read medical terms and to comprehend health-care documents (e.g., medication labels, patient bill of rights, appointment slips, informed consent, and disease information).

Nearly all health literacy research has used one of two reading tests to measure health literacy. (1) The Rapid Assessment of Adult Literacy in Medicine (REALM) is a medical word recognition test published in 1993 (Davis et al., 1991), (2) the Test of Functional Health Literacy in Adults, the TOFHLA, published in 1995, is a comprehension test using health-care documents (Parker, Baker, Williams, & Nurss, 1995). Research using these measures led to the most commonly used definition of health literacy published by the National Library of Medicine in 2000: several years after these reading tests became the accepted measures of health literacy.

> [Health literacy is] the ... capacity to obtain, process, and understand basic health information and services needed to make appropriate health decisions.
> — *U.S. Department of Health and Human Services, 2000*

In the quest for quick standardized screening tests, research has dropped the function from functional health literacy and shifted the focus back to basic technical skills and simple one-time reading skills tests using medical vocabulary and documents. This approach simplified the measurement of health literacy, a benefit for research, but limited the understanding of health literacy to reading in a clinical setting. Further, testing patients' literacy skills has been shown to induce shame and alienation in participants, with no offsetting benefits (Paasche-Orlow & Wolf, 2008).

HEALTH LITERACY INTERVENTIONS

Since health literacy has been framed and measured as ability to comprehend information from experts, health literacy practice has aimed at increasing patients' comprehension by reducing the cognitive demand of information and its delivery. Systems-level efforts to improve health and medical information have been part of a larger national Plain Language Movement that started in federal agencies following passage of the National Literacy Act of 1991 and is gaining popularity across the country as a means to increase compliance, safety, and consumer satisfaction in diverse arenas. Plain language has been supported as a matter of civil rights in several court cases, leading the majority of states to enact plain language laws. These policy-making activities illustrate the importance of efforts to improve health and medical information as well as public health messaging and disaster preparedness information.

Plain language and information improvement constitute a fundamental step toward a health literate society, but must be viewed as a partial solution. Information improvement strategies to address low literacy in patients presume that information equates to knowledge and that knowledge is all that patients need in order to maintain, regain, or promote health. This assumption contradicts theories of health education and behavior change.

Health literacy intervention studies are relatively rare. Most have examined the effect of improved information or its delivery on health knowledge and found mixed results. Limitations in study design, interventions tested, and outcomes assessed make it difficult to draw conclusions about the effectiveness of reported health literacy interventions. A clear association between low literacy and adverse health outcomes has been established. However, it remains unclear whether the association is mainly direct (meaning that outcomes would be improved by interventions designed to overcome limited reading skill, or by promoting other skills) or indirect (so that interventions addressing underlying causes such as poverty, racism and lack of access to care would be more effective). Reviewers have called for more rigorous methods and attention to important, longer-term health outcomes that matter to patients and families (e.g., tasks required for effective self-care and ability to perform those tasks). Three promising areas for continued efforts to improve health in persons with low reading skill are (1) access to and utilization of health care, (2) patient–provider interaction, and (3) self-management of disease, particularly chronic conditions.

CONTRIBUTIONS AND LIMITATIONS OF THE CLINICAL APPROACH TO HEALTH LITERACY

Clinical research on health literacy has improved access to health information for both skilled and unskilled readers. It has brought health literacy to local, state, national, industry, and professional agendas. Still, some scholars argue that the prevailing conceptualization and measurement of health literacy are too limited to achieve the vision of a health literate society. Critics suggest that beyond comprehension of health information, comprehensive research would require attention to cultural, social, political, and economic factors, and life skills. Frustration with lack of progress has led to discourse about the conceptual foundation of health literacy, alternative measures, and new directions for intervention (American College of Physicians Foundation (American College of Physicians and Institute of Medicine, 2008); Institute of Medicine (Institute of Medicine, 2009)).

THE HEALTH PROMOTION APPROACH: HEALTH LITERACY AS A PERSONAL AND COMMUNITY ASSET

An alternative approach to health literacy research and practice is documented primarily in the international public health literature, particularly in Canada, Australia, and the United Kingdom. The health promotion approach views health literacy as the ability to use information and services in ways that enhance health (Nutbeam, 1998; U.S. Department of Health and Human Services, 2000). In this approach, health literacy is seen as a personal and community asset to be promoted by developing people's interpersonal, social, and reflective ability to personalize relevant information and apply it in context for personal benefit. The model is applicable in both clinical and community settings. This asset-building approach to health literacy may be more relevant for social service providers who serve medically underserved populations in community settings.

The health promotion approach uses the World Health Organization's (WHO) definition of health literacy:

> Health literacy represents the cognitive and social skills which determine the motivation and ability of individuals to gain access to, understand and use information in ways which promote and maintain good health.
> —*Nutbeam, 1998, p. 358*

The WHO document goes on to say,

> Health literacy implies the achievement of a level of knowledge, personal skills, and confidence to take action to improve personal and community health by changing personal lifestyles and living conditions. Thus, health literacy means more than being able to read pamphlets and make appointments. By improving people's access to health information and their capacity to use it effectively, health literacy is critical to empowerment.
> —*Nutbeam, 1998, p. 357*

This definition takes a functional view. It is concerned with how people integrate information into their lives in order to maintain, regain, or promote health. In accordance with health promotion theory and practice, the goal of this approach to health literacy is to enable people to exert greater control over their personal, family, and community health and the factors that shape health (Nutbeam, 2008). This overarching goal is fundamentally different from the clinical goal of overcoming cognitive deficits in patients in order to improve their health and ensure efficiency in the system.

The health promotion approach incorporates additional categories or advanced levels of health literacy (Nutbeam, 2000), theories of health promotion and health education, and the concept of multiple functional literacies described above. The next section explores the levels or types of health literacy.

LEVELS OR TYPES OF HEALTH LITERACY

Literacy scholars describe three categories or levels of literacy that have been usefully applied to health literacy (Nutbeam, 2000). These are typically labeled (a) functional (basic, three Rs); (b) interactive (social); and (c) reflective health literacy. A reader could infer from the labels that the advanced health literacy skills (interaction and reflection) are not functional; that is, they are not necessary in order to function adequately in the health arena. However, the previously discussed concept of multiple functional literacies extends the idea of skills-enabling function to the array of health literacy skills so that more skills and more developed skills lead to more options and opportunities to enhance health. In this way, improved health literacy skills enable improved health functioning, for example, attitudes, actions, behaviors, and practices related to health. The following is a description of levels of health literacy.

Functional health literacy: Basic health literacy skills (the three Rs) are seen as "functional" in that they are assumed to enable a person to function at a minimal level in health-care contexts, for example, to read a brochure, find an appointment time in a document, and comply with prescribed behaviors. The prevailing approach to health literacy is limited to the basic level. The fundamental health literacy skills are useful; they are not necessary to engage in interactive and reflective health literacy.

Interactive health literacy refers to social skills such as speaking and listening needed for more complex health and health-care practices such as obtaining a referral or consulting with professionals. Individuals use interaction to make meaning from information, apply it in context for personal benefit, and gain experience. People use well-developed interactive skills to compensate for limited ability to read, write, and use numbers. A few studies have begun to address one aspect of interaction by experimenting with measuring "oral literacy" in order to identify patients with limited ability to comprehend spoken instructions (Downey & Zun, 2007).

Reflective health literacy (Freebody & Luke, 1990; Freire, 1994; McCaffrey, Merrifield, & Millican, 2007) refers to higher-order literacy skills such as synthesis and analysis used to exert control over one's health and health practices, for example, to evaluate risk, to weigh treatment options and lifestyle choices, and to change behavior. Using reflection to enhance health may or may not involve reading. Some literacy scholars (Charner-Laird, Fiarman, Park, Soderber, & Nunes, 2003) describe reflection as "the mind's strongest glue" for making connections essential for understanding, regardless of subject matter. They categorize reflection as a basic skill, one of the "four Rs": reading, "riting," rithmetic, and reflection.

Smith and Wollesen (2004) have described reflection as a repeating process of *Think, Link and Respond*. This three-part process of reflection corresponds to the three levels or categories of functional health literacy. Basic skills, the three Rs, are used for *thinking*, to understand health issues and information. Interactive skills (speaking and listening) are used for *linking*, to make meaning from information in real life contexts; and reflective skills (synthesis, analysis) are used to formulate a *response*, to decide what to do with the information. These theories suggest that interactive and reflective skills are as important as reading in the process of understanding health information in context, making appropriate health decisions, achieving optimal health functioning, and improving clinical outcomes.

Functional Measures are Experimental

The levels of health literacy described above reflect progressively greater autonomy, personal empowerment, and engagement in a wider range of health actions that extend from personal behaviors to health-care practices and lifestyle changes (health functioning) (Nutbeam, 2000). Therefore, improved functional health literacy (and so the impacts of intervention) can be measured as changes in health functioning. Health attitudes, motivations, self-efficacy, and actions are short-term health promotion outcomes and the immediate targets of health education and skills development. They lead to improvement in intermediate health outcomes (modifiable determinants of health) such as healthful behaviors and lifestyles, effective use of health information and health-care services, and maintenance of healthy environments. Intermediate outcomes lead to ultimate or end-stage outcomes (health status). Thus, the impacts of an intervention to promote functional health literacy can be measured as improvement in short-term health promotion outcomes, and intermediate health outcomes such as accessing information from a variety of sources, selecting reliable sources, and personalizing and appropriately applying relevant health information for personal benefit (Nutbeam, 2008). Smith (2009) first demonstrated the viability of assessing functional health literacy as an alternative to traditional measures of health literacy. Smith used the life skills progression (LSP) instrument (Wollesen & Pfeifer, 2006) to measure functional health literacy in 2532 parents and to assess the impacts of a home-based intervention on parental functional health literacy.

Smith derived from the LSP two scales to measure different aspects of functional health literacy: use of health information and services (functional health-care literacy) and self-management of personal and family health (functional self-care literacy). An analysis of these scales along with other LSP data captures the complex interrelationships of multiple factors (e.g., mental health and social support) that affect a parent's ability to achieve the two-part purpose of functional health literacy: (1) to use information and services and (2) to understand and exert control over their personal and family health. The LSP health literacy scales recognize both the clinical definition of health literacy as reading ability to understand health information and the broader health promotion definition of health literacy as ability to use information in ways that enhance health. Thus, the data capture the impact of systems-level efforts to improve information along with health promotion efforts to improve the use of information and services.

The LSP method of mapping pathways and monitoring progress from inadequate to optimal functioning can be used to assess longitudinal effects of social services programs that aim to develop life skills, particularly interactive and reflective health literacy skills, and may be adaptable for clinical use, especially for adults/families living with chronic conditions.

PRACTICE/INTERVENTION

The availability of the LSP functional health literacy scales makes the health promotion approach feasible for implementation. Smith (2009) first demonstrated that it is possible to promote functional health literacy through health promotion efforts in community settings.

An independent review of many lines of evidence summarized the intervention as follows:

> Six home visitation programs serving low-income, ethnically diverse pregnant women and new parents [$N = 2532$] use a reflective approach and easy-to-understand pregnancy and child care guides to improve functional health literacy. The reflective approach and curriculum, which includes regular assessments of functional health literacy to objectively chart a family's progress, are integrated into established home visitation programs promoting parent and child health and school readiness. The program led to significant improvements in functional health literacy scores after 6 months regardless of reading level, with scores continuing to improve over time. These gains, which were made across three ethnic groups, serve to empower participants to better manage their family's health and health care.
> —*AHRQ, 2009*

Statistical analysis eliminated the possibility that improvements were due to maturation or community events. The alternative functional approach to measuring and promoting health literacy as a personal and community asset is particularly promising for social services. Practitioners may find it necessary to develop functional health literacy in a service population to enable them to fully utilize and obtain the benefits of available services.

CONTRIBUTIONS AND LIMITATIONS

The health promotion approach to health literacy has established a strong theoretical foundation for functional health literacy as an asset that can be improved through health promotion efforts and measured as changes in health attitudes, actions, behaviors, and practices. Thus, the health promotion approach raises new issues to consider regarding the meaning and measure of health literacy. The first trial of this functional approach (Smith, 2009) demonstrated the viability of promoting people's ability to use information and services (functional health literacy) as a necessary complement to traditional information-improvement strategies.

The field test (Smith, 2009) also demonstrated the viability of the LSP as a meaningful measure of functional health literacy that increases our understanding of the interactions among multiple factors determining the ability of individuals to use the health-care system for taking care of themselves and others, and that can be used to evaluate interventions. This advance made the health promotion approach practical for implementation. Measurement matters, because it determines the range of possible solutions. What we measure determines what we find out about what works, what is worth doing, and who should do it.

The broader more practical understanding of functional health literacy in the health promotion approach opens new avenues for intervention both within and beyond the health-care system. It suggests new collaborations and partnerships between health-care and social services. Continued experimentation in the health promotion approach has the potential to advance long-standing health systems goals such as activated patients, and effective health-care consumers are not well supported by the prevailing deficit approach; to extend the benefits of the health-care system to currently underserved populations; to reduce disparities; and to bridge public health, health-care and social services.

Health promotion theory and strategies for developing health-enhancing skills and for supporting healthful practices and behavior change are well established. These strategies can be tailored to program and constituent goals, and integrated into the usual practices of social services providers to improve functional health literacy in economically and socially disadvantaged populations.

The health promotion approach represents a new way of thinking about health literacy. The health promotion model of health literacy has only recently been demonstrated to be feasible for implementation (AHRQ, 2009; Smith, 2009). The LSP as a measure of functional health literacy is experimental. However, the theoretical foundation is strong, and initial findings are very promising. More research is needed to hone measures and identify best practices in health literacy promotion for social services providers.

IMPLICATIONS FOR PRACTICE

Universal Precautions

Research has established that achieving health literacy is a complex challenge for almost everyone, regardless of reading ability. The Healthy People national health objectives call for "improving the health literacy of the population" in order to achieve the national vision of a health literate society. Therefore, a universal precautions approach is warranted. Practicing universal precautions for health literacy means providers anticipate that everyone has difficulty using information to enhance health. Social service programs should establish prudent standard practices to ensure comprehension of essential information, identify clients who lack fundamental skills and refer them to community-based literacy-enhancing services, and actively promote advanced health literacy skills. These precautions are necessary to ensure ethical and effective service, to achieve program goals, and to enable clients to achieve their goals and potential.

Improving Information

Social services providers can take lessons learned from clinical research on health literacy, particularly guidelines for evaluating, producing, and presenting information about health and health care. Attention to offering only information that is immediately applicable and useful, that is, attractive, acceptable, persuasive, and memorable *to the learner* (and not necessarily to the provider), will remove barriers to comprehension. At the same time, social services research and practice should aim at identifying and integrating health literacy-promoting practices into providers' usual activities in order to directly develop clients' ability to use information and services to protect or enhance their health.

Guidelines and Resources

Plain Language

Plain language is a strategy for making written and oral information easier to understand. It is an important tool for improving health literacy. Key elements of plain language include the following:

- Organizing information so that the most important points come first;
- Breaking complex information into understandable chunks;
- Using simple language and defining technical terms; and
- Using the active voice.

The importance of plain language is underscored by Government-wide directives requiring Federal agencies to incorporate plain language elements into all documents, presentations, and electronic communications intended for the public and to avoid jargon and highly technical language.

PLAIN LANGUAGE GUIDE FROM NATIONAL INSTITUTES OF HEALTH. This Guide offers tips for using plain language to provide Americans with health information they can use, and for evaluating materials for a particular audience. It includes links to additional government resources, including contact with National Institutes of Health (NIH) Plain Language Staff. http://www.nih.gov/clearcommunication/plainlanguage.htm

Clear and Simple: Developing Effective Print Materials for Low-Literate Readers

This guide outlines a process for developing publications for people with limited literacy skills. It features both proven principles and a discussion of the real-life issues that individuals developing low-literacy materials face, such as the constraints of time, budget, organizational pressures, and the Government publication process. (http://www.cancer.gov/aboutnci/oc/clear-and-simple)

How to Create and Assess Print Materials by Rima E. Rudd

An extensive collection of information, guidelines, and resources on reading skills, creating and assessing printed materials and websites and for teaching persons with low literacy skills. Harvard School of Public Health: Health Literacy Website: http://www.hsph.harvard.edu/health-literacy/materials.html

Plain Language Guide: Making the Transition from 10 Codes to Plain Language

This guide from the Department of Homeland Security outlines an approach for emergency response agencies, localities, and states to replace coded language radio transmissions with plain language. It includes reasons for adopting plain language, processes for making plain language a reality, and resources for transitioning to plain language.
http://www.safecomprogram.gov/NR/rdonlyres/5945AFE3-ADA9-4189-83B0-4D8218D0CA2F/0/PlainLanguageGuide.pdf

Strategies to Improve Health Literacy

The science of promoting functional health literacy is not as well developed as plain language and health communication. The following strategies are based on research on health education, health promotion, health behavior, and adult literacy and learning.

> Support the development of basic literacy skills. *Be alert about low basic literacy skills in all clients.* Be prepared to refer to community-based literacy-enhancing services. Low literacy crosses all boundaries. The number of years of education is not a reliable indicator of literacy level. There is a stigma attached to low literacy, and so persons who have difficulty in reading may be skilled in concealing that facts.
>
> *Screen for low literacy.* Recent research indicates that a single-question screen can identify many persons at high risk for low literacy without testing. Wallace, Rogers, Roskos, Holiday, and Weiss (2006) found that asking "How confident are you in filling out medical forms by yourself?" identified about 80% of participants who demonstrated limited literacy on the REALM. The researchers offered five possible responses (extremely, quite a bit, somewhat, a

little bit, or not at all) and used "somewhat" as the cutoff. Bennett, Robbins, and Haecker (2003) recommends following up a positive screen for low literacy with two questions to set up a referral: Do you think your reading could be better? Would you like to get some help with your reading? "Yes" answers are further indicators of low literacy. Plan carefully to support the client's participation in literacy classes, adult education, tutoring, or English Language Learning.

Support the Development of Advanced Literacy Skills

- To promote interaction and reflection, become interactive and reflective in practice. Remember that the purpose of improving health literacy is to empower the client to exert some control over personal or family health. This requires the ability to take action on one's own behalf. Rather than simply handing out information, it is important to interact with the client to make personal meaning from the information and create opportunities to practice developing interactive skills (speaking, listening, and self-advocacy). Reflect with the client to tap their experience and guide them to their own solution.

- Discover low-skilled clients' compensating abilities and their other functional literacies, and build on those. For example, a client may learn well by watching a demonstration and practicing, by looking at a picture, or by listening to instructions in his/her primary language.

- Keep clients in charge of their own learning. Adults learn in order to solve a current problem. To give dignity and confidence and build their health literacy skills, create opportunities to solve their own problem. Rather than giving expert advice, use your expertise to formulate questions that lead the clients to discover their information gaps. Then offer information to fill the gap; or discuss how the client could find the needed information. This positions you as a resource and positions the individual as a self-directed learner and problem solver. While it is sometimes more time consuming than simply supplying answers and expert advice, this practice builds skills and independence. Ultimately it is more effective and produces sustainable results.

- *Assist clients in personalizing and making meaning from information* in the context of their personal lives and current circumstance. Unskilled learners often miss the context of information on unfamiliar topics. For example, a learner may understand general information about "many people with this condition" but not apply it to them. Invite the client to read aloud a few sentences particularly relevant to the issue under discussion; or take turns reading with them. Discuss what the information means to them here and now.

- Help them apply information in context for personal benefit. Reflect on possibilities, options, and barriers. Lead the client to plan what to do with the new information. Have the client write out the plan, make a sketch, or create some other reminder. Collect information required to act on the plan (e.g., the counselor's name and phone number, questions to ask).
- Model use of information. For example, let the client watch you use an index, find a phone number, ask for a referral, or locate resources. Review and discuss what you did.
  - Take responsibility for the communication. Instead of "Do you understand?" ask "Have I been clear?" or "Is there something you would like to go over again?"
  - Use the "teach-back" method. Say something like: "This is important, so let's make sure we've got it straight. Tell me what you are going to do when ...." Or "Tell me how you will explain this to ____."

Resources

Questions are the Answer

The Agency for Health Care Research and Quality offers this "Question-Builder" to help people formulate questions in preparation for consulting with a health-care professional or pharmacist.
http://www.ahrq.gov/questionsaretheanswer/questionBuilder.aspx

Center for Health Literacy Promotion

This site reports research on promoting functional health literacy as a personal and community asset.
www.healthliteracy promotion.com

Health Literacy for Public Health Professionals

This free training program introduces participants to the fundamentals of health literacy and demonstrates the importance of health literacy within public health practice. The content spurs students to think about the significance of health literacy in the work done as public health professionals. It provides practical steps to apply the principles and strategies of health literacy in daily activities.

Centers for Disease Control and Prevention

http://www.cdc.gov/healthmarketing/healthliteracy/training/

Health Literacy Improvement

Department of Health and Human Services Office of Disease Prevention and Health Promotion. A resource for tools to improve health literacy, government resources, reports and research, and links to additional resources. http://www.health.gov/communication/literacy/

SUMMARY

Health literacy enables adults to obtain the benefits of the health-care system, for taking care of themselves and others, and to exert control over their personal, family, and community health. There are two approaches to health literacy research and practice: (1) the dominant clinical approach developed in U.S. academic medical centers and documented in the U.S. medical literature and (2) the emerging health promotion approach documented primarily in the international public health literature.

In the dominant view, health literacy is narrowly defined as the ability to obtain, process, and understand the information and services needed to make appropriate health decisions. Research focuses on "functional health literacy," such as reading and numeracy skills for acquiring knowledge about health. Most studies have measured health literacy as reading ability in a clinical setting. The goal of this line of research is to improve the health of persons with low literacy skills. Low literacy in a health-care setting is documented as a risk to patients and health-care systems that clinicians need to identify and manage. Health literacy intervention studies are relatively rare; most have aimed at increasing patients' comprehension by reducing the cognitive demand of information. This approach has raised awareness of literacy in health care and made health information more accessible to all. Critics argue that this prevailing clinical orientation to health literacy research is too narrow to improve the health literacy of the population and to achieve the vision of health literate society. Beyond the comprehension of health and medical information, critics argue, comprehensive research would require attention to cultural, social, political, and economic factors, and life skills.

An emerging alternative approach broadens the concept of health literacy as the ability to use information and services to enhance personal, family, and community health. This model interprets "functional health literacy" as one of the "multiple functional literacies," which enables adults to exert some control over their health and its determinants. In this view, functional health literacy involves the application of an array of basic (often called "functional"), interactive, and reflective skills used for managing health. Health literacy, as the ability to use information to enhance health, is seen as a personal and community asset that can be developed over time through health promotion efforts, notably health education, skills development, and various forms of social support. Measures of functional health literacy are experimental. This approach is applicable in both community and clinical settings and so may be more relevant for social services providers.

CONCLUSION

In whatever way it is defined, health literacy affects an individual's ability to access and obtain the benefits of health and social services. Factors that make persons and populations vulnerable (poverty, racism, physical and mental illness, and extreme age) are associated with low literacy and lower health literacy. Low health literacy increases vulnerability and may represent a significant barrier to achieving the goals of social service programs. Social services providers can play an important role in achieving the national vision for a health literate society by integrating into their practice and program strategies to improve health literacy. Successful programs will be those that take a multidimensional approach to provide clear information along with direct assistance to personalize and apply that information in context in ways that promote health.

REFERENCES

AHRQ Innovations Exchange. Innovation profile: *Home visits using reflective approach improve functional health literacy among low-income pregnant women and new parents.* In S. A. Smith (Ed.), AHRQ Health Care Innovations Exchange [Web site]. Rockville, MD: [cited December 04, 2009]. Available at www.innovations.ahrq.gov.

American College of Physicians & Institute of Medicine. (2008, November 19). New directions in health literacy national conference. Executive Summary retrieved March 25, 2009, from http://foundation.acponline.org/files/hcc2008_exsum.pdf.

Bennett, I. M., Robbins, S., & Haecker, T. (2003). Screening for low literacy among adult caregivers of pediatric patients. *Family Medicine, 35,* 585–590.

Charner-Laird, K., Fiarman, S., Park, F. W., Soderber, S., & Nunes, G. (2003). *Cultivating student reflection.* Boston, MA: Paul & Co.

Culligan, N. (2005). *Theoretical understandings of adult literacy: A literature review.* Wellington, NZ: Massey University.

Davis, T. C., Crouch, M. A., Long, S. W., Jackson, R. H., Bates, P., George, R. B., et al. (1991). Rapid assessment of literacy levels of adult primary care patients. *Family Medicine, 23,* 433–435.

Downey, L. V., & Zun, L. (2007). Testing of a verbal assessment tool of English proficiency for use in the healthcare setting. *Journal of the National Medical Association, 99*(7), 795–798.

Freebody, P., & Luke, A. (1990). Literacies programs: Debates and demands in cultural context. *Prospect, 5,* 7–16.

Freire, P. (1994). *Pedagogy of the oppressed.* New York, NY: The Continuum Publishing Co.

Hauser, R. M., Edley, C. F., Jr., Koenig, J. A., & Elliot, S. W. (Eds.). (2005). *Measuring literacy: Performance levels for adults, interim report.* National Research Council, Board on Testing and Assessment,Committee on Performance Levels for Adult Literacy. Washington, DC: The National Academies Press.

McCaffrey, J., Merrifield, J., & Millican, J. (2007). *Developing adult literacy.* Oxford: Oxfam.

National Research Council. (2005). Measuring literacy: Performance levels for adults. Committee on Performance Levels for Adult Literacy. In R. M. Hauser, C. F. Edley, Jr., J. A. Koenig, S. W. Elliott (Eds.), *Committee on performance levels for adult literacy.* Board on Testing and Assessment, Center for Education. Division of Behavioral and Social Sciences and Education. Washington, DC: The National Academies Press. Retrieved on March 12, 2009, from http://www.nap.edu/openbook.php?record_id= 11267&page=R2.

Nielsen-Bohlman, L., Panzer, A. M., & Kindig, D. A. (Eds.). (2004). *Health literacy: A prescription to end confusion.* Institute of Medicine, Committee on Health Literacy, Board of Neuroscience and Behavioral Health. Washington, DC: The National Academies Press.

Nutbeam, D. (1998). *Health promotion glossary. Health Promotion International, 13,* 349–364.

Nutbeam, D. (2000). *Health literacy as a public health goal: a challenge for contemporary health education and communication strategies into the 21st Century.* Health Promotion International, *15,* 259–267.

Nutbeam, D. (2008). The evolving concept of health literacy. *Social Science and Medicine, 67,* 2072–2078.

Parker, R. M., Baker, D. W., Williams, M. V., & Nurss, J. R. (1995). The test of functional health literacy in adults: A new instrument for measuring patients literacy skills. *Journal of General Internal Medicine, 10,* 537–542.

Paasche-Orlow, M. K., & Wolf, M. S. (2008). Evidence does not support clinical screening of literacy. *Journal of General Internal Medicine, 23*(1), 100–102.

Smith, S. A. (2009). *Promoting health literacy: Concept, measurement and intervention.* PhD dissertation, Union Institute and University, Cincinnati, Ohio. (Publication No. AAT 3375168).

Smith, S. A., & Wollesen, L. A. (2004–2008). *Beginnings guides life skills development curriculum implementation manual and home visitors handbook.* Seattle, WA: Practice Development Inc.

U.S. Department of Health and Human Services. (2000). *Healthy People 2010.* Washington, DC: U.S. Government Printing Office.

U.S. Department of Health and Human Services. (2009). *Developing Healthy People 2020. Healthy People 2020. Public Meeting 2009. Draft Objectives.* HC/HIT-1.

Wallace, L S., Rogers, E. S., Roskos, S. E., Holiday, D. B., & Weiss, B. D. (2006). Screening items to identify patients with limited health literacy skills. *Journal of General Internal Medicine, 21,* 874–877.

FURTHER READING

Measures of Health Literacy. (2009). *Measuring the function in functional health literacy.* Institute of Medicine, Washington, DC: National Academies Press.

CHAPTER TWENTY

Transformative Impact and Initiatives of the Mental Health Consumer/Survivor Movement

Harvey Rosenthal

INTRODUCTION

Inspired by the civil rights and psychiatric reform movements, as well as the 12-step addiction recovery and cross-disability community integration movements, the "mental health consumer/survivor/ex-patient movement" emerged in the 1960s. Its original mission was to take action against the dehumanizing personal and social impact of a psychiatric diagnosis and the damaging effects of psychiatric treatments and medications that had been the experience of thousands of individuals in the United States and internationally.

Since then, its focus has moved well beyond fighting against the loss of hope, meaning, connection, and wellness that resulted from contact with traditional mental health services, to innovative initiatives and values that are fundamentally transforming those systems. And as new health and behavioral health systems seek approaches that demonstrate measurable outcomes through cost-effective alternatives to costly emergency, inpatient, and lifelong stays in community programs, recovery-centered "peer-run" services are playing important and innovative roles.

This chapter will highlight some of the movement's key contributions and initiatives as it also recognizes the landmark efforts of some extraordinary pioneers. It includes web links describing the lives and contributions of leaders within this movement (see the References section to access these links). This chapter is meant to serve as an introduction to some of our field's most provocative challenges. It offers a resource of promising new innovations for further study and incorporation into modern practice.

BACKGROUND

First, let us discuss some important distinctions relating to terminology. Loosely and lightly put, the consumer/survivor/ex-patient movement consists of terms that characterize different reactions to having received mental health services and medications: *Consumers* describe some who receive services; *Survivors* are individuals who recount terrible experiences and want little to nothing to do with medications and services; *Ex-patients* are individuals who are just glad they got away. Most recently, many identify themselves as *Peers* in a "recovery movement" the term *peer-run services* is now widely used to describe services run by people who have been diagnosed and have experienced public mental health services.

While some prefer the term "people who experience mood swings, fear, voices, and visions," a great many have come to identify and accept the term *"person with a psychiatric disability."*

Historically, the movement has rejected a variety of terms connected with the medical model: Controversy exists over how accurate and helpful the broad array of psychiatric diagnoses have been, whether a biologically based illness is involved (i.e., many people experience symptoms and disabling reactions that result from traumas connected to aversive childhood and adult experiences, poverty, and deprivation). Even when people identify with a particular condition, they often object to being lumped into one homogeneous often negatively stereotyped group generally referred to as "the mentally ill."

The great aversion to the medical model comes from two major causes: The great harm that many people have experienced resulting from treatments, including brain damage from lobotomies, memory loss from electroshock; and movement disorders and numbing emptiness and agitation resulting from psychiatric medications. To this must be added the widely experienced "empty life" that so many have experienced as a result of the typically poor prognoses psychiatry has offered people diagnosed with "major mental illnesses." Society tends to confirm the verdict handed down by psychiatrists along with the diagnosis.

As a result, these individuals have been and continue to be routinely told that they will never be able to work, live independently, marry and have children, or, indeed, allowed the opportunity to experience most of life's gifts. In doing so, we have robbed people of their essential hopes and dreams. We have taken away the capacity of people diagnosed with mental illnesses to engage in the "normal" personal struggles that often bring out the best in a person.

A diagnosis of major mental illness has typically meant a life apart, forever segregated from the mainstream. It has meant a life of poverty, subsisting on public entitlements, riding in vans to programs that all too often unintentionally promote idleness, isolation, and apathy that then are ironically interpreted as "symptoms of the illness."

It also has frequently meant taking psychotropic medications, whether the individual wanted to or not. Fortunately, we now know that using medication is an active process that involves complex decision making and a chance to work through conflicts relating to those decisions. It requires a partnership between two experts: the client and the practitioner, rather than simply one of compliance strategies. Shared decision making provides a model for practitioners and clients to assess a treatment's advantages and disadvantages within the context of recovering a life after a diagnosis of a major psychiatric disability. (For more information, see Deegan, 2005; Deegan & Drake, 2006.)

Unfortunately, when many individuals reject these medications and services out of a desire for something better, some suggest that this is due to biologically caused noncompliance stemming from their unawareness or denial of their neurological deficit—a disorder known as *anosognosia*. Their solution is involuntary outpatient commitment (commonly known as "Kendra's Laws"), which permit courts to force people to accept many of the same medications and services that have failed them in the past.

Consequently, many public mental health system users prefer to identify themselves as *people with psychiatric disabilities*. Rather than providing lifelong maintenance, rehabilitation provides people with disabilities with ways to achieve acquisition of skills and supports that enable them to achieve self-defined goals.

This term also connects people with psychiatric disabilities with the broader disability community and their strong focus on a life in the "most integrated setting," which in turn has come to focus systems for the psychiatrically disabled on the goals of a home or apartment of one's own, a job, accessible transportation, and self-directed care.

RIGHTS, CHOICE, AND SELF-DETERMINATION

Fundamental to the consumer/survivor/ex-patient movement is the focus on the rights of individuals, both as human beings and as patients. The movement began in response to coercion, which was a central feature of the custodial care systems. Having had its origins in the state institutions created in the 1800s, the use of coercion continued within community systems even after deinstitutionalization began in the 1980s. These systems enforced the view that unorthodox behavior was an evidence of unremitting permanent "mental illness" from which recovery was impossible. Accordingly, most people, family members, doctors, and mental health professionals regularly devalued the capacity of people with psychiatric disabilities to make good judgments and know what they needed. It was as if snapshots of these people, taken at their worst emotional state and least stable time of life, were used to determine all that they could ever do or be. As a result, medications and services were routinely forced upon such individuals "for their own good" and for "the public's protection." People were expected to take prescribed medications and to live in and attend the residential and day programs to which they were assigned. Assistance and entitlements were often offered only as a condition of compliance with treatment and program regimens.

It was in this environment that Judi Chamberlin, called the "mother of the movement" emerged. She and other pioneers of the consumer movement will be briefly profiled over the following pages.

Judi Chamberlin

Judi Chamberlin grew up in Massachusetts, a state that claims an impressive number of leaders in the recovery and rehabilitation movements. Hospitalized for depression in a state institution when in her 20s, Chamberlin recalled her horror at its prison-like atmosphere and by her discovery that as a psychiatric patient she had no legal rights. She eventually found recovery in Vancouver at a crisis center run by others with psychiatric disabilities who had won government funding for alternative treatments. She subsequently helped found the Mental Patients' Liberation Front in Boston, and in 1975 the group won a landmark lawsuit that established the right of a patient to refuse treatment (Disability Social History Project, 2003).

Chamberlin's book *On Our Own: Patient-Controlled Alternatives to the Mental Health System* (McGraw-Hill, 1979) became the movement's manifesto. She joined forces with activists for people with physical disabilities, and was instrumental in the passage in 2006 of a United Nations treaty on the rights of disabled persons (Goldberg, 2009).

A fundamental underlying philosophy of the international disability rights movement was the concept of "Nothing about us without us." Indeed, Chamberlin (1999) bemoaned "the absence of people with mental and cognitive disabilities (in such efforts since)... these disabilities combine to make up the largest disability 'category'" and noted "that people with mental illness are the most discriminated against and the most isolated in their respective countries" (p. 124).

The substance use recovery and 12-step movements influenced the consumer/survivor movement, which began to adopt the concepts of recovery. Several years prior her death in 2009, Judi Chamberlin told an interviewer, "I was diagnosed with schizophrenia when I was 21 years old, and I'm a person who's recovered ... being told that you have schizophrenia is a devastating experience .... I was also told that I would always be ill, I was going to need treatment and it was terrifying .... I needed support, I needed someone to say that there are ways out of this morass you find yourself in and I wasn't hearing that" (Voices of Recovery, 2008).

"Howie the Harp"

While statistics from the National Coalition for the Homeless (2009) indicate that 16% of America's homeless may have psychiatric diagnoses, the streets produced several leaders who helped in giving rise to critical self-help support and innovative peer-run services. Howard Geld was born in New York City and spent a year in a school for emotionally disturbed adolescents.

"I've been diagnosed as a schizophrenic, as psychotic, as manic-depressive and as psychotic depressive," Geld said later. "I don't really believe in those labels, but there have been times in my life when I went into what can be called a manic episode, and when I went into severe depressions. What I'm doing with my life right now is trying to learn how to control what I call manic energy. If it can be controlled and directed and channeled, it could be really valuable and real powerful. I'd rather learn how to control it, rather than be cured of it" (Recovery Exchange, 2010).

To honor his skill as a harmonica player and the years he worked as a street musician in New York's Greenwich Village, Geld was given the affectionate title "Howie the Harp."

Geld's involvement in formal advocacy began in 1971 in Oregon and spanned years in New York and California. In 1993, he became the director of advocacy of Community Access, a significant housing and advocacy organization located in New York City. Today, under the auspices of Community Access, Howie the Harp Peer Advocacy and Training Center (HTH) in Harlem serves as a model peer-run resource for job training and placement for individuals with combined histories of psychiatric disability, homelessness, substance abuse, and incarceration. It provides classroom-based training, internships, job placement assistance, and alumni programs (Van Gelder, 1995).

Howie Geld, Sally Zinman, and Su Budd co-edited *Reaching Across: Mental Health Clients Helping Each Other* and *Reaching Across 2: Maintaining Our Roots/The Challenge of Growth*. They are nationally recognized manuals aimed at helping mental health clients and professionals to gain understanding and start self-help programs.

Edward L. Knight

Dr. Edward L. Knight was diagnosed with schizophrenia in 1969. He experienced homelessness and was hospitalized a number of times, the last time in 1981. He went on to become the founder of the Mental Health Empowerment Project, which helped to start over 600 self-help groups and nearly 35 self-help not-for-profit agencies that provided consumer-driven mental health services. They included drop-in centers, peer counseling, housing, case management, and mutual support. Today Dr. Knight infuses peer and recovery centered approaches into managed behavioral health designs as a Vice President with Value Options.

Joseph A. Rogers

Joseph A. Rogers was diagnosed with paranoid schizophrenia at age 19 and told that he was incapable of holding a job. But in 1984, under the auspices of a small agency, the Mental Health Association of Southeastern Pennsylvania (MHASP), he founded the Self-Help and Advocacy Resource Exchange Project (Project SHARE). Project SHARE ultimately became the umbrella organization for programs that provide such essential services as peer support, drop-in centers, housing, homeless outreach, mentoring, and job training for persons with psychiatric disabilities. Rogers transformed MHASP into a $14-million organization with 300 staff, the majority of whom have psychiatric disabilities.

In 1986, with federal funding, he founded the National Mental Health Consumers' Self-Help Clearinghouse, which provides thousands of U.S. mental health consumers and consumer-run organizations with the tools to be successful advocates and to establish and operate peer-run services (Schizophrenia.com, 2005).

Currently, Rogers and the MHASP, in collaboration with Magellan Health Services, Office of Behavioral Health, Delaware County, Pennsylvania and the University of Pennsylvania Collaborative on Community Integration, have piloted a transformative service design called *Self-Directed Care*. Key elements involve providing consumers with decision-making power over their own recovery plan, identifying appropriate services, and making decisions regarding their behavioral and health-care budget. By assuming responsibility for making and "owning" their choices, and making decisions regarding how to spend service dollars, Self-Directed Care advances independence and self-determination. For more information, see http://www.parecovery.org/advisory_materials/march_2010_handouts/Joint_CSIF_SDC.pdf.

Recently approved national health-care reform legislation contains improvements to the federal 1915.i Home and Community-Based Option that would permit states to establish self-direction programs for people with psychiatric disabilities. For more information, see http://www.familiesusa.org/issues/long-term-services/health-reform/changes-to-medicaids-1915.html.

Patricia Deegan

Patricia Deegan is one of the most prolific and inspired leaders in the survivor and recovery movements. After having been diagnosed as schizophrenic as a teenager, she went on to receive her doctorate in clinical psychology.

As cofounder and Director of Training of the National Empowerment Center Inc., a federally funded, national technical assistance center run by consumer/survivors, Dr. Deegan developed many self-help tools and resources to support people in their recovery, among them an audio-taped simulation of "hearing voices." The "voices curriculum" has received international acclaim and is used to train psychiatrists, mental health workers, family members, and police officers to work more compassionately with people diagnosed with mental illness. The curriculum can be accessed at http://www.power2u.org/mm5/merchant.mvc?Screen=PROD&Store_Code=NEC&Product_Code=Curricula-HearingVoicesDistressing&Category_Code=hearingvoices.

For more information on Patricia Deegan's work assisting persons with psychiatric disabilities to take an active informed role in treatment-related decisions with their psychiatrists, see http://www.power2u.org/downloads/ReclaimingyourPowerduringMedicationVisits.pdf and

"Shared Decision Making and Medication Management in the Recovery Process" (http://psychservices.psychiatryonline.org/cgi/content/full/57/11/1636).

Personal Assistance in Community

Developed by Dr. Daniel Fisher & Laurie Ahern of the National Empowerment Center, Personal Assistance in Community (PACE) has been used internationally to transform services and supports by emphasizing: the Development of trusting relationships; Dreams—regain valued social roles; Self-determination—Hope, Common capacity for recovery (mental distress temporary disruption); Have people who believe in, are concerned about and understand them; Emotionally and socially connected; Have self-care techniques; Understand that there is always meaning in emotional distress; Set personal goals/achieve them and Help others to recover dignity and rights through work.
http://www.power2u.org/

NATIONAL CONSENSUS STATEMENT ON MENTAL HEALTH RECOVERY

Thanks to the efforts of leaders such as these and many others, state and federal agencies began to take a closer look at issues of mental health diagnoses, treatment, and recovery. In 2004, the Substance Abuse and Mental Health Services Administration convened 110 expert panelists to craft a federal definition of mental health recovery and identify key elements that support it. Panelists included mental health consumers, family members, providers, advocates, researchers, academicians, managed care representatives, accreditation organization representatives, State and local public officials, and others.

The following consensus statement was derived from expert panelist deliberations on the findings.

The 10 Fundamental Components of Recovery (SAMHSA, 2004)

Self-Direction: Consumers lead, control, exercise choice over, and determine their own path of recovery by optimizing autonomy, independence, and control of resources to achieve a self-determined life. By definition, the recovery process must be self-directed by the individual, who defines his or her own life goals and designs a unique path toward those goals.

Individualized and Person Centered: There are multiple pathways to recovery based on an individual's unique strengths and resiliencies as well as his or her needs, preferences, experiences (including past trauma), and cultural background in all of its diverse representations. Individuals also identify recovery as being an ongoing journey and an end result as well as an overall paradigm for achieving wellness and optimal mental health.

Empowerment: Consumers have the authority to choose from a range of options and to participate in all decisions—including the allocation of resources—that will affect their lives, and are educated and supported in so doing. They have the ability to join with other consumers to collectively and effectively speak for themselves about their needs, wants, desires, and aspirations. Through empowerment, an individual gains control of his or her own destiny and influences the organizational and societal structures in his/her life.

Holistic: Recovery encompasses an individual's whole life, including mind, body, spirit, and community. Recovery embraces all aspects of life, including housing, employment, education, mental health and health-care treatment and services, complementary and naturalistic services, addictions treatment, spirituality, creativity, social networks, community participation, and family supports as determined by the person. Families, providers, organizations, systems, communities, and society play crucial roles in creating and maintaining meaningful opportunities for consumer access to these supports.

Nonlinear: Recovery is not a step-by-step process but one based on continual growth, occasional setbacks, and learning from experience. Recovery begins with an initial stage of awareness in which a person recognizes that positive change is possible. This awareness enables the consumer to move on to fully engage in the work of recovery.

Strengths Based: Recovery focuses on valuing and building on the multiple capacities, resiliencies, talents, coping abilities, and inherent worth of individuals. By building on these strengths, consumers leave stymied life roles behind and engage in new life roles (e.g., partner, caregiver, friend, student, and employee). The process of recovery moves forward through interaction with others in supportive, trust-based relationships.

Peer Support: Mutual support—including the sharing of experiential knowledge and skills and social learning—plays an invaluable role in recovery. Consumers encourage and engage other consumers in recovery and provide each other with a sense of belonging, supportive relationships, valued roles, and community.

Respect: Community, systems, and societal acceptance and appreciation of consumers—including protecting their rights and eliminating discrimination and stigma—are crucial in achieving recovery. Self-acceptance and regaining belief in one's self are particularly vital. Respect ensures the inclusion and full participation of consumers in all aspects of their lives.

Responsibility: Consumers have a personal responsibility for their own self-care and journeys of recovery. Taking steps toward their goals may require great courage. Consumers must strive to understand and give meaning to their experiences and identify coping strategies and healing processes to promote their own wellness.

Hope: Recovery provides the essential and motivating message of a better future—that people can and do overcome the barriers and obstacles that confront them. Hope is internalized, but can be fostered by peers, families, friends, providers, and others. Hope is the catalyst of the recovery process. Mental health recovery not only benefits individuals with mental health disabilities by focusing on their abilities to live, work, learn, and fully participate in our society, but also enriches the texture of American community life. America reaps the benefits of the contributions individuals with mental disabilities can make, ultimately becoming a stronger and healthier nation.

RESEARCH ON RECOVERY, NONVIOLENCE, AND PEER-RUN SERVICES

In the seminal longitudinal study *Maine and Vermont Three-Decade Studies of Serious Mental Illness* (DeSisto, Harding, McCormick, Ashikaga, & Brooks, 1995), the authors compared the long-term outcome of serious psychiatric disability in Vermont and Maine. The Vermont subjects participated in a model psychiatric rehabilitation program; the Maine group received more traditional care. Twenty-five years later, the Vermont subjects were found to be "more productive, had fewer symptoms, better community adjustment and global functioning than Maine subjects." DeSisto et al. concluded that "outcome differences may be due to Vermont's model programme and a policy of allowing an earlier opportunity for community life" (p. 331).

Violence by People Discharged from Acute Psychiatric Inpatient Facilities and by Others in the Same Neighborhoods (Steadman et al., 1998) found "no significant difference between the prevalence of violence by (mental) patients without symptoms of substance abuse and the prevalence of violence by others living in the same neighborhoods who were also without symptoms of substance abuse."

In fact, a later study found that people with psychiatric disabilities were 11 times more likely to be victims of violence (*Crime Victimization in Adults with Severe Mental Illness*) (Teplin, McClelland, Abram, & Weiner, 2005).

Consumer-Operated Services

The Consumer-Operated Services Program Multisite Research Initiative (1998–2004) was a randomized controlled study funded by the Center for Mental Health Services. The purpose of the initiative was to investigate the effectiveness and cost effectiveness of eight consumer-operated support programs for adults with psychiatric disabilities (four drop-in centers, two mutual support programs, and two educational/advocacy programs) when offered as an adjunct to traditional mental health services. At baseline, 4, 8, and 12 months, 1827 study participants were assessed using a common assessment protocol that measured outcomes such as employment, empowerment, housing, social inclusion, well-being, and satisfaction.

Participants who were randomly assigned to consumer-operated services programs of the drop-in type in addition to receiving their traditional mental health services were shown to have greater improvement in well-being over the course of the study than participants who were randomly assigned to receive only traditional mental health services (Campbell, 2004).

INNOVATIVE PEER-RUN PROGRAMS AND SERVICES

The following sections will briefly describe some innovative peer-run or developed programs, curricula, and media resources being used to advance the recovery and dignity of people with psychiatric disabilities.

WRAP: Wellness Recovery Action Plans

According to noted author, educator, and mental health recovery advocate Mary Ellen Copeland, Wellness Recovery Action Plans (WRAP) are "self-designed plans for staying well, and for helping you to feel better when you are not feeling well, to increase personal responsibility and control over your own life and help you make your life the way you want it to be" (Wrapworld.com, 2009). WRAP is transforming mental health systems by helping people define their struggles in their own terms and developing personalized strategies to heal and recover.

Informing the Public: Turning Experience into Art

When Willard Psychiatric Center, located in New York's Finger Lakes region, closed in 1995, workers discovered hundreds of suitcases in the attic of an abandoned building. They were the suitcases of institutionalized men and women that were abandoned and remained unopened for decades.

Darby Penney and Dr. Peter Stastny spent years uncovering the lives of a representative sample of the many individuals whose suitcases were discovered. Their extraordinary efforts resulted in a major New York State Museum exhibition in 2004, "Lost Cases, Recovered Lives: Suitcases from a State Hospital Attic." It has served to educate more than 600,000 visitors, as well as memorialize the lives that were lost. (For an in-depth discussion of this project, see http://www.suitcaseexhibit.org/indexhasflash.html)

Documentaries of Note

The Politics of Memory, a documentary by Dr. Deegan relating ex-patient perspectives on the history of mental health services, is one among the many projects developed by persons with psychiatric disabilities that expand society's understanding. Another documentary, *From Numbers to Names,* relates efforts to properly restore and memorialize individuals buried at state hospitals. (For more information about both documentaries, see http://www.patdeegan.com/cp_films.html.)

Peer Crisis Respite Programs

The Rose House in Milton, NY is an innovative and unique "hospital diversion" facility developed under the leadership of PEOPLe Inc's Steve Miccio, where individuals seeking temporary residential care/respite care. Services at The Rose House are designed to help "at risk" individuals to break the cycle of learned helplessness and recidivism through 24-hour peer support, self-advocacy education and self-help training. Guests are taught to use new recovery and relapse prevention skills and to move away from what are often long histories of cycling from home to crisis to hospital, year after year. The home-like environment is warm, friendly, safe, and supportive.

Peer Wellness Coaching

People with psychiatric disabilities currently die 20–25 years younger, primarily due to comorbid medical disorders. *Peer wellness coaching* helps individuals with psychiatric and major medical conditions to link to primary health care and improved health promotion activities, reducing high risk behaviors and health risk factors (Swarbrick, 2009). Larry Fricks of the Appalachian Consulting Group has done pioneering work in the development of Peer Support Whole Health workers that is currently the subject of national research. (For more information, see http://www.gmhcn.org/ACG/Core_Recovery_Curriculum_Agenda_with_notes_1_.doc)

Peer Bridger Supports

The New York Association of Psychiatric Rehabilitation Services (NYAPRS) (www.nyaprs.org) is a peer-run and staffed partnership of consumers and providers. Its aim is to improve social conditions and services for people with psychiatric disabilities by promoting their recovery, rehabilitation, and rights. One of its significant peer-supported programs is a "peer bridger model" of transitional peer support aimed at helping individuals transition from hospitals to communities. The model has been replicated nationally, in response to the nation's health care reform emphasis on improving outcomes and reducing costs by making integrated care more individualized and person centered. (For more information, see http://www.nyaprs.org/peer-services/peer-health-care-coaching/)

CONCLUSION

I hope this chapter has provided the reader with an opportunity to understand both the fundamental beliefs and the innovative contributions of the consumer/survivor/recovery community integration and disability rights movements over the past 50 years. More so, I hope that whether you identify as someone with a "history" or not, you are transformed by the courage, passion, and groundbreaking truths that are contained here and use it to inform your policy and practice to help bring hope, healing and dignity to people with psychiatric disabilities you will serve or support, professionally or personally.

RECOMMENDED RESOURCES

Asset Development

Self-Determination and Wellness through Innovative Asset Building Approaches
http://www.cmhsrp.uic.edu/nrtc/summit2009/Swarbrick.pdf

Rights and Recovery Advocacy

The National Coalition for Mental Health Recovery (www.ncmhr.org),

MindFreedom (http://www.mindfreedom.org/),

PsychRights (http://psychrights.org),

National Association for Rights Protection Advocacy (www.narpa.org),

Bazelon Center for Mental Health Law (www.bazelon.org),

We the People (http://www.theopalproject.org/),

NYAPRS (www.nyaprs.org),

CIAD (http://www.ciadny.org/) RIPPD (http://rippd.org/justice/),

Mental Health Association in NYS (http://www.mhanys.org/programs/pwpd/index.htm).

Alternative Healing

Will Hall and the Freedom Center (http://theicarusproject.net/),

Icarus Project (http://theicarusproject.net/),

Empathic Therapy Center (http://empathictherapy.org/),

MindFreedom (http://www.mindfreedom.org/mfdb/mfdb-search-form),

Spiritual Recovery (http://spiritualrecoveries.blogspot.com/2007/01/dr-edward-knight-recovery.html),

Center for Psychiatric Rehabilitation (http://www.ncbi.nlm.nih.gov/pmc/articles/PMC1447289/).

REFERENCES

Campbell, J. (2004). *Consumer-Operated Services Program (COSP) multisite research initiative overview and preliminary findings.* Retrieved from http://www.power2u.org/downloads/COSPVAREPORT.pdf. Accessed July 11, 2008.

Chamberlin, J. (1999). Nothing about us without us: Disability oppression and empowerment (Review of the book *Nothing About Us Without Us*). *Psychiatric Services, 50,* 124. Retrieved from http://psychservices.psychiatryonline.org/cgi/content/full/50/1/124. Accessed July 11, 2008.

Deegan, P. (2005). The importance of personal medicine: A qualitative study of resilience in people with psychiatric disabilities. *Scandinavian Journal of Public Health, 33*(66, suppl 29–35). Retrieved from http://sjp.sagepub.com/content/33/66_suppl/29. Accessed July 11, 2008.

Deegan, P., & Drake, R. (2006). Shared decision making and medication management in the recovery process. *Psychiatric Services, 57,* 1636–1639. Retrieved from http://psychservices.psychiatryonline.org/cgi/content/abstract/57/11/1636. Accessed July 11, 2008.

DeSisto, M., Harding, C. M., McCormick, R. V., Ashikaga, T., & Brooks, G. W. (1995). The Maine and Vermont three-decade studies of serious mental illness. II. Longitudinal course comparisons. *The British Journal of Psychiatry, 167,* 338–342. Retrieved from http://bjp.rcpsych.org/cgi/content/abstract/167/3/331. Accessed July 11, 2008.

Disability Social History Project. (2003). *Judi Chamberlin—Mental Patients' Liberation Activist (1944–).* Retrieved from http://www.disabilityhistory.org/people.html. Accessed July 11, 2008.

Goldberg, C. (2009). *A talk with Judi Chamberlin: Facing death, a plea for the dignity of psychiatric patients.* Boston Globe. Retrieved from http://www.boston.com/bostonglobe/ideas/articles/2009/03/22/a_talk_with_judi_chamberlain. Accessed July 11, 2008.

National Coalition for the Homeless. (2009). *Why are people homeless?* Retrieved from http://www.nationalhomeless.org/factsheets/why.html. Accessed July 11, 2008.

Recovery Exchange. (2010). *Howie the harp: Self-help.* Retrieved from http://www.recoveryxchange.org/HowietheHarp.html. Accessed July 11, 2008.

Schizophrenia.com. (2005). *Joseph Rogers, mental health advocate, wins $250,000 Heinz award.* Retrieved from http://www.schizophrenia.com/sznews/archives/001730.html. Accessed July 11, 2008.

Steadman, H. J., Mulvey, E. P., Monahan, J., Robbins, P. C., Appelbaum, P. S., Grisso, T., Roth, L. H., & Silver, E. (1998). Violence by people discharged from acute psychiatric inpatient facilities and by others in the same neighborhoods. *Archives of General Psychiatry, 55,* 393–401. Retrieved from http://archpsyc.ama-assn.org/cgi/content/abstract/55/5/393?maxtoshow=&HITS=10&hits=10&RESULTFORMAT=&fulltext=Steadman&searchid=1139212828284_30&FIRSTINDEX=0&journalcode=archpsyc. Accessed July 11, 2008.

Substance Abuse and Mental Health Services Administration. (2004). *National consensus statement on mental health recovery.* Retrieved from http://mentalhealth. samhsa.gov/publications/allpubs/sma05-4129/. Accessed July 11, 2008.

Swarbrick, P. (2009). *Peer wellness coach — A new role for peers.* Retrieved from http:// shrp.umdnj.edu/shrpnews/. Accessed July 11, 2008.

Teplin, L. A., McClelland, G. M., Abram, K. M., & Weiner, D. A. (2005). Crime victimization in adults with severe mental illness. *Archives of General Psychiatry, 62,* 911–921. Retrieved from http://archpsyc.ama-assn.org/cgi/content/abstract/ 62/8/911. Accessed July 11, 2008.

Van Gelder, L. (1995). *Howard Geld, 42, advocate for mentally ill, dies. The New York Times.* Retrieved from http://www.nytimes.com/1995/02/14/obituaries/ howard-geld-42-advocate-for-mentally-ill-dies.html. Accessed July 11, 2008.

Voices of Recovery. (2008). *Judi Chamberlin: Developing a recovery vision.* Retrieved from http://voices-of-recovery-schizophrenia.blogspot.com/2008/01/judi-chamberlin-developing-recovery.html. Accessed July 11, 2008.

Wrapworld.com. *Mary Ellen's Bio.* Retrieved from http://wrapworld.accountsupport.com/about/mary-ellens-bio/. Accessed July 11, 2008.

CHAPTER TWENTY-ONE

The Future of Managed Behavioral Health Care

Ann Boughtin and C. Richard Orndoff

INTRODUCTION

The United States has the highest health-care expenditures per capita of any industrialized nation, and this cost of care impacts government, employers, and everyone needing or paying for health care. Health-care payers, that is, employers, the government, and health plans, design their benefit plan and decide how much they will spend on health-care costs. These payers contract with managed care companies, to provide efficient, effective, and accessible services to their members. Managed care is a health-care management approach that brings together the payer (the employer, health plan, or government entity that is paying for the health-care coverage), plan members, and plan providers. The role of the managed care organization is to balance the needs and interests of the three stakeholders by coordinating care, assuring quality, managing the health-care benefit, and maintaining a network of providers to meet care needs. To more fully understand managed care requires examining its core components: health-care *benefit* management; *quality management* of services delivered; and provider *network management*. This chapter will focus on managed behavioral health care, particularly Medicaid managed care, and will also provide historical and operational information regarding the functions of managed care organizations, plan design, reimbursement and payment structures, and emerging trends.

431

MANAGED CARE HISTORY

Managed care models began to emerge as early as the 1920s, but there was limited managed care penetration until the 1990s. Since then enrollment in managed care has grown. "In 1991, 2.7 million beneficiaries were enrolled in some form of managed care. By 2004, that number had grown to 27 million." (August 6, 2009—9:30 am ET | by Anne Zieger (Fierce Healthcare)). Much was happening in health care at the end of the last century. The behavioral health industry was firmly committed to community-based care; psychiatric treatment philosophies included rehabilitation and recovery; and new antidepressants and antipsychotics were coming to the market. At the same time, health-care costs grew dramatically over the decade, and the economic downturn renewed the interest in improving the management of the health-care benefit and maintaining access to care. Payers turned to managed care to add value to the health-care dollars they were spending. Managed care provided an approach that improved quality of care and access to needed services through more efficient and effective service delivery. The federal government, the single largest payer of health care in the United States, recognized that managed care was a model that could improve the quality of care and contain costs. This was reflected in the Medicare Advantage programs and the Medicaid waivers that allowed Medicaid managed care to emerge in numerous states. The core of these programs reflected efforts to build networks and negotiate rates that were sometimes more innovative and financially rewarding than more traditional fee for service models. Additionally with a large repository of data on members, managed care companies were able to implement quality initiatives that provided enhanced supports to individuals with chronic conditions or co-occurring healthcare needs.

In 2009, concerns central to the health care reform discussions included the rising cost of health care and the increasing number of people without health insurance. For every 1% increase in unemployment, the Medicaid roles swelled by more than 1 million people. In addition, the number of people losing employer-sponsored health insurance increased. Spending on mental illness rose faster than spending on any other category of health care. The cost for treating mental disorders rose from $35 billion (in 2006) to nearly $58 billion between 1996 and 2006, according to data from the Agency for Healthcare Research and Quality (AHRQ) (August, 2009—HHS Agency for Healthcare Research and Quality). As the largest payers of health-care costs, the federal government, and in turn the state governments, engaged managed care companies in supporting and implementing state health and fiscal policy to improve clinical outcomes for consumers, especially for high-risk/high-cost/high-need members; assure that members can choose their provider and have timely access to services; promote the appropriate use of clinical services; and contain the rate of growth of health-care costs. Employers, health plans, and the government contract with managed care organizations to promote wellness and recovery, and spend health-care dollars to improve access to the right service at the right time for plan members.

MANAGED CARE AS A HEALTH-CARE TOOL

Components of Managed Care

There are two types of manage care organizations (MCOs): health maintenance organizations (HMOs) and managed behavioral health organizations (MBHOs). Sometimes, MCOs employ MBHOs to manage the behavioral health benefit, because the behavioral health needs of members are complex and management of care for these services is different from medical services. The special focus on managed behavioral health care acknowledges the special needs of people diagnosed with mental illness and reflects the fact that spending on mental illness grew faster than for heart disease, cancer, trauma-linked disorders, and asthma (AHRQ) as researchers noted. (August 6, 2009—9:30 am ET | by Anne Zieger (Fierce Healthcare)).

Managed care is an organized system of care that includes the payer, the provider of care, and the members receiving services. The *payer* (the employer, health plan, or government entity that is paying for the health-care coverage) wants value, that is, good clinical quality at a price that will reduce health-care spending trends and improve outcomes for members. The *provider* delivers services to promote wellness and maintain functioning by treating and/or referring the member to the right service, at the right time. The *member* receives health-care services based on the benefits or covered services in the plan, their needs, and individually developed plans of care.

In managed care, the customer is the payer, and the payer defines the benefit available to the members. In addition, the payer determines how much money is available to spend on care for members. The primary relationship between the managed care organization and the purchaser, for example, the health plan, the employer, or the government, is defined in a contract. The payer determines and builds into the contract the terms related to member eligibility for services, the benefits or covered services in the plan, standards related to the network, member satisfaction, and quality outcomes. Most importantly, the contract includes the amount of money the payer is willing to expend to support the cost of care and development of the network. The managed care company does not define the benefit or the dollars available for the cost of care. Rather, the managed care company is responsible for managing the benefit plan and the cost of care dollars, and implementing processes and networks that support the terms of the contract with the payer.

Purchasers/payers take different approaches to contracting for managed care. A commercial purchaser, for example, a company purchasing managed care for their employees, relies on the expertise of the managed care company to recommend a benefit design that would provide a good health-care benefit to their employees at a reasonable cost. Ultimately, the purchaser/payer makes the final decision on the scope of benefits offered to members and how much they are willing to pay for services. When governmental units purchase managed care for Medicare or Medicaid recipients, the staff involved in the contracting process usually are health-care policy makers, and they bring that experience to health-care delivery. Generally, public sector administrators and policy makers will define what the benefit will be, the types of services to be offered, and the types of providers to be included in the network. They are also more likely to set benchmarks for clinical outcomes and develop the types of quality management and financial reports they want delivered. All of this is embedded in the contract between the public sector payer and the MCO/MBHO. This contrast between the "commercial" business and "public sector" business has evolved into separate market sectors within the managed care world, to reflect the different needs of the members and the interests of the payer.

Operations

Whether managing medical services or behavioral health services, the operational functions of the MCO are to manage the use of services (assuring timely access to medically necessary services); measure the performance of health-care providers; bring together health-care financing and health-care delivery into one operating system; and manage large databases to better serve members, improve quality, pay providers, and be accountable to the stakeholders. Today the managed care companies partner with states, health plans and employers to improve health-care outcomes for members and provide access to medical and specialty services. Contracts with their customers will require managed care organizations to meet or exceed many performance indicators, for example, geo-access to services, managing the health-care benefit to achieve the payer's objectives for financial performance, and quality management focused on clinical outcomes and other key indicators.

Utilization Management

Utilization management has a variety of definitions. Generally it is a tool used by managed care organizations on a case by case basis to work with providers to consider appropriate care alternatives that will meet the needs of the individual.

In consultation with the treating provider, a UM review is conducted to determine if the treatment is covered by the member's benefit plan. In addition, UM applies level of care criteria to each case to determine medical necessity. Level of care criteria includes definitions and guidelines that reflect state and federal regulations, elements of evidence-based practices, and philosophy of care, for example, psychiatric rehabilitation and recovery. Ultimately, the purpose of UM is to help members receive the right service, at the right time, to ameliorate their condition and facilitate recovery.

In the late 1980s, efforts were made to develop uniform standards for UM. National organizations, like URAC, developed standards for level of care criteria for, for example, mental health and substance abuse, inpatient and outpatient services.

UM is divided into two segments: prior authorization and continued stay reviews. In prior authorization, a licensed clinician from the MBHO consults with the treating practitioner regarding the medical needs of the member, the treatment plan, expected time for discharge, and the wishes of the member. Using the information supplied by the practitioner and applying the level of care criteria, the UM reviewer decides if an authorization for payment will be granted for admission to the service. Likewise, as the member continues in care, the clinician will periodically consult with the practitioner to review the clinical progress of the member, and expected date of discharge. Once again, using the information supplied by the practitioner and applying the level of care criteria, the UM reviewer decides if an authorization for continued stay will be granted. The managed care organization does not deny care or treatment. The decision regarding admission, treatment planning, continued stays in treatment, and discharge planning rests with the treating professional.

Today, MCOs and MBHOs voluntarily invite accrediting bodies to review their UM operations, as a way to demonstrate their compliance with national standards and commitment to quality.

Networks

The plan benefits are delivered through a network of providers organized to effectively and efficiently deliver the benefit defined by the payer. Managed care companies build networks of hospitals, general practitioners, and specialists that are geographically distributed to assure that members have access to services that are relatively close to their homes. Networks are built to meet "geo-access" requirements and include providers who have historically served the members.

The network is established through the contractual relationship between the provider and the managed care company, whereby the network providers are under contract to the managed care company. The core components of the network contract include the description of services to be provided, the location and hours of operation of the provider; capacity to serve any of the plan members who need/request services offered by the provider; current licensure and/or accreditation, liability insurance; and the fees that will be paid for the services. The availability of a network of providers that affords accessibility and a choice of providers to members is important for achieving the goals of the payer. If members do not have access to quality primary care to maintain wellness or get early treatment for their health-care needs, the clinical outcome may be a worsening of a condition resulting in an avoidable visit to the emergency rooms or inpatient stay. Payers want value from dollars spent, and the provider network is a key component of the value proposition offered by the managed care company. Payers want to know whether provider practices and clinical outcomes are measured so that there are data to show that the services provided are clinically effective. Likewise payers want the plan members to be satisfied with the care received. This customer satisfaction is reflected in how providers interact with members, for example, person-centered practice and an orientation to recovery from mental illness and/or alcohol/substance abuse. It is through the network that the MBHOs assure access to medically necessary services that are accessible, affordable, and effective.

Quality Management

To improve the efficiency and effectiveness of care for members enrolled in managed care, MCOs and MBHOs use data to track and trend clinical processes and clinical outcomes.

Quality reviews are also conducted to track and trend practice patterns and utilization to identify continuous opportunities to manage the health-care benefit. For example, as part of the quality review, the managed care company may identify people who have had multiple visits to the emergency room without ever seeing practitioners after discharge. The MBHO can reach out to the member to assist in making appointments and connecting them with a community-based provider. With reviews like this, consumers are more likely to receive timely, targeted interventions that can result in better clinical outcomes.

To provide accountability to the customer/payer, the MCOs report on several functions including the performance of the network, member satisfaction, and expenditures related to the cost of care. As part of their infrastructure, MCOs maintain large data repositories with real-time information on episodes of care, member service utilization, clinical improvement, and recovery of members. Once tracked, numerous analytic tools are used to identify trends, improve clinical outcomes, assist members in using the right service at the right, and manage cost. Some managed care companies have introduced "pay for performance" models in which providers can receive additional payments based on the achievement of certain quality outcomes related to care coordination and clinical practice.

The Healthcare Effectiveness Data and Information Set (HEDIS) is a tool used by more than 90% of America's health plans to measure performance on important dimensions of care and service, according to the National Council on Quality Assurance (www.ncqa.org). In addition, the major managed care companies voluntarily participate in rigorous quality reviews to attain accreditation by national bodies. Also, to maintain accreditation by national bodies, all managed care companies conduct ongoing studies and evaluations, as part of continuous quality improvement.

MEDICAID MANAGED CARE PLANS: DESIGN AND TRENDS

Eligibility, Benefits, and Network

Medicaid managed care has continued to grow over the past decade. Medicare is the federal health-care program for the aged, blind, and disabled. Medicaid is a joint federal–state program that pays for medical assistance provided to low-income people. Medicare and Medicaid enrollees include people with routine health-care needs, that is, temporary assistance to needy families (TANF) recipients, who use services at about the same level as people enrolled in commercial plans. Medicare and Medicaid enrollees also include people with disabilities and/or severe or chronic health conditions. Payers have become increasingly concerned with this latter group, since their health-care costs tend to be higher. These are high-risk/high-need individuals, many with comorbid health conditions, who can benefit from case management and care coordination to improve wellness. As the federal and state governments who pay for Medicare and Medicaid recognized these trends, they turned to managed care in an effort to hold down the rate of health-care spending and improve the health profile of their enrollees.

The services that are available to members under any managed care plan are called benefits. Unlike commercial managed care where payers rely on managed care companies to design the benefit plan, in the public sector, the Medicaid benefit plan is drafted by the States and approved by the Federal government. The benefit plan is generally consistent with the approved Medicaid inpatient and outpatient services, and in the case of behavioral health may include some state-funded behavioral health benefits.

Acknowledging that there are different service levels that are needed for the TANF population and those with more complex needs, the government payer may construct a plan that has a basic and extended benefit. The basic behavioral health-care benefit for the Medicaid TANF population is generally 30 inpatient days and 20 outpatient visits for mental health and alcohol/substance use treatment. Specialty services for high-risk populations like people diagnosed with serious mental illness may be bundled separately within the plan or carved out into a separate benefit, outside of the managed care benefit. Examples of more intensive services used by high-risk behavioral health populations include intensive outpatient services, partial hospitalization, and support services, for example, case management, psychiatric rehabilitation, and peer services.

From the network perspective, providers who serve TANF populations may or may not work with people diagnosed with *serious* mental illness. In general, public-sector TANF networks are characterized by health clinics, private practitioners, hospitals, and emergency rooms. Network providers who work with high-risk/high-need populations include hospitals, licensed mental health clinics, case management and specialty service providers offering peer support, residential services, etc. Networks are designed to meet geo-access standards, for example, a hospital must be available to a member within 60 minutes or 60 miles of their home and be large enough to offer members a choice of providers. As discussed in the previous section, network providers are paid a fee consistent with the contract negotiated between the managed care company and the service provider. Generally, in exchange for the potential for referrals from the managed care companies, providers will receive a negotiated payment that is either a fixed fee for service, or a case rate, with service guarantees, for example, an inpatient case rate that will not be paid again if the member is readmitted to inpatient within a certain period of time. The differences in benefits, networks, and payments are summarized in Table 21.1.

THE CHANGING CHARACTERISTIC OF MEDICAID MANAGED CARE: TRENDS AND THE FUTURE

High-Risk/High-Need/High-Cost Populations

With the recent downturn in the economy, Medicaid rolls have grown dramatically. For every 1% increase in the unemployment rate, 1 million people are added to Medicaid and SCHIP (State Children's Health Insurance Programs). With 63 million Medicaid members in the United States, the government is now spending $361B per year on health care, making it the dominant health-care purchaser in the United States. From a mental health perspective, 27% of total mental health costs are financed by Medicaid *(Source: CHCS—Center for Health Care Strategies—Dianne Hasselman—March 2009)*. The states also pay for inpatient care for adults between the ages of 19 and 65 at Institutes for the Mentally Disabled (IMDs), for example, state psychiatric hospitals.

In addition to the growth in Medicaid rolls, it is also worth noting that people diagnosed with a serious mental illness have changing and more complex needs. People with serious mental illness have a high incidence of comorbid health conditions and have a shorter life expectancy than the general population. It has been widely published that people diagnosed with serious mental illness are now dying 25 years earlier than the general population, and have numerous co-occurring medical conditions that put them in a high risk/high need category. High-risk/high-need individuals are among the most expensive 1% of Medicaid beneficiaries. In this group, using diagnostic and pharmacy data over a one year period, 87% had *three or more* chronic conditions, and 67% had *five or more* chronic conditions. And, 75% of the total Medicaid costs were associated with individuals with 3 or more chronic conditions (Kronick et al., 2009).

TABLE 21.1
Differences in Benefits, Networks, and Payments

Populations	Network	Benefits and Services	Payment Structures
TANF			
Utilization is relatively comparable to healthier, employed populations covered in employer-sponsored health plans	Public health clinics Hospitals and Emergency Rooms	Basic benefits for annual exams, labs, and for mental health (30 inpatient days and 20 outpatient visits) *Services*: They use individual services for routine care, prevention and treatment for particular episodes of illness	Managed care (fee for services)
High-Risk/High Need			
Among the top 1% of Medicaid recipients, comorbid chronic health conditions occur frequently, especially for those with serious mental illness	Hospitals and ERs Public health clinics Licensed mental health clinics Case management Intensive outpatient Support services, e.g., psychiatric rehabilitation and peer services Specialty services, e.g., residential services, etc.	All basic benefits plus access to a broader array of specialty services, e.g., behavioral health and HIV/AIDS *Programs*: Due to the presence of co-morbid conditions, they are often enrolled in ongoing programs of support and rehabilitation to achieve recovery goals Recovery approaches improve behavioral and physical health as well as other quality of life interests for the consumer Complex care management with medical providers and other support systems for people with high costs/high needs and co-morbid medical and behavioral health issues	Fee for service or case rates

From a cost perspective, a recent McKinsey study reported that the costliest 5% of people drove 45% of Medicaid spending. This was in one state with 1.4 million enrollees in all aid categories over a period of 2 years (*Source*: Blinded single-state data, McKinsey analysis). In New York State, the Chronic Illness Demo Project serves the high-risk/high-need/high-cost population. In New York, eligible patients have significant medical needs: 76% have chronic disease, 52% have multiple chronic diseases, 69% have a history of mental illness, 73% have a history of substance abuse, and 54% have a history of mental illness and substance abuse. Despite these needs, they are not well connected to the delivery system: 24% have had no primary/specialty care visit in the prior 12 months and 65% have had at least one emergency room visit in the past 12 months (Bachrach, 2008).

Like New York, other states are increasingly interested in providing health-care dollars to providers willing to engage in providing specialized services to people with chronic and comorbid health and behavioral health conditions. The goal is to improve the overall health-care status of this high-need group, and reduce their total cost of health care.

Data Analytics

Managed care organizations have robust data sets, and use a variety of analytic tools to track and trend member utilization, provider practice, and the costs of care. Using claims data and other information, the data sets are analyzed using the following: *Algorithms* to define special populations, *Disease Burden Indicators*, and *Predictive Modeling*.

Algorithms have been used by public payers and managed care companies to identify existing high-risk/high-cost consumers through retrospective reviews of claims, for example, diagnoses, the use of the emergency room, inpatient stays, length of stay in a service, etc. In recent years, these data have prompted the development of disease management programs. Disease management models provide education and coaching to plan members who have a specific, chronic condition, for example, diabetes or asthma, to help improve self-management of that condition and promote early intervention when necessary. Like physical health care, Medicaid MBHOs use data-driven health management to identify members with complex care needs, and then work in partnership with network providers to coordinate person-centered care, and to promote wellness and recovery.

A review of utilization patterns of high-risk/high-need individuals indicates that they are not well connected with community providers of physical or behavioral health care. For many individuals with high needs, their lack of active, consistent engagement with a provider of choice is reflected in the use of emergency rooms and inpatient units. To improve clinical services to these individuals the MBHOs and the public sector behavioral health community are increasingly interested in the

"Medical/Behavioral Home" as a strategy to better integrate physical and behavioral health care. Whether these Accountable Care Organizations (ACOs), as they were called by the Massachusetts Special Commission on the Health Care Payment System, or "Medical Homes" are virtual or based with behavioral or physical health providers, their responsibility will be to provide and coordinate care that is needed by an individual enrollee. This is a model that shows promise, so providers, payers, and managed care companies are increasingly likely to use the Medical/Behavioral Home model.

Predictive modeling is a strategy to identify prospectively those who are likely to become high-cost/high-risk consumers. Using the most recent data available, managed care companies will use utilization histories, age, comorbidity, prescription use, etc. to identify people for interventions before their health-care needs make them high cost. The goal in predictive modeling is to effectively manage the risks associated with the person's health history trajectory to intervene earlier, appropriately reduce health-care costs, and improve clinical outcomes for members.

Disease Burden is another analytic tool that shows the impact of a health problem measured by financial cost, mortality, morbidity, or other indicators. The disease burden is sometimes measured in Quality Adjusted Life Years (QALYs) or Disability Adjusted Life Years (DALYs) that link death and morbidity in a manner to predict the possible impact of health interventions. The World health Organization (WHO) measures disease burden as years lost due to disability (YLD). From the perspective of behavioral health care, the leading cause of YLD worldwide for both men and women was *unipolar depressive disorder* (2004). With these data, the impact of effectively managing behavioral health conditions can have an impact not only on the cost of health care, but also on employers concerned with productivity and absenteeism.

Because managed care companies have some of the most robust and contemporary databases on health care, managed care organizations are uniquely positioned to work with consumers and providers. Rarely will a provider have real-time knowledge of a consumer, for example, when a behavioral health consumer is admitted to the hospital; or is seeing another clinician; or is taking prescription drugs that are contra-indicated. Managed care companies can review UM information and claims payment data to work with consumers and providers to coordinate and enhance care, for example, letting consumers and providers know that prescriptions may need to be reviewed, or assisting with timely access to aftercare appointments following discharge from the hospital. The use of data will continue to shape the work of the managed care companies, the services offered by network providers, the quality of care received by members, and payments to providers that focus on value measured by practice and clinical outcomes.

INNOVATIVE FUNDING THAT FOCUSES ON PROCESS AND PRACTICE

All purchasers are seeking value for limited health-care dollars and are expecting managed care companies (and their network providers) to deliver value reflected in clinical outcomes, services for special needs populations, and continuous review of the data to find opportunities for cost containment. Outcomes may include identification of life improvements, for example, community tenure, decreased length of stay or admissions to inpatient or residential programs, decreased use of emergency rooms and member satisfaction with goal achievement (FierceHealthcare.com, 2009). The payers are seeking accountability from the MCOs and MBHOs regarding outcomes and cost of care. To support this focus on outcomes, and to foster the use of evidence-based practice, in the future payments to providers will see more performance-based models, rather than fee for services. Among the financial models that are emerging, especially in the public sector, are the following:

1. *Pay for performance*, which focuses on the provision of bonus payments to providers who meet quality benchmarks related to improved clinical outcomes, timely access to aftercare services, and/or enhanced services to target populations.
2. *Subcapitation or global payment* provides a fixed payment to providers for most or all services delivered to a defined population. In this model, the providers manage the clinical risk associated with managing the care for the defined population.
3. *Case rates* are all inclusive payments for an episode of care for an individual needing service at a single level of care, for example, inpatient. The provider agrees that no additional payments will be made for any readmissions to that level of care within a fixed period of time, for example, 90 days.
4. *Braided funding* is used primarily for people in the public sector who receive services from multiple care sectors, for example, a person whose needs are addressed by a mental health clinic, a community health clinic, aging services, and public housing. In the braided model, dollars are combined so that duplicate efforts are reduced, for example, multiple case managers for each person are eliminated, and care is

coordinated in a manner that reduces the overall cost of health care and social supports for people with complex needs.

5. The PROMETHEUS Payment model presents a blueprint for physician payments based on packaging a comprehensive "episode" of medical care that covers all patient services related to a condition. The model uses an "Evidence-informed Case Rate®" (ECR), which creates a patient-specific, severity-adjusted prospective budget for a patient with a chronic condition. Each patient is assessed a budget based on his/her condition and its relative severity. These budgets can be added up across a specific patient population and represents a global budget for the physicians caring for these patients, irrespective of whether the physicians are incorporated in a "system." Patients access care as they do now; physicians who care for the patients get paid under their current negotiated fee schedules; and all claims get accumulated against the prospective budget for each patient. At the end of the year, the actual costs are compared with budgets, and any excess is the upside opportunity for the physicians. This model is a variation of the episode of care payment, in that it can be operationalized without any major disruption to payer or provider operations. According to the Robert Wood Johnson Foundation, in "Sustaining the Medical Home" (May 8, 2009) it also does not necessitate forced integration into "accountable care organizations," to yield significantly improved margins for physicians that deliver coordinated, patient-centered care ("Sustaining the Medical Home", 2009).

In the future, MBHOs will make greater use of provider payment models that link clinical performance and outcomes to payments. This will happen incrementally and in response to the demands of payers for additional value and accountability relative to quality outcomes and cost containment.

CONCLUSION

Managed Behavioral Health Care has grown in membership, impact, and focus over the past 20 years. Managed care:

- Uses data and data analytics to identify ways in which the managed care tools can have the most impact on achieving positive clinical outcomes and reducing costs.
- Targets interventions to consumers who are high risk and high cost.

■ Focuses management interventions and provider incentives on quality practices, which may lead to cost savings as the natural result of quality and utilization goals.

In identifying specialized high-risk/high-need populations, MBHOs will turn to network providers to use evidence-based practices; to integrate behavioral health and medical strategies for people with comorbid conditions; and to attain positive results for enrolled consumers. The overarching goals of managed behavioral health-care organizations continue to be to improve the quality and consistency of behavioral health practice based on nationally recognized evidence-based practice; improve patient outcome through the use of person-centered service plans with recovery goals; and ultimately to reduce the rate of spending on behavioral health services. It seems likely that while managed care tools may change in the future, the fundamental goals of this health-care management strategy will remain the same well into the next decade.

REFERENCES

Agency for Healthcare Research and Quality (AHRQ) Home. (n.d.). *Agency for Healthcare Research and Quality (AHRQ) Home.* Retrieved from http://www.ahrq.gov/

Hasselman, D. (n.d.). Center for Health Care Strategies (CHCS): Improving medicaid quality and cost-effectiveness. *Center for Health Care Strategies (CHCS): Improving medicaid quality and cost-effectiveness.* Retrieved from http://www.chcs.org/

Healthcare Industry, Healthcare News, Healthcare Companies FierceHealthcare. (n.d.). *Healthcare Industry, Healthcare News, Healthcare Companies FierceHealthcare.* Retrieved October 8, 2009, from http://www.fiercehealthcare.com/

Kronick, R. G., Bella, M., & Gilmer, T. P. (2009). *The Faces of Medicaid III; Center for Healthcare Strategies; Center for Healthcare Strategies, Inc.* p. 5. (for more details see http://www.chcs.org/publications3960/publications_show.htm?doc_id=1058416)

Sustaining the Medical Home—RWJF. (2009). *The Robert Wood Johnson Foundation: Health and Health Care Improvement—RWJF.* Retrieved from http://www.rwjf.org/qualityequality/product.jsp?id=42555

Zieger, A. (n.d.). Healthcare Industry, Healthcare News, Healthcare Companies FierceHealthcare. *Healthcare Industry, Healthcare News, Healthcare Companies FierceHealthcare.* Retrieved from http://fiercehealthcare.com

Index

CPSIA information can be obtained
at www.ICGtesting.com
Printed in the USA
LVOW05s0123070117
520028LV00014B/357/P